ADVANCE PRAISE FOR *A PRACTICAL GUIDE TO EMERGENCY TELEHEALTH*

"Dr. Sikka has edited an outstanding and very important guide to the basics of telemedicine and telehealth, and its wide variety of applications. This excellent text will serve the practitioners with a ready reference as telehealth continues to grow in importance and utility in the aftermath of a global pandemic, as well as the enlightened community of scholars with currency in this rapidly evolving paradigm."
—**Charles R. Doarn, MBA, FATA, FAsMA**, Research Professor,
Department of Environmental and Public Health Sciences,
MPH Program Director, College of Medicine,
University of Cincinnati

"While telehealth as a method of providing care is not new, pre-COVID growth accelerated by the response to COVID-19 has been remarkable. Dr. Sikka and his colleagues have provided us with the most comprehensive body of work to date on this important subject. While technological advances and clinical use cases may broaden telemedicine utilization in even more new ways, *A Practical Guide to Emergency Telehealth* provides the comprehensive view needed now by the increasing number of organizations for whom telehealth is a critical part of their care delivery systems."
—**B. Tilman Jolly, MD, FACEP,** Chief Medical Officer, Aveshka, Inc.,
Clinical Professor of Emergency Medicine,
The George Washington University

"Emergency telehealth has grown substantially since the onset of the COVID-19 pandemic in the United States. It is likely here to stay given the durability of many of the changes in reimbursement policy. This book provides an excellent summary of the contemporary issues in emergency telehealth, and is a must read for clinicians interested in this topic. Telehealth will undoubtedly be an evolving topic over time that will change the way we practice emergency care."
—**Jesse Pines, MD**,
National Director of Clinical Innovation,
US Acute Care Solutions

A Practical Guide to Emergency Telehealth

NEAL SIKKA

OXFORD
UNIVERSITY PRESS

Oxford University Press is a department of the University of Oxford. It furthers
the University's objective of excellence in research, scholarship, and education
by publishing worldwide. Oxford is a registered trade mark of Oxford University
Press in the UK and certain other countries.

Published in the United States of America by Oxford University Press
198 Madison Avenue, New York, NY 10016, United States of America.

Library of Congress Cataloging-in-Publication Data
Names: Sikka, Neal, author.
Title: A Practical Guide to Emergency Telehealth / editor Neal Sikka.
Description: New York, NY : Oxford University Press, [2021] |
Includes bibliographical references and index. |
Identifiers: LCCN 2021027764 (print) | LCCN 2021027765 (ebook) |
ISBN 9780190066475 (paperback) | ISBN 9780190066499 (epub) |
ISBN 9780190066505 (online)
Subjects: MESH: Telemedicine | Emergency Medical Services | Emergencies
Classification: LCC R855.3 (print) | LCC R855.3 (ebook) | NLM WX 215 |
DDC 610.285—dc23
LC record available at https://lccn.loc.gov/2021027764
LC ebook record available at https://lccn.loc.gov/2021027765

DOI: 10.1093/med/9780190066475.001.0001

9 8 7 6 5 4 3 2 1

Printed by Marquis, Canada

CONTENTS

In 2012, I had the opportunity to work with Drs. Hartmut Gross, Bob Galli, and John Rodgers to create the American College of Emergency Physicians Emergency Telehealth Section and serve as its founding chair. The Section represents a robust and growing number of emergency physicians who are working to define our roles as leaders in the emerging field of emergency telehealth.

In just a few short years, the profile of emergency telehealth has grown. For example, fellowship training programs, a telehealth quality framework, and telehealth training for all levels have been developed. Much hard work has resulted in improved access to care for patients across the country as well as contributions to the scientific literature related to telehealth. Ingenuity, interdisciplinary collaboration, and the entrepreneurial spirit of the emergency medicine community have led to the creation of a strong cadre of academic and community-based emergency telehealth services and digital health companies. Interest in emergency telehealth applications, their implementation, and operations continues to expand.

In 2018, the need for a practical guide to assist persons exploring opportunities in the field of emergency telehealth became apparent, and this book is designed to fulfill that need. The ensuing three years have seen the growth of emergency telehealth, in a variety of formats, such as direct patient evaluations, clinician-to-clinician consultations, remote physiologic monitoring, as well as further integration with electronic records, health information exchanges, clinical decision support, and artificial intelligence. Much of this growth happened in 2020 as a direct result of COVID-19, one of the largest disruptive forces of our lifetime. While the pandemic's impact on the health of individuals and families has been devastating, public health mitigation efforts to slow the spread of infections called for rapid and widespread deployment of telehealth solutions.

Enabled by sweeping regulatory waivers to long-standing telehealth legislation that had historically impeded the use of telehealth, some health systems saw the majority of their patients virtually for months. The COVID-19 pandemic-induced growth of telehealth allowed for experimentation with virtual care by patients and clinicians who may have never considered it an option before. During this time, clinicians realized that there were numerous use cases for which they could safely care for their patients. Many also realized that they were unprepared to provide care via telemedicine. The importance of training our current and future health care workforce to practice medicine in a technology-enabled environment has now been fully recognized. Additionally, it is clear that strategies to drive patient engagement in telehealth should be encouraged so that patients and families can access care when and how they need it. Providing simple training for telepresenters, those family and community members who may help a patient during a virtual visit and advocate for them to get the care they need, could be transformative.

Health disparities became increasingly obvious during the pandemic, further raising our awareness of the impact of the digital divide. This means that telehealth, as a field, must be concerned with equitable access to technology and connectivity. The ability to deliver the skills, motivation, comfort, and trust is important for encouraging patients to utilize technology to improve their health. At this writing, vaccination programs are rolling out, and there is a hope that COVID-19 rates will be decreasing. There is optimism for reopening society. Lessons learned from the pandemic regarding telehealth should have a long-term impact on care delivery. However, there is much uncertainty about the future, as it is unclear if new legislation enabling widespread access to telehealth will be enacted.

Most telehealth programs today are increasing patient access to clinicians. However, emerging models will lead to more highly coordinated and patient-centered care that will rely on secure and integrated telehealth (digital health) platforms, data, and real-time clinical decision support. Improving population and individual health-utilizing technology can spur the creation of digital ecosystems for patients and clinicians seeking and providing emergency care. Future services will be a continuum of technology-enabled care services that can integrate with in-person care and lead to more effective service delivery while reducing cost.

This book is an effort to reveal new opportunities for emergency medicine to meet the demands of an evolving health care environment. Emergency clinicians will be asked to provide highly coordinated and cost-effective care, leveraging technology, and effective communication, all in the context of social determinants of the individual patients' health. Each chapter provides a view into well-established or novel emergency telehealth programs or concepts and seeks to provide the reader with some context as to the state of emergency telehealth. As one of the first books to compile the experience of emergency telehealth, I hope to germinate a larger conversation and further collaboration from payers, clinicians, health care organizations, and patients that will support the wider implementation of emergency telehealth.

ACKNOWLEDGMENTS

It is clear that the COVID-19 pandemic catalyzed the completion of this book. The COVID-induced growth in telehealth created the right time to share ideas, projects, programs, and a vision for emergency telehealth to improve patient care and access.

I want to extend my appreciation to each of the telehealth experts and chapter authors, many of whom are practicing clinicians managing the stress of COVID-19 response while writing and editing. Each author demonstrated great dedication to work with me through multiple revisions and a rapidly evolving telehealth environment to ensure that the content and concepts of emergency telehealth are delivered in a consistent and useful manner.

The completion of this book could not have been possible without the hard work and collaboration of my two section editors, Hartmut Gross (Originating Site Services) and Dean Smith (Telehealth Operations). Their thoughtful feedback and critique were vital in shaping the story of each chapter they edited.

It definitely takes a village of people, beyond the authors, to complete a book project. I received many hours of help with organizing drafts, communicating with authors, and editing help from Jacob Keller and Lavanya Nawlakhe. Marta Moldvai and Tiffany Lu from the OUP team provided me timely direction, feedback, encouragement, and reassurance throughout this long process.

Finally, I want to say a special thank you to my wife and partner in everything, Anjum (whom I don't thank often enough) for being so supportive of writing this book. She managed the kids, two guinea pigs, the house, her full time job, and kept our household safe during a global pandemic, allowing me to hide away in the basement to work on this project. Thank you.

Ahmad A. Aalam, MBBS
Assistant Professor of Emergency Medicine
Department of Emergency Medicine
King Abdulaziz University
Jeddah, Saudi Arabia
Telemedicine and Clinical
    Informatics Fellow
Department of Emergency Medicine
George Washington University, School
    of Medicine and Health Sciences
Washington, DC, USA

Yasser Ajabnoor, MBBS
Department of Emergency Medicine
University of Jeddah
Telemedicine, and Medical Education
    Fellow
Department of Emergency Medicine
George Washington University, School
    of Medicine and Health Sciences
Washington, DC, USA

Hana Akselrod, MD, MPH
Associate Professor of Medicine
George Washington University, School
    of Medicine and Health Sciences
Division of Infectious Diseases
Washington, DC, USA

Ksenya K. Badashova, MD
Research Instructor of Emergency
    Medicine
ED Medical Leadership and
    Operations Fellow
George Washington University, School
    of Medicine and Health Sciences
Washington, DC, USA

Keith Boniface, MD
Professor of Emergency Medicine
Chief, Emergency Ultrasound Section
Department of Emergency Medicine
George Washington University, School
    of Medicine and Health Sciences
Washington, DC, USA

Ethan Booker, MD
Medical Director
MedStar Telehealth Innovation Center
    and MedStar eVisit
MedStar Institute of Innovation
Washington, DC, USA

**Marie L. Borum, MD, EdD, MPH,
MACP, FACG, AGAF**
Professor of Medicine
Director, Division of Gastroenterology
    and Liver Disease
George Washington University, School
    of Medicine and Health Sciences
Washington, DC, USA

Guenevere Burke, MD, MBA
Assistant Professor
Department of Emergency Medicine
George Washington University, School
    of Medicine and Health Sciences
Washington, DC, USA

Elias G. Carayannis, MBA, PhD
Professor of Science, Technology,
   Innovation and Entrepreneurship
Director, European Union
   Research Center
George Washington University, School
   of Business
Department of Information Systems
   and Technology Management
Washington, DC, USA

Tearsanee Carlisle, DNP,
FNP-BC, FAANP
Director, Clinical and Advanced
   Practice Operations
UMMC Center for Telehealth
Assistant Professor, UMMC School of
   Nursing
University of Mississippi
   Medical Center
Jackson, MS, USA

Bill Wayne Chan, MD Candidate
Department of Emergency Medicine
George Washington University, School
   of Medicine and Health Sciences
Washington, DC, USA

Davin T. Combs, BS
MD Candidate
Virginia Tech Carilion School of
   Medicine
Roanoke, VA, USA

Elizabeth Dearing, MD
Assistant Professor
Department of Emergency Medicine
George Washington University, School
   of Medicine and Health Sciences
Washington, DC, USA

Thomas E. Dell, BA
Research Program Coordinator
Johns Hopkins University School of
   Medicine
Baltimore, MD, USA

Krista Drobac
Partner, Sirona Strategies Executive
   Director
Alliance for Connected Care
Washington, DC, USA

Damien J. Drury, LLB (Hons), MB
BChir (Hons)
Foundation School, Morriston Hospital
Swansea Bay University Health Board
Swansea, UK

David G. Ellis, MD
Associate Professor of Emergency
   Medicine
Jacobs School of Medicine and
   Biomedical Sciences
State University of New York at Buffalo
Buffalo, NY, USA

Kyle Y. Faget, Esq. Partner, Foley and
Lardner LLP
Boston, MA, USA

Javad John Fatollahi, MD
Department of Psychiatry and
   Behavioral Sciences
George Washington University
   Chief Resident in Psychiatry and
   Behavioral Sciences
Washington, DC, USA

Robert Galli, MD
Professor of Emergency Medicine
University of Mississippi Medical Center
Jackson, MS, USA

Alexis S. Gilroy, JD
Jones Day
Washington, DC, USA

Jason C. Goldwater, MA, MPA
Senior Research Scientist, Index
   Analytics, LLC
Laurel, MD, USA

Anika Goodwin, MD, FACS
Co-founder & CEO
EYEmergencyMD, Inc.
Oro Valley, AZ, USA

Peter Greenwald, MD, MS
Assistant Professor of Clinical
   Emergency Medicine and
Director Telemedicine, Weill Cornell
   Department of Emergency Medicine
NewYork Presbyterian Hospital-Weill
   Cornell
New York, NY, USA

Hartmut Gross, MD, FACEP
Professor of Emergency Medicine and
  Neurology
Assistant Professor of Pediatrics
Department of Emergency Medicine
Medical College of Georgia
Augusta University
Augusta, GA, USA

Tenagne Haile-Mariam, MD
Assistant Professor of Emergency
  Medicine
Department of Emergency Medicine
George Washington University, School
  of Medicine and Health Sciences
Washington, DC, USA

Greg Hall
Director of IT
Center for Telehealth, University of
  Mississippi Medical Center
Jackson, MS, USA

Mark A. Hanson, PhD
Adjunct Assistant Professor
George Washington University
Washington, DC, USA
Co-Founder and Chief Product Officer
Heartbeat Health
New York, NY, USA

Lisa Haynie, PhD, RN, FNP-BC
Professor, School of Nursing
University of Mississippi
  Medical Center
Jackson, MS, USA

Judd E. Hollander, MD
Senior Vice President, Healthcare
  Delivery Innovation
Thomas Jefferson University
Associate Dean for Strategic Health
  Initiatives
Sidney Kimmel Medical College
Vice Chair, Finance and Healthcare
  Enterprises
Department of Emergency
  Medicine, SKMC
Philadelphia, PA, USA

Colton D. Hood, MD, MBI
Assistant Professor of Emergency
  Medicine
Department of Emergency Medicine
George Washington University, School
  of Medicine and Health Sciences
Washington, DC, USA

Ewald Horwath, MD, MS, LFAPA
Professor and Chair
Department of Psychiatry
MetroHealth System
Case Western Reserve University
  School of Medicine
Cleveland, OH, USA

Robert Jarrin, JD
Managing Member, The Omega
  Concern, LLC
Adjunct Assistant Professor of
  Emergency Medicine
Department of Emergency Medicine
George Washington University, School
  of Medicine and Health Sciences
Washington, DC, USA

Aditi U. Joshi, MD, MSc, FACEP
Sidney Kimmel Medical College of
  Thomas Jefferson University
Department of Emergency Medicine
National Academic Center for
  Telehealth
Philadelphia, PA, USA

Simranjit Kaur, MBBS
Internal Medicine PGY-1
MedStar Washington Hospital Center
Washington, DC, USA

Newton E. Kendig, MD
Clinical Professor of Medicine
George Washington University, School
  of Medicine and Health Sciences
Washington, DC, USA

Chloe T. L. Khoo, MD
Department of Ophthalmology
George Washington University School
  of Medicine and Health Sciences
Washington, DC, USA

Natalie Lynn Kirilichin, MD, MPH, FACEP
Co-director, GWU MFA Health Policy
  Fellowship and the SMHS Health
  Policy Scholarly Concentration
  Program
Assistant Professor of Emergency
  Medicine
Department of Emergency Medicine
George Washington University, School
  of Medicine and Health Sciences
Washington, DC, USA

Paul Knight, OT, MBA
Chief Information Officer
Symbria
Warrenville, IL, USA

Anita Kumar, MD
Assistant Clinical Professor of Medicine
George Washington University, School
  of Medicine and Health Sciences
Division of Gastroenterology and Liver
  Disease
Washington, DC, USA

Matthew Laghezza, MS, MBA, PA-C
Director of Practice Operations
Instructor of Physician Assistant Studies
  in Emergency Medicine
New York Presbyterian Hospital-Weill
  Cornell
New York, NY, USA

Susie Q. Lew, MD
Professor of Medicine
George Washington University, School
  of Medicine and Health Sciences
Division of Renal Diseases and
  Hypertension
Washington, DC, USA

Jared Lucas, MD
Research Instructor
Telemedicine and Digital Health Fellow
Department of Emergency Medicine
George Washington University, School
  of Medicine and Health Sciences
Washington, DC, USA

Claire Marblestone
Partner, Foley & Lardner
Los Angeles, CA, USA

Aaron Martin
Managing General Partner of
  Providence Ventures and Executive
  Vice President
Chief Digital Officer
Providence Seattle, WA, USA

Jason McKay, MPA, NRP, FP-C
Adjunct Instructor
Department of Emergency Medicine
George Washington University, School
  of Medicine and Health Sciences
Washington, DC, USA

L. Kendall McKenzie, MD
Professor and Chair
Department of Emergency Medicine
University of Mississippi Medical Center
Jackson, MS, USA

Andrew C. Meltzer, MD, MS
Associate Professor of Emergency
  Medicine
George Washington University, School
  of Medicine and Health Sciences
Department of Emergency Medicine
Washington, DC, USA

David Mishkin, MD, FACEP
Assistant Medical Director, Department
  of Emergency Medicine
Medical Director, Telemedicine
Baptist Health South Florida
Miami, FL, USA

Ameer Mody, MD, MPH, FAAP
Associate Division Director, Pediatric
  Emergency Medicine
Director of Emergency Department
  Clinical Informatics
Division of Emergency and Transport
  Medicine | Children's Hospital Los
  Angeles
Associate Professor of Pediatrics
  (Clinician-Educator)
Keck School of Medicine
University of Southern California
Los Angeles, CA, USA

Deborah Ann Mulligan, MD, FAAP, FACEP
Assistant Professor
Osteopathic Medicine, Kiran C. Patel
  College
Founder and Director, NSU Institute for
  Child Health Policy
Nova Southeastern University
Fort Lauderdale, FL, USA

M. Omar Chohan, MD, FAANS
Associate Professor
Neurosurgical Oncology, Epilepsy
  Surgery, Stereotactic Radiosurgery
Department of Neurosurgery,
  Neurology and Radiation Oncology
University of Mississippi
  Medical Center
Jackson, MS, USA

Obinna M. Ome Irondi, MD Candidate
George Washington University,
  School of Medicine and Health
  Sciences
Washington, DC, USA

Cameron Onks, JD
Director of Innovations in Health
  Technology
Texas Tech University Health
  Sciences Center
Lubbock, TX, USA

Kareem A. Osman, BS
George Washington University,
  School of Medicine and Health
  Sciences
Washington, DC, USA

Kimberly L. Rockwell, MD, JD
Jones Day
Detroit, MI, USA

Adam Rutenberg, DO, MBA
Assistant Professor of Emergency
  Medicine
Quality Director, GW Maritime
  Medical Access
Department of Emergency Medicine
George Washington University, School
  of Medicine and Health Sciences
Washington, DC, USA

Zeina Saliba, MD
Assistant Professor and Medical
  Director for Hospital Mental Health
  Services
George Washington University
Department of Psychiatry and
  Behavioral Sciences
George Washington University School
  of Medicine and Health Sciences
Washington, DC, USA

Ariel Santos, MD, MPH, FRSCS, FACS, FCCM
Associate Professor of Surgery
Director of Telemedicine
Chief, Acute Care Surgery Service
Principal Investigator, Texas-Louisiana
  Telehealth Resource Center
Texas Tech University Health
  Sciences Center
Lubbock, TX, USA

Rahul Sharma, MD, MBA
Professor and Chairman
Department of Emergency Medicine
New York Presbyterian Hospital-Weill
  Cornell
New York, NY, USA

Shailendra Sharma, MD
Sparrow Medical Group Nephrology
Lansing, MI, USA

Robert Shesser, MD, MPH
Chair
Department of Emergency Medicine
Professor of Emergency Medicine
Professor of Medicine
Department of Emergency
  Medicine
George Washington University,
  School of Medicine and Health
  Sciences
Washington, DC, USA

Marc O. Siegel, MD
Associate Professor of Medicine
George Washington University, School
  of Medicine and Health Sciences
Division of Infectious Diseases
Washington, DC, USA

Neal Sikka, MD, FACEP
Professor of Emergency Medicine
Director, Telemedicine and Digital
  Health Fellowship
Chief, Innovative Practice and
  Telehealth Section
Department of Emergency
  Medicine
George Washington University,
  School of Medicine and Health
  Sciences
Washington, DC, USA

Dean L. Smith, MD, MBI
Principal, Cascade Clinical
  Informatics, LLC
Consultant Chief Medical Officer,
  GlobalMed, LLC
Consultant Chief Medical Officer,
  Planned Systems International
Redmond/Bend, Oregon

Martina Stippler, MD, FACS, FAANS
Assistant Professor of Neurosurgery,
  Harvard Medical School
Cambridge, MA, USA

**Jeffrey A. Switzer, DO, MCTS,
FAHA, FAAN**
Professor and Chair of Neurology
Director of Telestroke and
  Teleneurology
Department of Neurology
Medical College of Georgia
Augusta University
Augusta, GA, USA

**Sam P. Tarassoli, BSc (Hons), MSc,
MB, BChir**
Foundation School, Morriston Hospital
Swansea Bay University Health Board
Swansea University College of Medicine
Swansea, UK

Kylie Taylor, MSN, CPNP
Pediatric Nurse Practitioner—III
Division of Emergency and Transport
  Medicine
Children's Hospital Los Angeles
Los Angeles, CA, USA

Renoj Varughese, MD
Clinical Instructor of Emergency
  Medicine
Jacobs School of Medicine and
  Biomedical Sciences
State University of New York at Buffalo
Buffalo, NY, USA

Sylvan Waller, MD
Principal, Sylvan Waller, MD LLC
Adjunct Assistant Professor of
  Emergency Medicine
George Washington University, School
  of Medicine and Health Sciences
Washington, DC, USA

Denise Wassenaar, RN, MS, NHA
Principal, Wassenaar Consulting, LLC
Surprise, AZ, USA

Susy Salvo Wendt
Telehealth Specialist
Summit Healthcare Regional
    Medical Center
Show Low, AZ, USA

Jeffrey D. Wessler, MD, MPhil, FACC
Assistant Professor of Medicine
Columbia University
Co-Founder and Chief Executive
    Officer
Heartbeat Health
New York, NY, USA

Howard Yonas, MD
UNM Distinguished Professor and
    Professor Emeritus
Department of Neurosurgery
University of New Mexico
Wilmington, NC, USA

PART I

Telehealth Operations

(Section Editor: Dean Smith)

Telemedicine Basics

GUENEVERE BURKE AND JARED LUCAS ■

INTRODUCTION

Telemedicine is a rapidly growing field in health care and emergency medicine. The terms *telemedicine*, *telehealth*, and *virtual health* are often used interchangeably, but they have unique definitions. Collectively, they refer to the use of telecommunications technology and electronic information to support health and provide care over distance (Nesbitt, 2020).

The terms *telehealth* and *telemedicine* both describe the "use of medical information exchanged from one site to another via electronic communications to improve the patient's health status" (Institute of Medicine, 2012, p. 3). Telemedicine is generally limited to direct clinical provider-to-patient care, whereas telehealth services include but are not limited to clinical care, health screening and prevention, health maintenance, professional health-related education, public health, and health administration (Sikka, 2019).

The terms *virtual health*, *e-health*, and *digital health* refer to an even broader array of digital information tools. Their definition includes telehealth and extends further into other categories such as health information technology (IT), medical device data systems, electronic health records (EHRs), and clinical decision support tools (Office of Health Policy, Office of the Assistant Secretary for Planning and Evaluation [ASPE], 2016; U.S. Food & Drug Administration, n.d.; Telligen and the Great Plains Telehealth Resource and Assistance Center, 2020).

In practice, telehealth terms (Figure 1.1) have various definitions across different settings, and many of these terms are used interchangeably. The definitions provided in this chapter are adapted from the American Telemedicine Association and the Center for Connected Health Policy; these are commonly cited sources, given the inability of lawmakers and health care providers to reach consensus on definitions (Congressional Research Service, 2016).

Telemedicine has been used to improve access to health care in geographically remote areas for decades, but its use and recognized benefits have expanded considerably over the years. These benefits include the ability to reduce health care costs, improve the efficiency of health care resource utilization, promote better health

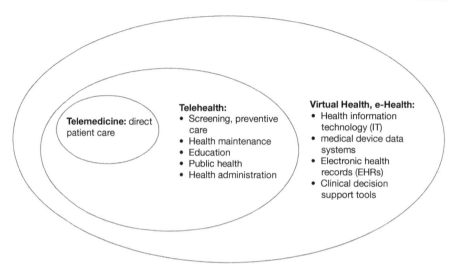

Note: In practice, telehealth terms have various definitions across different settings, with many terms being used interchangeably.

Figure 1.1 Definitions of telehealth terms

outcomes, and enhance patient satisfaction. As with any emerging technology or novel care delivery model, the expanded use of telehealth has also presented unique challenges. This chapter introduces telehealth and telemedicine basics, including key terms, history, and modern applications, with a focus on emergency care.

A BRIEF HISTORY OF TELEHEALTH

Distance communication for health care has existed for centuries, but the foundations of modern telehealth are most commonly traced to the 1950s. Since that time, telehealth services have expanded rapidly.

Since telehealth's origins predate emergency medicine, it is not surprising that other specialties pioneered its first use cases. Teleradiology appeared in the late 1950s when the telephone was used to transmit radiologic images. The first interactive video for neurologic examination was used for educational purposes around this time as well. Advances were made in emergency care as first responders in Miami began sending cardiac monitoring results to emergency physicians in the late 1960s and a medical station in Boston was created to provide long-distance primary and emergency services to airport staff and travelers (Nesbitt, 2020).

In the 1990s–2000s, telehealth continued to develop and mature. Academic health centers began pioneering telehealth programs to address limited rural health care access, and large national networks, including the Veterans Health Administration and Kaiser Permanente, launched telehealth pilots. Funding for telehealth began to emerge within health systems and at the state and federal levels during this period. A notable example includes the Telemedicine Development Act of 1996 in California, which advanced telehealth reimbursement and became a model for other states. The

Balanced Budget Act of 1997 mandated Medicare reimbursement for telehealth in rural counties designated as health professional shortage areas and for demonstration projects to examine the use of telemedicine in the management of diabetes and chronic diseases.

Emergency telehealth also saw a significant expansion during this timeframe. Telestroke services to administer thrombolytic therapy were implemented, and pediatric emergency care telehealth delivery models were established in remote facilities without specialty care (Nesbitt, 2020).

Today, telehealth continues to mature and broaden due to multiple factors. Location and provider restrictions by payers have been gradually lifted, allowing for expanded services. Telecommunication infrastructure and broadband access continue to improve, supporting more widespread use. Additionally, the rise of e-commerce has changed people's day-to-day activities, as well as their expectations for accessing health care and interacting with providers. In one analysis, six major drivers of telehealth adoption were identified: policy, financing, evidence, technology, health system transformation, and consumer demand (Figure 1.2; Center for Connected Health Policy, 2014). Yet, to many industry observers, telehealth remains in the early stages of adoption despite recent accelerated growth.

The most rapid expansion in telemedicine use in the modern era was spurred by the global coronavirus pandemic, which began in late 2019. Concerns regarding disease transmission fueled widespread adoption of telemedicine, aided by emergency legislation at the state and federal levels. Despite these trends, telehealth's full potential remains unrealized, though it is anticipated that it will continue to transform health systems into the future. Internationally, adoption of telehealth has also

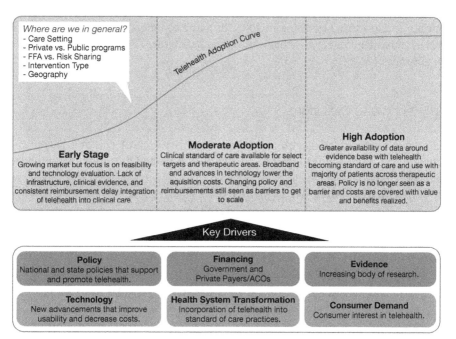

Figure 1.2 Key drivers of telehealth adoption. Reprinted with permission from CCHP/ www.cchpca.org.

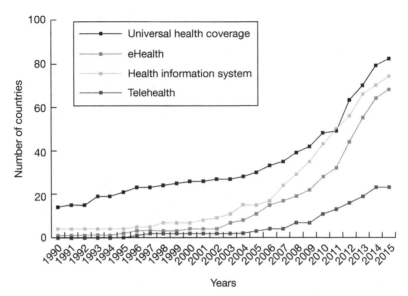

Figure 1.3 Number of countries with UHC, eHealth, HIS, and telehealth policies or strategies, cumulatively by year of adoption (1990–2015). From Global diffusion of eHealth: Making universal health coverage achievable. ISBN -92-4-151178-0. https://apps. who.int/iris/bitstream/handle/10665/252529/9789241511780-engpdf;jsessionid=7465F00 9AFB4C7AAF2075E5AB207A15B?sequence=1
Reproduced with permission.

been rapidly increasing, with the World Health Organization (WHO) establishing eHealth as a priority beginning in 2005. In many countries, telehealth adoption is part of a broader strategy to achieve universal health care (Figure 1.3; World Health Organization, 2016).

Key Terms and Definitions

As previously noted, telehealth and telemedicine are broad terms and encompass different approaches and technologies. A few key terms and definitions are provided here for reference.

Telehealth Modalities. According to the U.S. Department of Health and Human Services (HHS), there are four basic telehealth modalities: synchronous, asynchronous, remote patient monitoring, and mobile health (Office of Health Policy, Office of the ASPE, 2016).

> *Synchronous (live interactive)*—the delivery of a live audiovisual interactive consultation between any person and a health care provider. The person may be a patient, caregiver, or even another provider requesting specialist assistance. This communication occurs in real time and can often substitute for an in-person encounter. (American Telemedicine Association, 2019; Center for Connected Health Policy, 2019)

Asynchronous (store and forward)—the transmission of recorded health history (diagnostic images, vital signs, video clips) via a secure electronic communications system to a health professional (typically, a specialist) to later diagnose or render a service. This service occurs outside of a real-time, live interaction and most commonly utilizes email communications. (American Telemedicine Association, 2019; Center for Connected Health Policy, 2019)

Remote Patient Monitoring—the use of digital devices and technologies to remotely collect and securely send medical data from individuals to remote health care providers or to a remote diagnostic testing facility (RDTF) for interpretation. Examples include patient vital signs, blood glucose, ECG, and weight. Numerous platforms exist for telemetry and arrhythmia detection via remote monitoring with increasingly advanced interpretation capabilities (Siwicki, 2020). Such services can be used to augment the management of chronic medical conditions requiring frequent monitoring, allowing individuals to remain at home or in their long-term health care facility. (Center for Connected Health Policy, 2019; American Telemedicine Association, 2019; Congressional Research Service, 2016)

Mobile Health—the provision of health care services and personal health data via mobile devices (cell phones, tablet computers). These devices typically download and use application software (apps) designed to foster health. Examples include messaging to encourage healthy behaviors, alerts about disease outbreaks, reminders to adhere to care regimens, and peer-to-peer support. These apps may also use mobile device features (camera, microphones) or other sensors that use remote physiologic monitoring (RPM) as input. (American Telemedicine Association, 2019; c, 2015)

Telehealth Location. In discussing remote care delivery via telemedicine, two specific terms are used to identify the location where care is taking place: the *originating site* and the *distant site*.

Originating Site—the site where the patient and/or the patient's clinician requesting the telehealth service is located during the telehealth encounter or consult. (Other common names include spoke site, patient site, remote site, and rural site; Institute of Medicine, 2012.)

Distant Site—the telehealth site where the provider/specialist is seeing the patient at a distance or is consulting with the patient's provider. (Other common names include hub site, specialty site, provider/physician site, and referral or consulting site; Institute of Medicine, 2012.)

TELEHEALTH MODELS OF CARE

Hub-and-Spoke: This model utilizes networked programs to link a tertiary or quaternary care hospital or clinic (hub) to outlying clinics or community health centers in rural areas or urban areas with little access to care (spokes). Telecommunication links between sites occur via dedicated high-speed lines or the internet. Given the rapid expansion of telemedicine, isolated hub-and-spoke networks have become less common, and a network of networks is increasingly described (Telehealth Resource Center, 2018). Tele-ICU care was one of the earliest hub-and-spoke models of care, as centrally located intensivists provided care to patients at outlying facilities. More recently, teletriage has been deployed at multiple emergency centers, provided via a hub-and-spoke model and utilized to intentionally maintain physical distance during the COVID-19 outbreak. (Joy, 2020)

Point-to-Point Connections: Used by both hospitals and clinics, this model describes the outsourcing of specialty services to independent medical service providers. Like hub-and-spoke, this type of service connection lets smaller or understaffed clinics outsource medical care to specialists at other locations, but the specialty service does not have to exist within the same health care network. Examples include radiology, stroke assessment, mental health, and intensive care services. (Rheuban, n.d.)

Specialty Consultation: Long representing the traditional model of telemedicine, specialty consultations are intended to improve access to specialty expertise for patients and providers. In this model, a provider (most commonly a primary care provider) or patient may request guidance from a clinical specialist. Specialty consults are used for a variety of purposes both within and across medical centers. A wide variety of applications exist today for almost every medical specialty, including dermatology, gastroenterology, orthopedics, and obstetrics. When specialty consultations are not real time, they are called e-consults. *E-consults* describe consultative provider-to-provider or provider-to-patient communications (i.e., secure email or portal communications) within a shared network or web-based platform. (Rheuban, n.d.; Vimalananda, 2015)

Monitoring Center Links: This model describes the use of digital connections between the patient's location (e.g., house or assisted living center) and a remote monitoring facility. Communication links occur via landline, wireless, or internet connections and use remote patient monitoring modalities to facilitate the patient's care by remote health care providers. Examples include cardiac, pulmonary, and fetal monitoring. (Rheuban, n.d.)

Direct-to-Consumer: This model of care refers to platforms that provide immediate on-demand care by health care providers directly to patients (consumers). In this model, visits are initiated by the patient. There is no intermediary clinician or facilitator present, and care typically occurs outside the patient's primary care medical home. (Rheuban, n.d.; Elliott, 2019)

CURRENT TOPICS IN EMERGENCY TELEHEALTH

The American College of Emergency Physicians (ACEP) recently supported the development of a working definition of emergency telehealth. In the ACEP commissioned report, emergency telehealth was defined as "remotely caring for acute illness, injury and exacerbations of chronic diseases, including the initial evaluation, diagnosis, treatment, prevention, coordination of care, disposition and public-health impact of any patient requiring expeditious care, irrespective of any prior relationship" (Sikka, 2019, p. 2).

As reflected in this definition, telehealth has been described at each stage of the emergency care spectrum—from prehospital interventions to triage, diagnosis, treatment, disposition, and follow-up. It has also been utilized in closely related fields and subspecialties such as disaster preparedness, critical care, and emergency pediatrics.

The telephone has been used to avoid unnecessary medical visits since 1879, just three years after the technology was patented in the United States (Institute of Medicine, 2012). Today, emerging telehealth technology is increasingly utilized to guide appropriate patient transport from home, nursing, or correctional facility to the emergency department (ED).

On arrival to the ED, a virtual provider in triage facilitates decreased wait times and reduces the number of patients who leave without being seen or completing a medical screening exam. Telemedicine can increase emergency provider capacity via remote connection, augmenting clinical staffing and allowing remote supervision of advanced practice providers (see Chapter 17 for more information). Specialty applications and e-consults can also support emergency care of complex patients.

Finally, after treatment, telemedicine may be used to support discharge planning, care coordination, and follow-up care. Remote patient monitoring has proven especially useful in a broad array of clinical conditions requiring emergency treatment, including hypervolemia and hypoxemia. These and many more topics in emergency telehealth are described in greater detail in subsequent chapters.

SUMMARY

Use of telemedicine, telehealth, and virtual health is rapidly growing in health care and emergency medicine. These related terms refer to the use of telecommunications technology and electronic information to support health and provide care over distance.

Despite emergency applications being described since the 1960s and more recent exponential growth, adoption of telehealth in the United States remains at an early stage. It is characterized by four primary delivery modalities (synchronous, asynchronous, remote patient monitoring, and mobile health) and an ever-expanding number of care models.

Telehealth applications described in emergency medicine already span the full spectrum of care from preparedness and prehospital care to acute care and disposition. Emergency telehealth has the potential to improve access and quality of care for patients, while decreasing health care costs and improving the patient experience. As emergency practitioners continue to pioneer emerging technologies and develop telehealth knowledge and experience, health system transformation is achievable.

KEY TAKEAWAYS

- *Telemedicine* and *telehealth* are often used interchangeably. However, telemedicine generally refers to direct clinical provider-to-patient care. Telehealth services include clinical care as well as health screening and prevention, health maintenance, professional health-related education, public health, and health administration. *Virtual Health*, *e-health*, and *digital health* refer to an even broader array of digital information tools.
- Four basic telehealth modalities are generally described: synchronous, asynchronous, remote patient monitoring, and mobile health.
- Telehealth care models include hub-and-spoke, point-to-point, specialty consultation, and direct-to-consumer models. Specific applications and adoption have been growing for decades and continue to expand rapidly, with the potential to improve access and quality of care, decrease health care costs, and improve the patient experience.
- Emergency telehealth is "remotely caring for acute illness, injury, and exacerbations of chronic diseases, including the initial evaluation, diagnosis, treatment, prevention, coordination of care, disposition, and public-health impact of any patient requiring expeditious care, irrespective of any prior relationship." (Sikka, 2019, p. 2)

REFERENCES

American Telemedicine Association. (2019, October 5). *Telehealth: Defining 21st Century Care*. Retrieved from https://www.americantelemed.org/resource/why-telemedicine.

Center for Connected Health Policy. (2014). *Recommendations from the CCHP Telehealth and the Triple Aim Project: Advancing Telehealth Knowledge and Practice*. Sacramento: Center for Connected Health Policy. Retrieved from https://www.cchpca.org/sites/default/files/2018-09/Telehealth%20%20Triple%20Aim%20 Report%202_0.pdf.

Center for Connected Health Policy. (2019, October 7). *About Telehealth*. Retrieved from https://www.cchpca.org/about/about-telehealth.

U.S. Congressional Research Service. (2016, March 29). *Telehealth and Telemedicine: Description and Issues*. R44437.

Elliott, T., Shih, J. (2019). Direct to Consumer Telemedicine. *Current Allergy and Asthma Reports*, 19(1): 1.

Institute of Medicine. (2012). *The Role of Telehealth in an Evolving Health Care Environment: Workshop Summary*. Washington, DC: National Academies Press.

Joy, K. (2020, April 30). How "Tele-Triage" Models Work to Keep Patients and Clinicians Safe. *Health Tech Magazine*. Retrieved from https://healthtechmagazine.net/article/2020/04/how-tele-triage-models-work-keep-patients-and-clinicians-safe-perfcon.

National Telehealth Policy Resource Center. (2014). *Recommendations from the CCHP Telehealth and the Triple Aim Project:Advancing Telehealth Knowledge and Practice.* Sacramento: Center for Connected Health Policy.

Nesbitt, T. S., Katz-Bell, J. (2020). History of Telehealth. In K. S. Rheuban and E. A. Krupinski, *Understanding Telehealth*. New York: McGraw-Hill. Retrieved July 11, 2021, from https://accessmedicine.mhmedical.com/content.aspx?bookid=2217&sectionid=187794434

Office of Health Policy, Office of the Assistant Secretary for Planning and Evaluation (ASPE). (2016). *Report to Congress: E-health and Telemedicine*, August 12, 2016. Washington, D.C.: U.S. Department of Health and Human Services.

Rheuban, K. Shipman, S. (n.d.). Workforce, Definitions, and Models. In K. S. Rheuban and Elizabeth A. Krupinski, *Understanding Telehealth*. New York: McGraw-Hill. Retrieved October 23, 2020, from https://accessmedicine-mhmedical-com.proxygw.wrlc.org/content.aspx?bookid=2217&sectionid=187794500.

Sikka, N. G. (2019). Defining Emergency Telehealth. *Journal of Telemedicine and Telecare*, 135.

Siwicki, B. (2020, May 6). *A Guide to Connected Health Device and Remote Patient Monitoring Vendors*. Retrieved from Healthcare IT News: https://www.healthcareitnews.com/news/guide-connected-health-device-and-remote-patient-monitoring-vendors.

Telehealth Resource Center. (2018, February). *Telehealth: What Do I Need to Know*. Retrieved from Telehealth Resource Center: https://www.interoperabilityshowcase.org/sites/interoperabilityshowcase/files/white_paper_-_telehealth_-_what_do_i_need_to_know.pdf.

Telligen and the Great Plains Telehealth Resource and Assistance Center. (2020, October 23). *Telehealth Start-Up and Resource Guide*. Retrieved from HealthIT.gov: https://www.healthit.gov/sites/default/files/telehealthguide_final_0.pdf.

U.S. Food & Drug Administration. (n.d.). *What Is Digital Health?* Retrieved from https://www.fda.gov/medical-devices/digital-health-center-excellence/what-digital-health.

Vimalananda, V. G., Supte, G., Seraj, S. M., Orlander, J., Berlowitz, D., et al. (2015). Electronic Consultations (e-consults) to Improve Access to Specialty Care: A Systematic Review and Narrative Synthesis. *Journal of Telemedicine and Telecare*, 21(6): 323–330.

World Health Organization. (2016). *Global Diffusion of eHealth: Making Universal Health Coverage Achievable. Report of the Third Global Survey on eHealth*. Retrieved from https://apps.who.int/iris/bitstream/handle/10665/252529/9789241511780-eng.pdf;jsessionid=7465F009AFB4C7AAF2075E5AB207A15B?sequence=1.

2

Telemedicine Technologies

DEAN L. SMITH ■

INTRODUCTION

Telemedicine is the use of technology to connect clinicians, or clinicians and patients, who are geographically or temporally separated. It comes in many forms, reflecting the complex ways health care is delivered. The earliest examples of telemedicine were simply phone calls between clinicians. Now, telemedicine encompasses live videoconferences involving the full spectrum of stakeholders in the health care continuum, a wide array of diagnostic devices, as well as an ever increasing number of patient-driven modalities, all benefiting from improving communication technology. with the goal of delivering timely, cost-effective health care.

As discussed in Chapter 1, the terms *telemedicine*, *telehealth*, and *virtual health* are frequently used interchangeably, yet they have discrete meaning unto themselves. Telemedicine is typically used to denote direct clinician-to-clinician encounters, whereas telehealth expands on this to include "ancillary" health care measures such as health maintenance, patient education, and public health activities. Virtual health is generally used as an umbrella term to encompass telemedicine and telehealth, as well as other applications of technology in health care, such as artificial intelligence, chatbots, and machine learning.

Let's take a closer look at the tools that make telemedicine, telehealth, and virtual health a reality.

TELEHEALTH HARDWARE

Carts and More

Telehealth hardware comes in a wide array of sizes and configurations, tailored to specific uses, clinical scenarios, and requirements (Figure 2.1). This includes clinical cart stations, wall-mounted systems, and, increasingly, portable solutions that scale to any offsite transport scenario, from first responder units to overhead bins in aircraft to backpacks in austere locations. At the core of these platforms is an integrated

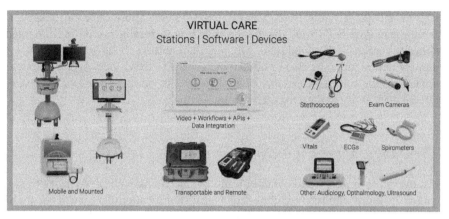

Figure 2.1 Virtual care: stations, software, and devices. Reprinted with permission from GlobalMed.

audiovisual conferencing system that allows for secure two-way communication between the sending station and the receiving clinician.

Mobile Telemedicine Stations for Hospitals and Clinics

Mobile stand-alone telemedicine stations are ideal for use in "brick-and-mortar" settings such as emergency departments (EDs), outpatient clinics, and in-patient hospital wards. Their mobility makes them easy to store away when they're not in use. Some are robotically controlled and typically find use in the intensive care unit (ICU) and other high-acuity care settings. Other configurations include laptop or tablet devices mounted on carts, ideal for supporting clinical teams who require ease of access, such as the ED, or while conducting in-patient rounds. The core functionality of these and other telehealth systems is an audiovisual conferencing capability, which allows for real-time synchronous telehealth consultations, as well as data capture for store and forward asynchronous telehealth encounters. Most of these devices can interface with a wide array of peripheral devices to facilitate the clinical evaluation process. These peripherals include vital sign devices that capture blood pressure, temperature, oxygen saturation, as well as examination cameras, ultrasound probes, ophthalmoscopes, electrocardiograms, and a host of other devices as dictated by the clinical setting. These devices are explored in more detail later in this chapter.

Wall-Mounted and Kiosk Devices

Wall-mounted and kiosk telehealth devices have many of the same features of the mobile cart stations listed above, again with a core functionality of audiovisual (AV) conferencing capability augmented with peripheral devices. They are ideal for clinical situations where the equipment is stationary. In addition, their narrow profile makes them less obtrusive. As the name implies, these devices are fixed in location, typically in a hospital or clinic. Many EDs have found them to be ideal, and in fact some have deployed both fixed, wall-mounted systems and mobile cart telemedicine stations. Another setting that has been finding increasing use of wall-mounted telehealth stations is the retail space, where wall mounting creates a kiosk-like environment and reduces the chance of theft or damage to the device. Again, users can supplement the core AV capability of these devices by adding a wide variety of peripheral devices as required for each specific setting.

Transportable Units and Backpacks

Advances in technology and communication networks have allowed telehealth systems to "do more with less" and thus deploy in austere locations far outside the traditional clinical realms of hospitals and clinics. One specific telehealth use case is first responders, who have a requirement for highly mobile platforms weighing a fraction of the hospital and clinic systems discussed above. To meet this need, suitcase-sized transportable telehealth stations weighing less than 50 pounds have been developed. These readily fit into "grab-and-go" ruggedized containers to withstand the rigors of travel and exposure to physical elements. They also interface with a large number of peripheral devices (see below), as dictated by the clinical use case, integrated around a core AV platform. Recently, backpack telehealth solutions weighing less than 20 pounds have been deployed. These have many of the clinical capabilities of their larger cousins and are ideal for emergency medical technicians in the field, home health care providers, and others such as military personnel, who provide clinical care in medically austere, remote locations with high mobility requirements.

PERIPHERAL DEVICES

Virtually every examination and data capture device used in traditional acute and ambulatory care is now available as a digital peripheral device that can be tethered to one of the telehealth hardware platforms cited above. The most common of these devices, particularly in the emergency setting, capture the full range of vital signs, including real-time blood pressure, pulse, heart rhythm, and oximetry. Other frequently used devices are described in more detail below. This is by no means an exhaustive list, and telehealth systems can be outfitted by an ever-increasing number of devices as dictated by the clinical requirements. Each of these devices connects to the telehealth station or directly to the communication network by one of following technologies—USB, Bluetooth (BT), or wireless internet. Some connect by more than one modality, providing connection redundancy. It should also be noted that many of the peripheral devices cited below are sized specifically for adult or pediatric patients.

General Examination Cameras

Although the camera integrated into the core AV system of the telehealth station can be used to visualize the patient, a camera tethered to the system (again via

USB, BT, or wireless) adds significant flexibility of use. This general examination camera allows the examining clinician to obtain gross and focused images of the patient—for example, examination of the patient ambulating, followed by examination of the painful extremity that generated the clinical encounter. General examination cameras also have exchangeable heads that can be used to examine the ears (including tympanic membranes), nares, and oropharynx. Some also accommodate skin examination (see the section "Dermatoscopes" below). One common clinical use case for the general examination camera in the emergency setting is for telestroke, as the camera allows for real-time visualization and assessment of the patient's motor skills, a focused examination of cranial nerve function, and other neurologic assessment as required by the receiving neurologic stroke specialist.

Stethoscopes

Auscultation of the heart and lungs is finding increasing use in telehealth encounters. The clinical value has always been there, but advances in soundwave capture capabilities and communication networks are making the digital stethoscope an important, if not critical, tool in the telehealth suite of peripheral devices. Now, a nurse in a remote emergency clinic in Alaska can transmit breath sounds and cardiac tones to a critical care specialist hundreds of miles away, in real time, without loss of clinical fidelity. Telehealth stethoscopes can be easily configured to both bell and diaphragm settings, and specific frequencies can be amplified or muted as required to allow the receiving clinician to make a diagnosis. Sounds can also be captured and stored for incorporation into the digital health record as needed.

Expert Tip
Many clinicians find that auscultation is the most challenging aspect of a telemedicine remote encounter. We recommend use of high-quality digital stethoscopes, dedicated audio channels, and most importantly, high-quality headphones that do not use so-called noise-canceling technology.

Pan-Tilt-Zoom (PTZ) cameras

Pan-tilt-zoom (PTZ) cameras are typically mounted on the top of the telehealth platform and allow for a wide-angle view of the clinical encounter. This permits the receiving clinician to zoom in and observe the patient up close and also zoom out to observe some of the subtleties of the clinical encounter, such as the body language of the patient and interaction with others who may be present in the examination room. Moreover, the receiving clinician can remotely control the specific view they are receiving, allowing them to see what they feel is important in the encounter without asking the sending clinician to adjust the view and thus interrupt the flow of care. This functionality has particular value when the sending site is a busy emergency department.

Point-of-Care Ultrasound

Point-of-care ultrasound (POCUS) has many uses in telehealth, both real-time (synchronous) and store-and-forward (asynchronous). Ultrasound (US) probes that interface directly with the telehealth platform can be used for abdominal examinations—for example, Focused Assessment with Sonography in Trauma (FAST) examinations in the ED. Since these devices can transmit live ultrasound images to clinical specialists anywhere in the world, a clinician who is inexperienced in POCUS can be guided through an examination, and perhaps more importantly, through an invasive procedure. Ultrasound probes for obstetrics, vascular, and ophthalmic use cases are also available and "plug-and-play" into the telehealth platform. Increasingly, these are being consolidated into single multiprobe devices, some of which interface directly with the clinician's smart phone or other portable device.

Dermatoscopes

Dermatology was one of the first medical specialties to widely adopt telehealth technology, in large part due to the image quality and ease of use of telemedicine dermatoscopes. These peripheral devices allow the clinician to get a magnified view of the skin and to add measurements and other mark-ups that are useful for sequential and follow-up care. In addition, some dermatoscope devices have polarization capability that allows the clinician to view into deeper layers of the epidermis, a particularly useful modality for diagnosing some cutaneous malignancies. Telehealth skin imaging is amenable to both synchronous and asynchronous use cases.

Miscellaneous Peripheral Devices

As noted above, a large number of additional peripheral devices can be connected to the fixed or mobile telehealth station. Notable among these devices are ophthalmoscopes with lenses for imaging the anterior chamber and retina. These find use in emergency settings for assessing the causes of acute vision loss such as retinal hemorrhages and detachments, as well as routine use for diabetic retinopathy screening. Digital electrocardiograms can be utilized by emergency medical technicians (EMTs) and other emergency responders to quickly assess patients with chest pain, ensuring that those with acute coronary syndrome receive immediate interventional care. Electroencephalograms are used by neurologists to remotely monitor seizure patients. Similar peripheral devices for dental and audiometry use cases are now in common use in telehealth.

Remote Patient Monitoring and Patient-Driven Devices

Remote patient monitoring is another growing area within the telehealth sphere. Monitoring devices such as glucometers and spirometers can provide the remote health care team with real-time and longitudinal data regarding a patient's chronic conditions. The real-time capability is particularly useful in disaster settings, where victims with exacerbated medical conditions, such as diabetes or chronic lung disease, can be identified and triaged to early care response. Remote patient monitoring of temperature, oxygen saturation, and other vital signs has proven very useful during the COVID-19 pandemic. In addition, as peripheral devices have become smaller and ease-of-use improved, companies such as Tyto and MedWand have developed patient-driven devices that meet the growing consumer demand for personalized telemedicine evaluations. These devices allow the patient to conduct their own in-home telemedicine examination concurrent with a synchronous consultation with a clinician.

TELEHEALTH SOFTWARE

The telemedicine hardware described above relies on software programs, which are an increasingly important part of the telehealth platform and clinical encounter. Indeed, it is the integrated, configurable software that unlocks the key benefits of telehealth—access to care, efficiency of care, cost reduction, and most importantly, clinical outcomes.

Scheduling and Secure Messaging

Telehealth software increasingly incorporates a variety of scheduling modalities. These include appointment scheduling by both the provider and patient. On the provider side, acute visits can be scheduled as well as follow-up appointments. A patient with a subacute complaint can thus be triaged to the appropriate specialist in the right timeframe for their condition. Patients in turn can request appointments with their primary care providers or call in to an urgent care telehealth "waiting room" for an immediate appointment, using an app on their smart phone or home computer (see Figure 2.2). Note that messages between patient and clinician are fully encrypted in transit as well as on the respective device(s), ensuring all Health Insurance Portability and Accountability Act (HIPAA) requirements for protection of personal health information are met.

Clinical Documentation

The clinical care delivered in the telehealth encounter can be captured and documented in a variety of ways. Clinicians can document their care in a separate charting system (either paper or electronic) following the encounter, but that option creates duplication of work and unnecessary inefficiency, and also introduces the possibility of erroneous charting. Most telehealth platforms solve these problems in one of two ways: (1) interfacing directly with the clinician's native electronic health record (EHR) system or (2) documenting the care directly into a documentation database intrinsic to the telehealth platform. The latter permits upload to an EHR at a later time if needed. Direct EHR interface has the added

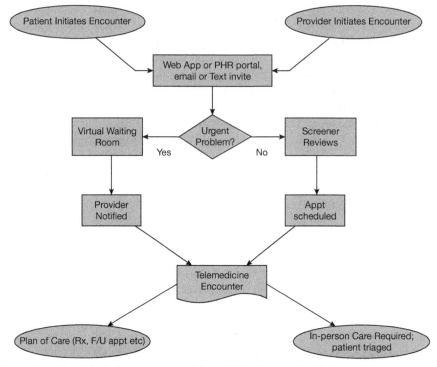

Figure 2.2 Simplified telemedicine workflow. PHR= Patient Health Record, Rx = Prescription, F/U = Follow-up, appt= appointment

benefit of not only pushing telehealth encounter data to the EHR, but pulling data from the EHR to the telehealth platform as well. The key driving force here is that clinicians do not like to duplicate clinical documentation efforts—any telehealth program workflow that is predicated on inefficient duplication of documentation will ultimately fail.

Billing

Just as with clinical documentation, billing for the telehealth encounters can occur with a billing application integrated into the telehealth platform, or through the clinician's EHR and practice management system if that is the preferred workflow. As with clinical documentation, a single "source of truth" for billing should be implemented.

Reporting and Analytics

Telehealth encounters utilizing even the basic hardware and software modalities capture a very robust clinical dataset—vital signs, examination images, and stethoscope sounds, as well as POCUS, point-of-care labs, clinician documentation, and any other artifacts captured during the encounter. Recall that virtually every peripheral device currently in clinical use can be tethered to the telehealth station and thus add to the clinical data set. This rich source of data can then be digested and analyzed by the user's native EHR or increasingly by the telehealth platform itself. This data can be used for a variety of reporting and analytics uses, including work-load optimization, quality care measurement and improvement, population health, biosurveillance, and customer satisfaction.

> **Quick Fact:**
> As a result of the COVID-19 pandemic, Dr. Joseph Kvedar, president of the American Telemedicine Association (ATA) and professor, Harvard Medical School, projects that Mass General Brigham providers will go from approximately 1,500 virtual visits per month pre-COVID to 250,000 per month. Pre-pandemic, only 0.2% of all ambulatory outpatient visits were conducted via telehealth. Dr. Kvedar now anticipates that 60% of ambulatory care will be delivered remotely (Kvedar, 2020).

OPERATIONS

Staffing

A key decision point to consider when setting up any telehealth program is how to provide the necessary clinical staffing, both at the sending (originating) and receiving sites if within health care facilities. Many factors must be considered in this equation, and a more detailed discussion of complex issues such as provider credentialing, licensing, and quality oversight is found later in this book. But a central decision is whether to use (and train) existing clinical staff or to outsource the telehealth program to another entity. This issue is analogous to the "build versus buy" decision that health care systems implementing telehealth programs must also consider pertaining to deploying required hardware and software for their program.

Network Infrastructure

Telehealth is the connection of a patient and a clinician or clinicians who are geographically separated from each other. As such, it is intrinsically dependent on a communication network. Even store-and-forward asynchronous encounters require at least email or other connectivity between the sending and receiving sites. For real-time synchronous telehealth, a dependable and preferably redundant communication network is needed. Redundancy can be achieved through fail-over from hardwired and wireless network connections (e.g., long-term evolution [LTE] and broadband internet) and even satellite communications. Modern telehealth encounters can be conducted with surprisingly little bandwidth; although broad-band networks are preferred, some platforms support real-time encounters with 256 kbps with minimal pixilation or other degradation in content. Network latency is another determinant of transmission quality and also needs to be considered and assessed before a telehealth program is deployed. Concurrent users on the network must also be taken into consideration. Forthcoming network technologies such as high-speed 5G wireless and low-Earth orbit satellite internet hold great promise in furthering the adoption and use of telehealth technologies.

Systems Integration

As discussed previously, clinicians will not tolerate duplication of effort, nor should they. Before deployment of a telehealth program, existing health IT systems should be inventoried, especially any EHRs in use within the clinical network, and due diligence should be given as to how the telehealth system will interface with these. Application Programming Interfaces (APIs), the Fast Healthcare Interoperability Resources (FHIR) standard, and other interoperability technologies can then be used to ensure the new telehealth system integrates seamlessly into the existing clinical information technology (IT) systems, as well as future IT systems that might be deployed.

Emergency Management

The mobility and scalability of telehealth systems make them an ideal platform for emergency management. Hospital carts and wall-mounted stations can be deployed in the emergency department or emergency management center, and mobile transportable exam and backpack solutions can be deployed in the field by emergency responder personnel. These can be readily moved to where they are needed, thus permitting delivery of care when it is needed, as well as workload balancing. Telehealth systems purchased and deployed as part of an emergency management program can also be utilized for nonemergent purposes, including mass casualty training scenarios, as well as routine telehealth primary care. This has the dual benefit of leveraging the investment as well as ensuring that clinician users are proficient in using the telehealth system when the emergency arises. In the early weeks of the COVID-19 pandemic, ED visits dropped by 42%, attributed in large part to the public's concern about exposure to the COVID virus. According to the CDC, this underscores the need for health care systems to deploy virtual health technologies for triage and treatment for conditions not requiring in-person care (Hartnett et al., 2020).

CLINICAL USE CASE STUDIES

A growing body of medical literature demonstrates that telemedicine improves health care outcomes in emergency and a wide variety of other clinical care settings:

- A systemic literature review published in *Health Affairs* (Mueller et al., 2014) noted that telemedicine use in rural emergency care settings "improves clinical quality, expands the care team, increases resources during critical events, shortens time to care, improves care coordination,

- promotes patient-centered care, improves the recruitment of family physicians, and stabilizes the rural hospital patient base."
- A study by Kaiser Permanente (Sauser-Zachrison et al., 2016) showed a significant increase in the timely use of thrombolytic therapy following a telemedicine consult with a stroke specialist. In stroke care, "time is neurons," and minutes can make the difference between little or no impairment versus devastating paralysis and other stroke complications.
- A peer-reviewed analysis of Nemours Children's Health System's pediatric telemedicine program in *Telemedicine and e-Health Journal* (Vyas, Murren-Boezem, & Solo-Josephson, 2018) found that telemedicine decreased visits to "brick-and-mortar" facilities such as emergency departments, urgent-care centers, or ambulatory clinics, and resulted in an estimated net savings of $113 million. Another benefit of telemedicine demonstrated by this study is that patients with communicable diseases can often be treated at home, limiting exposure to others and thus reducing transmission of illness.
- In another study, telemedicine resulted in a reduction in Pediatric Intensive Care Unit (PICU) admissions and triage of pediatric patients to a more clinically appropriate level of care (Harvey et al., 2017).
- Telemedicine improves access to specialized care and lowers barriers to screenings for diabetic retinopathy, resulting in earlier diagnosis and treatment.
- Although telemedicine has "potential to add value to the delivery of emergency care in rural emergency departments," Zachrison et al. (2020) noted that it may be underused, chiefly due to the cost of implementing the technology.

VENDOR-PROVIDED TECH—OPPORTUNITIES AND RISKS

Build vs. Buy: Hardware, Software, and Staffing

Any clinical entity planning to implement a telehealth program must decide whether to build their own system. In so doing, they must identify and procure various hardware, software, and peripheral device components then assemble these into a cart or other configuration as required. Prior to doing so, due diligence requires that all components are protocol compatible and thus readily interface with one another. This requires a significant amount of internal expertise and effort, not to mention life-cycle support. System users also need to be trained, either internally or outsourced externally.

The alternative is to buy a "preassembled" telehealth system, and there are a number of commercial vendors in the telehealth marketplace with a full range of integrated telehealth hardware, software, and peripheral device offerings, as described above. Most telehealth vendors also provide life-cycle support and maintenance for the hardware and software they sell, as well as user training and round-the-clock help desk support. Some vendors allow the purchasing health care system to "white label" their telehealth equipment, thus branding it to their specific health care system or network.

In addition, some telehealth vendors provide clinical staffing, thus freeing the deploying health care system from the burden of telehealth staffing, which includes training, credentialing, licensing, and other administrative duties unique to managing a telehealth program. These duties are discussed in more detail in a later chapter.

SUMMARY

Telehealth is gaining ever-increasing acceptance across the clinical landscape, including in EDs and emergency management programs. The COVID-19 pandemic has greatly accelerated its adoption. Increased reimbursements and reduced regulatory restrictions are also factors in this trend. This has been concurrently driven by advances in telemedicine hardware, software, and an ever-growing armamentarium of peripheral exam devices, supported by improvements in the communication networks that telemedicine depends on. These advances are helping to realize the key benefits telehealth brings to the health care equation—improving access to care, increasing efficiency of care, reducing health care costs, and, most importantly, improving clinical outcomes.

TELEHEALTH PROGRAM DEPLOYMENT CHECKLIST

- ✓ Determine if cases are fixed site or mobile use —for example, ED, first responders, disaster response.
- ✓ Define other clinical requirements—for example, primary or specialty care, dental work, audiometry.
- ✓ Assess network capabilities and infrastructure.
- ✓ Define other technical requirements.
- ✓ Confirm security requirements—HIPAA and enterprise-specific regulations.
- ✓ Develop a training plan—including assessing and sustaining telemedicine skills.
- ✓ Develop a budget—start-up, training, and sustaining skills, life-cycle costs.
- ✓ Obtain stakeholder buy-in

Key Takeaways

- ➤ Telemedicine hardware comes in a wide array of configurations meeting almost all clinical use cases, including those of emergency departments and first responders.
- ➤ Telemedicine software, when integrated with hardware and interoperable with EHR systems, allows users to complete a wide spectrum of clinical

as well as administrative tasks, including scheduling, secure messaging, clinical documentation, billing, and data analytics.

➢ Adoption of telemedicine technology has been greatly accelerated by the COVID-19 pandemic, and continued advances in technology and communication networks will ensure it plays a key role in the health care continuum, alongside in-patient and ambulatory medicine.

➢ In addition to improving access to care and reducing costs, peer-reviewed studies confirm that telemedicine improves health care quality.

REFERENCES

Kvedar, J. C. (2020). President, the American Telemedicine Association (ATA) Professor, Harvard Medical School Senior Advisor, Virtual Care, Mass General Brigham (Partners HealthCare) Senate Committee on Health, Education, Labor and Pensions Telehealth: Lessons from the COVID-19 Pandemic.

Hartnett, K. P., Kite-Powell, A., DeVies, J., et al. (2020). Impact of the COVID-19 Pandemic on Emergency Department Visits—United States. *Morbidity and Mortality Weekly Report, 69,* 699–704. doi:http://dx.doi.org/10.15585/mmwr.mm6923e1external icon

Harvey, J. B., Yeager, B. E., Cramer, C., Wheeler, D., & McSwain, S. D. (2017). The Impact of Telemedicine on Pediatric Critical Care Triage. *Pediatric Critical Care Medicine, 18*(11), e555–e560. doi:10.1097/PCC.0000000000001330. PMID: 28922271.

Mueller, K. J., Potter, A. J., MacKinney. A. C., & Ward, M. M. (2014). Lessons from tele-emergency: Improving care quality and health outcomes by expanding support for rural care systems. *Health Affairs (Project Hope), 33*(2), 228–234.

Sauser-Zachrison, K., Shen, E., Sangha, N., et al. (2016). Safe and effective implementation of telestroke in a US community hospital setting. *The Permanente Journal, 20*(4), 15–217. doi:https://doi.org/10.7812/TPP/15-217.

Vyas, S., Murren-Boezem, J., & Solo-Josephson, P. (2018). Analysis of a pediatric telemedicine program. *Telemedicine and e-Health, 24,* 993–997.

Zachrison, K. S., Boggs, K. M., Hayden, E. M., Espinola, J. A., & Camargo, C. A. Jr. (2020). Understanding barriers to telemedicine implementation in rural emergency departments. *Annals of Emergency Medicine, 75*(3), 392–399. doi:10.1016/j.annemergmed.2019.06.026. Epub 2019 Aug 29. PMID: 31474481.

3

Telehealth Training and Education

ADITI U. JOSHI AND NEAL SIKKA ■

INTRODUCTION

Telehealth is an increasingly common offering of physician practices and health care systems designed to improve patient access. As health care providers consider providing telehealth services, they must have the skills needed to effectively and safely utilize this modality of providing care. In 2014, more than half the respondents to a national survey of family practitioners reported training as a key barrier to telehealth adoption (Moore, 2016). Prior to the COVID-19 pandemic, telehealth programs developed slowly with considerations to the various aspects required for success, which included training. During the spring of 2020, the pandemic-induced need for physical distance to decrease exposure required health care providers across the United States and the rest of the world to rapidly adopt telehealth with minimal onboarding. Many clinicians found a new opportunity to connect with patients and learned that evaluations they had previously not considered suitable could be completed over telehealth. However, this rapid adoption of telehealth also revealed the value of formal training regarding effective practice via telehealth. Further, as the telehealth originating site shifts from in-facility to the home, patients need guidance on optimizing their virtual visits as well. Despite this need, there are few validated training programs for telehealth and little consensus on training skills and competencies. Recognizing this gap, the American Association of Medical Colleges (AAMC) convened an expert consensus panel that developed and published telehealth competencies to guide programs for training creation. The guide was published in September 2020, and so time will determine its utility.

While we consider telehealth to be only a modality of care, it still requires common understanding and strong communication between providers, telepresenters, patients, and carepartners. Telehealth programs touch many parts of an organization; therefore, education and training programs need be developed for all stakeholders and levels of learners, with varied emphasis on theoretical, didactic, and practical training (Edirippulige, 2016; Gifford, Niles, Rivkin, Koverola, & Polaha, 2012; Papanagnon et al., 2018; Papanagnon, Sicks, & Hollander, 2015). The focus of this chapter is on practical training for the implementation of emergency telehealth and will examine clinician, telepresenter, and patient training.

Training Goals and Objectives

Many training programs are created to meet the need of onboarding physicians for organization-specific telehealth programs. For example, telemedicine companies selling direct-to-consumer platforms and services have specific onboarding processes related to their technology and clinical pathways. Healthcare institutions may develop training that meets the scope of their telehealth offerings. As telehealth services expand, it has become necessary to ensure the training of all stakeholders within the organization in order to maximize adoption and ensure quality, provide a consistent patient experience, and enable troubleshooting. Stakeholders include leadership, administrative staff, clinical learners, nursing and other ancillary staff, advanced practice providers, physicians, telepresenters, and patients. Collecting program-specific data on current telehealth practice, the regulatory landscape, operations, quality assurance, and patient satisfaction can inform the development of a training program.

TRAINING CLINICIANS

Clinician engagement is critical to the success of telehealth programs. Clinicians must recognize the benefits of telehealth and its appropriate use, understand how to provide the service, and be able to support patients through the telehealth visit. Training topics vary by organization but typically include areas such as onboarding to the organization's specific program and technology platform, basic technology troubleshooting, web etiquette, as well as performing a virtual physical exam, quality assurance, and care delivery (Box 3.1). Using a consensus method, the AAMC also

---

Box 3.1

SAMPLE LIST OF TELEHEALTH TRAINING TOPICS

Telehealth Basics: Definitions, background, history, efficacy and quality.
Telehealth liability, risk management, malpractice, licensure, and regulation
Reimbursement
Appropriate complaints and conditions
Conducting a virtual physical exam
Documentation requirements
Technology platform overview, onboarding and basic troubleshooting
Escalation and contingency planning
Telehealth ethics and professionalism
Telehealth and health equity
Web etiquette

Box 3.2

ASSOCIATION OF AMERICAN MEDICAL COLLEGES TELEHEALTH COMPETENCIES[6]

Patient Safety and Appropriate Use of Telehealth
Data Collection and Assessment via Telehealth
Communication via Telehealth
Ethical Practices and Legal Requirements for Telehealth
Technology for Telehealth
Access and Equity in Telehealth

*Competencies in these 6 domains are graded by levels, as follows: (1) Entering Residency; (2) Entering Practice; (3) Experienced Faculty Physician.

created six domains to assess competency in telehealth that can be used to inform existing or future training programs (Box 3.2).

Basics of Telehealth and Onboarding

Telehealth stakeholders need to understand the terminology related to telehealth, as well as basic historical context and common use cases. Clinicians need to be familiar with the available telehealth modalities, such as video, phone, chat or text, and synchronous or asynchronous, as well as why and when to use each. Additionally, they should learn how telehealth fits into their practice, specifically understanding which patient visits in their practice are appropriate for telehealth. The expected benefits for patients, health care professionals, and the organization as a whole should be clear.

Telemedicine Liability, Licensure and Regulation

Clinicians are often hesitant to begin providing telehealth services due to perceived risk of liability. It is important to clearly articulate that malpractice risk is low and how the organization will ensure coverage for services delivered through telehealth. Many clinicians may not be aware of the complex web of regulation associated with telehealth. Topics to cover include licensure requirements, any state-specific rules regulating telehealth practice, prescribing policies, and payer restrictions. For those in organizations with cross-state practice, it will be important to convey frameworks that accommodate the rules for multiple jurisdictions.

Telehealth Reimbursement

All stakeholders should have a general understanding of reimbursement issues related to telehealth. It is important to consider the different requirements for reimbursement and coverages for commercial payers, Medicaid, and Medicare. Many payers have specific requirements for consent, documentation, disclaimers, reporting, and location of services. Additionally, clinicians who submit billing codes should learn about telehealth-specific billing codes and modifiers.

Clinical Pathways/Patient Selection

Many clinicians new to telehealth are unclear as to which patients and complaints are appropriate for telehealth visits. Almost any patient can start their evaluation with telehealth recognizing that they may require escalation to an in-person visit. However, depending on the service and specialty, clinicians may elect to define a list of complaints that are preferentially routed to telehealth. Shared experience among the practice is a powerful tool for expanding use cases based on a colleague's positive experience.

A set of clinical pathways can be helpful to aid clinicians new to telehealth. Pathways can be created by using current clinical decision-making tools and tailoring them to telehealth. Many are based on current practice for in-person care or other currently published guidelines (Figure 3.1). Of note, there are no validated guidelines specific to telehealth as of this publication. Most telehealth clinical pathways are based on common practice or guidelines established from in-person encounters. These pathways outline current guidelines on history, tips on exam, and treatment, and they point out red flags requiring an in-person visit. Using telehealth forces clinicians to think more clearly about guidelines, tests that may or may not be necessary, and whether a patient needs to be seen in person.

Guidelines can also serve to improve clinical practice and quality, and help clinicians extend the limits of their virtual practice. Providers who have more experience may feel comfortable with using telehealth more broadly; having pathways can give those new to the practice a way to understand what their practice can and should entail.

Telehealth offers uninterrupted online counseling time with patients that can be invaluable. This time provides the opportunity to ask questions, better understand their disease process and progression, and have a better sense of what is normal and abnormal. In a time when in-person care is stressful and time sensitive, telehealth can allow patients to feel they have more control over their health.

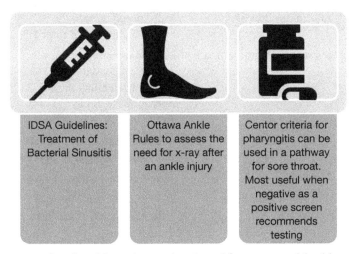

IDSA Guidelines: Treatment of Bacterial Sinusitis

Ottawa Ankle Rules to assess the need for x-ray after an ankle injury

Centor criteria for pharyngitis can be used in a pathway for sore throat. Most useful when negative as a positive screen recommends testing

Figure 3.1 Examples of guidelines that can be adapted for use over telehealth

Technology Platforms and Basic Troubleshooting:

Organizations should train clinicians to understand the features and basic troubleshooting for all utilized software and hardware. Synchronous visits may require real-time troubleshooting to ensure that appointments are not missed, canceled, or lost. Training will be unique to the use case and platform. For example, if a direct-to-consumer platform is in use, the clinician may be required to help a patient navigate the patient facing interface of the platform to ensure optimal use of video or audio. The provider should also understand how to set up an account and know its barriers, in case it is necessary to help a patient or family member. A provider-to-provider or teletriage encounter will likely have a telepresenter also trained in using the software and hardware. The clinician and telepresenter can work collaboratively to resolve technical problems and enable optimal consultation.

Telehealth patient satisfaction is intimately tied with working technology. While a robust IT department is necessary to set up the technology and help with complicated issues, all clinicians should have a good sense of what issue they can troubleshoot and when to escalate to IT support (Table 3.1).

Most of the basic issues are part of training and using the technology, although not all issues are evident at implementation and the learning will be iterative. In general, a good plan in tandem with IT will help develop a comprehensive workflow to deal with technology issues.

Table 3.1 BASIC TROUBLESHOOTING TIPS

Problem	Troubleshooting
Cannot access the app or program or download and setup an account	App store Patient portal Program website
Turning on/off the video or camera and common audio connection issues	Restart the device or application Video on/off buttons Ensure neither side is muted
Optimizing the camera image	Positioning the camera Adding a second device Avoid backlighting Appropriate lighting Switch to back or front camera
Issues with electronic prescriptions	Able to find pharmacy contact Understand controlled substance rules
Connectivity Issues	Able to contact patient via phone or email
Escalate to right party when a higher level of help is needed	IT support or vendor support depending on the application or hardware
Bluetooth(R) connectivity	Direct to Bluetooth settings in device Toggle Bluetooth setting

Webside Manner

Translating in-person care bedside manner to virtual care is referred to as *webside manner, virtual presence,* or *telemedicine etiquette.* These terms refer to the basic behavioral and environmental factors of a professional virtual visit, and their importance in producing a successful encounter cannot be overstated. The basics of webside manner include:

- Professional background: office, clinic, or neutral background that is private
- Appropriate lighting—enough light to see the provider's face and avoidance of backlight. For telepresenters, having enough light to appropriately examine the patient.
- Looking at camera—making eye contact through camera, informing patients when looking in other directions such as to the chart or at pictures.
- General demeanor and comfort in speaking over camera: getting practice with it as a medical encounter, having appropriate greetings to all parties, developing general comfort with virtual care on camera.
- Appropriate closing and goodbye: understanding that an abrupt ending over camera is detrimental to the provider–patient relationship

Generally, the points of a good webside manner are similar to those historically associated with a good bedside manner. Optimizing environmental factors and engaging behaviors improves trust, empathy, communication, and professionalism. These factors are critical for patient satisfaction and require an understanding of nonverbal communications skills as transmitted and perceived over video (Gifford et al., 2012; Papanagnon et al., 2018; Papagagnon, Sicks, & Hollander, 2015; Ishikawa, Hashimoto, Kinoshita, & Yano (2010). While strong observational skills and history taking are keys to effective clinical practice, during a telehealth encounter it is essential to use simple and clear language, pause for questions, avoid speaking over the patient, and ensuring that patients understand the treatment and follow-up plan.

For some clinicians, improving their webside manner will be a struggle. However, with continued practice, tips from experienced providers, appropriate training and support, practice cases, and seeing more patients, webside manner will improve. While those with a good bedside manner may find it easier to convert this behavior to video, it should be noted that almost anyone can still find engagement over video harder and more awkward than anticipated.

For this reason, training and practice in virtual presence is a necessary and critical component of a comprehensive telehealth training program. The Master Interview Rating Scale (MIRS) can be a useful tool in providing clear and objective feedback to clinicians as they learn these communications skills (Wagner, Pfeiffer, & Harrington, 2011). The scoring allows learners to track their progress over time and potentially measure competency. At George Washington University, the MIRS questionnaire was adapted to telehealth and utilized to evaluate students and faculty during observed telemedicine visits. Research presented at the 2017 SEARCH conference shared the results of using adapted MIRS questions to evaluate 20 teleneurologists in mock stroke scenarios (Table 3.2).

Table 3.2 EVALUATION OF 20 MOCK TELESTROKE CONSULTS BY TELENEUROLGIST
AND RATINGS ON QUESTIONS ADAPTED FROM MASTER INTERVIEW RATING SCALE
(JARED LUCAS AND NEAL SIKKA)

Question	Result (Mean or %) (*Variance*)
Background	3.68
Professional Appearing, minimizes distracting clutter (Scale 1-5)	(1.56)
Professional Attire	
White Coat Optional (Yes/No)	85%
Lighting	80%
Minimizes backlighting (Yes/No)	
Camera Positioning	80%
At or above eye-level (Yes/No)	
Opening	3.63
Patient ID/preferred name, MD name, state role (Scale 1-5)	(0.35)
Adequate History	70%
HPI, Rx, Allergies, Risk Factors (Yes/No)	
Questioning	4.42
Starts with open ended questions (Scale 1-5)	(0.59)
Pacing	4.89
Minimizes pause, avoid interruption (Scale 1-5)	(0.1)
Duplication	4.94
Minimizes unnecessary repeat questions (Scale 1-5)	(0.05)
Summarizing	3.58
Gives patient a summary of provided info (Scale 1-5)	(0.59)
Jargon	4.1
Minimizes medical terminology (Scale 1-5)	(0.43)
Verbal Facilitation	4.0
Provides verbal encouragement (Scale 1-5)	(0.44)
Non-Verbal Facilitation	3.16
Open body language, eye-contact with camera (Scale 1-5)	(0.58)
Empathy	3.58
Supportive and avoids criticism (Scale 1-5)	(0.37)

History and Physical Exam

A concern among clinicians when beginning telehealth is how to successfully complete a history and physical exam. Training on completing a history and physical exam should be differentiated from training on webside manner.

Generally, taking a history over video is straightforward. It requires asking the same questions providers would normally ask in person. In the virtual environment, the clinician should begin with an introduction, as well as confirm the patient's identity, location, and callback number in the event of a connectivity issue. Any additional participants in the encounter, for example, family caregivers and learners working with the clinician, must also be introduced. Before history taking, the clinician should verbally review telemedicine consent information as required by local regulations.

It is a myth that clinicians do not conduct physical examination over telehealth. The physical exam over telehealth takes more practice and nuance. There are specific skills to completing a virtual physical exam that include directing the patient or telepresenter to perform selected tasks, in addition to close observation of the patient's movements and speech patterns. There is much to be learned by observing their living environment and surroundings. Clinicians can have patients move their joints, assess pain with specific actions or areas of the body, move the camera to see the eyes, throat, skin rashes, and other areas as needed. Patients can be directed to take their own pulse and to use home monitors such as blood pressure cuffs, thermometers, or scales as available. Family members can also be recruited to examine the patient. For example, under the clinician's guidance, the family caregiver can assist with an abdominal or neurological examination. Not only does this add valuable information to the physical examination, it aids the patient in being an active part of their health care. In the above example, having the patient understand where the right lower quadrant is and why it is important to know whether the pain localizes in that region helps them realize when and why they might need further evaluation.

Parts of the examination, such as auscultation of heart and lung sounds, may be unavailable without a remote monitoring device. Currently, the rate of use of these remote devices is low; however, in the future they will be more readily available. The goal for the clinician is to gather actionable information and be able to effectively communicate a plan to the patient or caregiver and ensure their understanding of their current status and potential red flags.

Telehealth physical exam skills can be taught, and there are available online training programs and continuing medical education (CME) that can be part of the training process. Jefferson Health created a basic telehealth examination course in 2017 and added more courses during the pandemic in 2020, due to the crucial need that had arisen. Like any new medical skill or procedure, practice is required to improve this skill. It should be noted that those who have more clinical experience are more likely to easily translate these skills to telehealth evaluations.

Contingency Planning

Telehealth clinicians should be familiar with protocols that address the escalation of care from virtual to in-person. Whether physical or psychiatric, clinicians should know when and how to call emergency services, and plans should be specific to the modality of telehealth. It is critical that patient identification and location are confirmed at the beginning of the consultation so that if an emergency occurs, the clinician has accurate information to provide to emergency dispatch personnel. Emergency situations may entail recognizing impending worsening clinical symptoms, an acute change in condition like syncope, the need for emergency psychiatric evaluation, and other difficult situations.

For difficult or angry patients, having scripting to help defuse situations can improve patient care and clinician satisfaction. While most clinicians with any experience will have their own strategies, tailoring these strategies to telehealth with scripts for specific situations can be helpful. In cases where deescalation is not possible, clinicians should be given instructions on how to disengage from visit, how and to whom to escalate, and appropriate charting.

TRAINING OF UNDERGRADUATE AND GRADUATE MEDICAL STUDENTS

There is currently little formal education regarding the practice of telehealth in undergraduate or graduate medical education. The new AAMC Telehealth Competencies contain a leveled approach that can help guide medical schools and residency programs. A survey of 316 medical students from the United States and Canada in 2016–2017 revealed that they received little exposure in the clinical years to telehealth, mobile health, or remote patient monitoring (Figure 3.2). Additionally, in a review of 104 residency program milestones, only child adolescent psychiatry mentioned telehealth (Pourmand et al., 2020). During the COVID-19 pandemic, rapid implementation of telehealth has increased awareness, participation, and clinical engagement of trainees in telehealth. It is likely that curricula will soon include more formal training and participation in telehealth.

It is technically complicated to use standard teaching models from in-person care in telehealth; however, simulation can be valuable to create realistic and useful experiences. Telehealth training can be further integrated during the modules teaching the physical exam: teaching in-person physical exam maneuvers while also including how those same findings might be elicited over video. Additionally, standardized patient (SP) encounters are a mechanism to improve virtual interdisciplinary practice. Where the use of SPs is not feasible, telehealth electives, seminars, and integration into the business of medicine or innovation courses is also common. These venues offer trainee exposure to telehealth business models, operations, implementation challenges, and clinical use cases and provide a deep look at regulations, use case selection, and technology platforms.

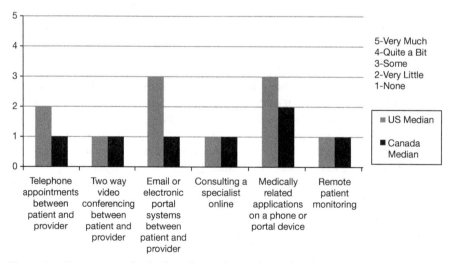

Figure 3.2 Frequency with which students observed specific telemedicine areas in use in clinical rotations; 12 medical schools in United States and Canada, 2016–2017 (*n* = 316)

One barrier to teaching telehealth lies in converting the current model of a trainee seeing and then presenting a patient to an attending. It would be redundant and require a callback, none of which are realistic alternatives in telehealth encounters. Measures to alleviate this include:

- Direct supervision: The student or resident conducts the visit with an attending next to them who can jump in when needed.
- Third-party call-in: This allows both trainees and attending to be on call from two remote locations.

Admittedly, this process can be stressful for trainees and take extra time for supervising faculty; however, it can also allow for quick feedback and improvement.

TRAINING FOR TELEPRESENTERS

A telepresenter functions as an extension of the hands of the clinician as they are onsite with the patient. There are two types of telepresenters: clinical and layperson. The clinical telepresenter may be an advanced practice provider (APP), nurse, medical assistant, emergency medical technician (EMT), paramedic, or medical student, all of whom have baseline familiarity with clinical care and the health care system. As clinical telepresenters typically have medical skills, training can be tailored to the level of clinical experience and the telemedicine use case. For example, telepresenters assisting with endocrinology or neurology teleconsults were taught how to conduct monofilament testing or how to collect data to complete a neuropathy scale, something with which many ancillary clinical team members have less familiarity (Wilson et al., 2020). The focus of training for clinical telepresenters is helping them understand the telemedicine modality, webside manner, and utilization of good communication with the distant site clinician.

The layperson telepresenter (LTP) may be a community health worker, an activated community member, or a family carepartner. This type of telepresenter will be a growing part of the telehealth ecosystem as increased care will occur at home or in the community. Since the layperson has less knowledge of the health system and clinical care experience, the training curriculum needs to be more in depth to their needs. For layperson telepresenters, clinical skills are one of the most anxiety-provoking content areas, as they have limited knowledge of anatomy, are less comfortable with digital tools like digital stethoscopes and otoscopes, and may have limited experience with clinical interactions with patients. LTPs must be trained so they can demonstrate the ability to collect and document vital signs, place the digital stethoscope over the heart and lungs as directed by the clinician, utilize a digital otoscope or dermatoscope, palpate the abdomen in four quadrants and evaluate the lower extremities for edema as directed by the clinician. They should also practice introducing the patient and serving as a patient advocate if they feel the distant clinician is not able to adequately perceive the patient's concerns. Table 3.3 presents some of the topics covered in one innovative program developed between an academic medical center and a community-based house of worship for layperson telepresenter training (Sikka, Combs, Lum, & Curry, 2020).

Table 3.3 LAYPERSON TELEPRESENTER TRAINING MODULES

Module 1	Didactics
	What is telemedicine? Key definitions and brief history
	Telemedicine utility and benefit(s) for all stakeholders
	Role of the telemedicine clinical presenter
	Environmental considerations and web etiquette
	How to capture and document vital signs
	How to assist with the physical examination
	How to communicate with patients and providers
	HIPAA privacy and security
	Technology training (telemedicine, video, laptop)
Module 2	Vital signs (yes/no/other)
	Places blood pressure cuff correctly
	Identifies and records blood pressure
	Places thermometer correctly under the tongue
	Identifies and records temperature
	Places pulse oximeter correctly
	Identifies and records pulse oxygen saturation
	Identifies and records heart rate
Module 3	Physical examination (yes/no/other)
	Identifies four locations for heart sounds
	Identifies six locations for lung sounds
	Identifies four quadrants of the abdomen
	Shines light in the eye to check for pupil reactivity
	Places the otoscope in the ear while pulling up and out
	Applies pressure to shins to assess edema

For both clinical and layperson telepresenters, it can be helpful to add prompts and pictures to the training content and within the clinical space. For example, Figure 3.3 demonstrates the appropriate position of the stethoscope on the heart and lungs, as well as the four quadrants of the abdomen.

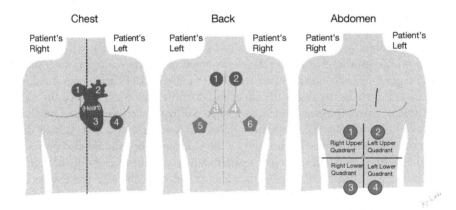

Figure 3.3 Poster sample that can be hung at originating site for telepresenter and clinician reference. Printed with permission from Jay Sikka (2016).

TECHNIQUES FOR TRAINING

In-person Training

In-person training can either be set up as one-on-one or in groups, depending on the number of learners. This is likely the most useful for those running onsite training for in-house programs. Learners may need to train on the platform, do practice calls, and go through basic troubleshooting under the guidance of teachers. The trainers should be well versed in telehealth, whether they are clinicians conducting telehealth visits or a team dedicated to training.

Remote Training

Remote training refers to similar training done in person but over video. It may be tailored for a group of remote learners or for an online course with live teachers (differentiated from a CME-type video course). Remote training was relied on heavily during the COVID-19 pandemic. There are benefits of conducting training via the same technology platform that will be used for clinical care; when clinicians are viewed online, teachers can provide feedback regarding environmental issues such as lighting, cluttered workspace, eye contact, and other virtual presence tips that may not be recognized unless the learner is on video. After clinicians have completed some patient encounters, doing scheduled follow-up or refresher training can be very helpful in further improving telehealth skills.

Adjunct Training

It is valuable to create training manuals, audio or video materials, and other such resources that decrease the need for live teachers. These resources can be helpful for refresher training as well. They should be housed with other organizational training resources, such as those for the electronic health record. Some training programs require learners to asynchronously complete the online content and then complete one-on-one or group training on the platform.

Simulation Training

Simulation education has become a standard part of emergency medical education, allowing learners to have an immersive experience with patient care. Simulation can also be used similarly to practice telehealth calls for both clinical experience and technology troubleshooting.

Remote Presenter Training

Remote presenters and EMTs can be trained similarly using the above types of models. As EMTs will likely also be on an ambulance and clinical telepresenters will be remote, their simulation (SIM) based education modules should reflect these differences. Aside from this, the types of training are similar, requiring troubleshooting, practice encounters, and basics of telehealth.

COMPETENCY EVALUATION AND CONTINUING EDUCATION

Quality programs, such as peer review, patient safety conferences, patient satisfaction surveys, and patient complaints, are used as adjuncts to improve care. In formal didactic settings, like medical schools and residency training, competency can be assessed through the variety of educational settings already in place, including direct observation, simulation cases, and standardized patients. These same tools may be more difficult to implement in a small practice of experienced clinicians starting telehealth. In these situations, using modular asynchronous training should be considered. Ensuring that clinicians share strategies that they have found effective and challenges that they frequently face can be helpful. Until the AAMC publication, there had been no consensus recommendations for telehealth competencies for education as evaluation of competency is a potentially challenging and time-consuming endeavor. These competencies can now be used to create and improve existing education.

Telehealth training programs need to provide continuing education to maintain credentialing on a regular basis. A quality assurance/process improvement (QA/PI) process may require physicians to change practice and require reassessment. Some focus areas for continuing education include:

- CME maintenance as per state medical board
- Compliance with any QA/PI process intervention
- Maintenance of credentialing, including practice calls, adjunct videos
- Training in new utility added to institution since initial onboarding
- Reimbursement and regulatory updates

PREPARING YOUR ORGANIZATION FOR TELEHEALTH

Adoption of telehealth requires awareness of the telehealth program across the clinical enterprise. Each business unit within the organization will be impacted by the addition of telehealth services and must adhere to goals, objectives, policy, and procedures that guide the program. Staff will need periodic refreshers regarding relevant aspects of the telehealth program, and mechanisms should be in place to monitor adherence (AHIMA Telemedicine ToolKit, 2017). A comprehensive education program for all parts of that team is essential for success.

CONCLUSION

Telehealth training and education for stakeholders across an organization are critical for effective use of this modality of care. Much of the focus is on clinician training to ensure they understand the goals of offering telehealth, legal, and regulatory constraints, as well as optimal patient evaluation. They must also recognize the importance of practicing good web etiquette to portray professionalism and improve patient engagement. However, administrative, billing, and technical teams must also be trained to ensure telehealth implementation works for patients, clinicians, and the practice as a whole. Improved training will increase quality of care, engagement, and efficient use of telehealth and therefore requires a comprehensive plan for initial and ongoing delivery.

KEY TAKEAWAYS

- ➤ All stakeholders supporting or participating in delivery of care via telehealth require training.
- ➤ There are a variety of skills that clinicians must be aware of, practice, and improve to provide optimal care via telehealth.
- ➤ Telehealth education and training can be delivered in a variety of formats, customized for the organization's program, and should be ongoing.
- ➤ Clinicians often need specific training and support to improve webside manner and perform virtual physical exams.
- ➤ Training for telepresenters can expand the capabilities of telehealth services.

REFERENCES

AAMC. (2021). *Telehealth Competencies Across the Learning Continuum.* AAMC New and Emerging Areas in Medicine Series. Washington, DC: AAMC. https://www.aamc.org/system/files/2020-09/hca-telehealthcollection-telehealth-competencies.pdf

AHIMA Telemedicine ToolKit. (2017). https://healthsectorcouncil.org/wp-content/uploads/2018/08/AHIMA-Telemedicine-Toolkit.pdf.

Edirippulige, S., & Armfield, N. R. (2017). Education and training to support the use of clinical telehealth: A review of the literature. *Journal of Telemedicine and Telecare,* 23(2), 273–282. doi:10.1177/1357633X16632968.

Gifford, V., Niles, B., Rivkin, I., Koverola, C., & Polaha, J. (2012). Continuing education training focused on the development of behavioral telehealth competencies in behavioral healthcare providers, *Rural Remote Health, 12,* 2108.

Ishikawa, H., Hashimoto, H., Kinoshita, M., &Yano, E. (2010). Can nonverbal communication skills be taught? *Medical Teacher, 32*(10), 860–863.

Moore, M. A., Coffman, M., Jetty, A., Petterson, S., & Bazemore, A. (2016). Graham Center Policy One-Pagers: Only 15% of FPs Report Using Telehealth; Training and Lack of Reimbursement Are Top Barriers. *American Family Physician, 93*(2), 1–101.

Papanagnou, D., Stone, D., Chandra, S., Watts, P., Chang, A. M., & Hollander, J. E. (2018). Integrating telehealth emergency department follow-up visits into residency training. *Cureus, 10*(4), e2433.

Papanagnou, D., Sicks, S., & Hollander, J. E. (2015). Training the next generation of care providers: Focus on telehealth. *Healthcare Transformation, 1*(1), 52–63. doi.org/10.1089/heat.2015.29001-psh

Pourmand, A., Ghassemi, M., Sumon, K., Amini, S. B., Hood, C., & Sikka, N. (2020). Lack of telemedicine training in academic medicine: Are we preparing the next generation? *Telemedicine and e-Health*, ahead of printhttp://doi.org/10.1089/tmj.2019.0287 Online Ahead of Print: April 15, 2020.

Sikka, N., Combs, D., Lum, N., & Curry, K. E. (2020, May 18). Layperson telepresenters: increasing capacity for telehealth in underserved communities. *Telemedicine and e-Health*, Epub ahead of print. Jan 2021. 99–101. PMID: 32423355.

Wagner, J. A., Pfeiffer, C. A., & Harrington, K. L. (2011). Evaluation of online instruction to improve medical and dental students' communication and counseling skills. *Evaluation and the Health Professions*, 34(3), 383–397.

Wilson, A. M., Jamal, N. I., Cheng, E. M., et al. (2020). Teleneurology clinics for polyneuropathy: A pilot study. *Journal of Neurology*, 267, 479–490.

4

Telehealth Adoption and Patient Engagement

AHMAD A. AALAM, KAREEM A. OSMAN, AND AARON MARTIN ■

INTRODUCTION

Emergency department (ED) providers and hospital administrators eager to bring telehealth services to their practice should incorporate engagement strategies to maximize the utilization and benefit of telehealth for their patients. As the use of teletriage and direct-to-consumer telehealth grows, among other use cases, the best practices for engagement and retention are evolving (O'Connor et al., 2016; Pearl, 2017).

Health care engagement has been defined as "patients, families, their representatives, and health professionals working in active partnership at various levels across the health care system" (Gillespie, 2016). This can have a significant positive impact on health care utilization. In a tele-emergency study measuring the partnership between senior living community members and physicians, the most engaged communities had a 28% decrease in annualized ED visits compared to no significant change in ED use among control communities (Gillespie, 2016). To better describe where the engagement benefit comes from, this chapter divides health care engagement into the constitutive parts of clinician engagement, patient engagement, and administrator engagement. Additionally, we consider how better digital patient engagement, as can be seen in other industries, lowers costs and improves revenues (Westerman & McAfee, 2012). In health care, digital patient engagement, which occurs continuously, can make population health more effective and deliver better clinical outcomes (Ming Tai-Seale, 2019).

CLINICIAN ENGAGEMENT

Clinician engagement is paramount to the growth of a telehealth program (Freed Associates, 2019). In a 2015 Gallup study, physicians who were considered as "engaged" or "fully engaged" were 26% more productive than their peers (Kamins, 2019). However, many clinicians view telehealth programs as disruptive to their clinical practice and workflow. This necessitates the use of engagement strategies to motivate clinicians. The key strategies outlined in this section include establishing the "why," developing sponsorship, and reinforcing implementation.

Establishing the "Why"

Clinicians are driven toward change, understanding the value it will bring to their patients. To establish the "why," clinical leaders must identify and convey a clear problem statement through a needs assessment to demonstrate relevance (Kamins, 2019; Ground, 2019; Roga, 2019). Furthermore, telehealth program managers can leverage telehealth pilots to build clinician confidence that telehealth will benefit, rather than disrupt, their practice. The Jefferson Health e-health team held multiple meetings with all clinical department chairs and administrators, where they identified problems, areas for improvement, selected appropriate solutions, and tasked physicians to conduct at least twelve video visits each over a one-year period (Ellimoottil, 2018).

Identifying, quantifying, and providing supporting data to a problem that may be addressed by telehealth is critical to achieving clinician buy-in. However, evidence-based problems may still not engage clinicians, and they may require motivation tied to individual or peer metrics, such as patient visits, relative value units, or charges.

Identifying Sponsors

The second, and arguably most important, strategy to foster clinician engagement in telehealth is sponsorship. A sponsor takes on tasks that cannot be delegated to the personal management of clinicians or even the departmental head (Ground, 2019). Sponsors' tasks include resource allocation, reinforcement, and addressing resistance to change as it arises (Ground, 2019). Employees tend to follow the behavior of their colleagues with similar level positions (Ellimoottil, 2018). Therefore, cascading sponsorship, or sponsorship at every staff level, is required to establish champions at all levels affected by a telehealth innovation.

Often known as change champions, sponsors need to be empowered with the authority to cultivate an environment for practice improvement, express clear vision for the larger organization, and actively and enthusiastically promote the innovation. Furthermore, sponsors who integrate telehealth into their workflow doubly amplify the success of implementation over those who only express their commitment (Alsher, 2019). In some cases, identifying a champion for a telehealth initiative may be a challenge. Experts recommend noticing which clinicians are enthusiastic and who advocates for the advancement of new service delivery models. Selecting a sponsor from this group is an easy way to recruit effective telehealth champions (Wolverton, 2019).

An interesting example of clinician engagement is the collective health care response to the COVID-19 crisis, which made many organizations realize the importance of quick and organized change of pace to rapidly expand or introduce a new telehealth program. The response was driven by extensive clinician engagement from every part of a practice to expedite this process with patient care continuity in mind.

Reinforcement

The next principle essential to driving utilization of telehealth takes root from change management. Periodic and ongoing training for providers is essential to ensuring program goals are achieved and to fostering a departmental culture of telehealth. MDLIVE is a direct-to-consumer (DTC) telehealth company offering urgent care, behavioral health, and dermatology consults for health systems, health plans, and private consumers (MDLIVE, 2019). MDLIVE uses a learning management system with a 10-module provider onboarding curriculum and on-going training (Folino, 2019). Clinicians learn telepresence skills and the curriculum of medical virtualism. Similarly, the American Telemedicine Association lists four accredited training programs for clinicians and program managers (ATA, 2019).

The next step in provider reinforcement is to link desired behaviors to the goals of the program (Expert Program Management, 2018). Positive reinforcement should precede punishment during the early phases of the program (Ground, 2019). When physicians know they will not be penalized in time, cost, or convenience for offering telehealth to their patients, they are more likely to embrace telehealth (Pearl, 2017). Lastly, from an organizational perspective, rewards need not be exclusively monetary. Jefferson Health gives annual telehealth awards to involved staff members, presented by the CEO or senior executive vice president of the health system (Ellimoottil, 2018). Awards and accolades promote the view of telehealth involvement as a career differentiator and reinforce an engagement culture.

PATIENT ENGAGEMENT

Patient engagement is the most differentiated form of engagement in telehealth as user adoption is dependent on many factors, such as usability of the platform, awareness of available services, required payments, and perceptions of privacy. Emergency telehealth programs across the United States have gathered experience in engaging previously nonestablished patients through their telehealth platforms (AHA, 2017). New York-Presbyterian provides an excellent example of direct patient engagement through its ED-based Telehealth Express Care Service and suite of OnDemand services, including self-service kiosks and a mobile application, an approach that leverages digital tools inside and outside the facility (NYP, 2019). After analyzing telehealth program successes and failures, it is evident that telehealth plays a significant role in supporting organization-wide patient engagement strategies by enhancing patient access to care (PatientEngagementHIT, 2018).

A normalization process theory framework has been used to identify two major themes that define key engagement criteria and better understand how telehealth

Table 4.1 EXAMPLES OF PATIENT ENGAGEMENT STRATEGIES TELEHEALTH INITIATIVES

Strategies	Integration with patient's relational network	Artificial Intelligence (AI) integration
Cases	When Hurricane Irma hit Florida in 2017, the Neymours Children's Health System advertised their Care Connect service on social media and news outlets to offer free emergency teleconsultations and set up carts at shelters near providers that had access to Neymours pediatric specialty care (Wicklund, 2018; Bryant, 2019). This social media outreach received an "unprecedented number of shares and feedback," and the program had more encounters in a three-day period than typically seen in three months	CareAngel is an AI nurse assistant that uses voice-powered health monitoring over the phone to collect patient-reported biometrics, physical and mental health, and general well-being data (CareAngel, 2019a). In effect, the tool acts as a virtual nurse to collect repetitive data like medication adherence and vital signs. CareAngel can also send notifications to loved ones within the patient's "care circle" to involve them more actively in patient care (CareAngel, 2019b.) A case study of the use of CareAngel has produced a 63% reduction in hospital readmissions and an 85% patient engagement rate as measured by their remote and physical interaction with the health care system (CareAngel, 2019c).
Strategies	Customized Approaches	Digital marketing and social media
Cases	Providence St. Joseph Health developed a Patient and Provider Engagement Center (PEC) as part of its Virtual Health System in 2018 (PSJH, 2018). The PEC is a call center used to connect patients to their integrated virtual care system, including providers, education, and channels for feedback (PSJH. Patient Engagement Center, 2019). Implementation of the PEC has increased the call-in appointment rate from 28% to over 70% for one hospital in the Providence St. Joseph Health system (Comstock, 2019).	MDLIVE uses robust outreach protocols to drive registration and utilization of their virtual visits, with digital marketing and social media driving 24% of all virtual consultations (Folino, 2019). Examples of strategic best practices include targeted messaging based on seasonality (flu season, summer travel, etc.), annual updates on engagement metrics, including net promotor score (84.7 in 2019 [Power], 2019]) as part of their marketing tactics, and education on key messaging strategies to drive home the value of telemedicine for employees and patients. "Sophie" is an AI chatbot developed to drive 50% more registration for clients. Engagement statistics like these, along with incentives outcomes such as zero co-pay for a virtual visit, results in a 20% increase in utilization and are frequently communicated to their partners and patients (Folino, 2019).

initiatives affect patient retention and engagement (Mair et al., 2012). First, the engagement approach used must incorporate an understanding of the patient's personal motivation, values, and support system (O'Connor et al., 2016). Second, taking a telehealth initiative from pilot to scale requires a modification in recruitment and engagement strategy (Table 4.1) (Mair et al., 2012).

Reinforcement

There are a number of creative ways to reinforce patient engagement in telehealth initiatives. Incentives are used to engage patients at all stages in telehealth. Table 4.2 provides an overview of successful incentive models.

The responsibility to engage and reinforce patients in telehealth initiatives is an organization-wide concern. While clinicians are tasked with direct engagement through patient care (AHA, 2019), program managers are responsible for indirect engagement including advertisement, messaging, sponsorship, and support (O'Connor et al., 2016).

Table 4.2 REINFORCEMENT APPROACHES FOR PATIENT ENGAGEMENT

Referral Incentives	A telehealth and texting pilot demonstrated the successful use of a $25 participant incentive for both the referring participant and new participant to improve HIV care engagement (Wootton, Legnitto, & VA, 2019).
Multimodal Outreach Channels	MDLIVE reinforces exposure to their program through at least seven communications channels, including benefits events, newsletters, webinars, and wellness program integration. They demonstrate that "increased exposure through these channels builds brand/benefit recognition, keeps the benefit top of mind, encourages clinically appropriate use, and addresses key barriers to adoption" (MDLIVE, 2018).
Gift Certificates	In 2015, DocChat became the first telemedicine company to offer "Digital Doctor Gift Certificates" for up to a year's worth of telemedicine visits (PRWeb, 2015). This move to increase customer engagement in the fast-growing direct-to-consumer telemedicine market was called an "industry-first" and was a bold marketing strategy to increase buy-in from patients (Wicklund, 2015).
Health Coaching	Telehealth Services iCare Navigator uses gamification and health coaching to motivate patients to take an active role in their recovery (Telehealth Services, 2019).

Developing a Digital Engagement Strategy to Support Telehealth

Telehealth by itself is not a sustainable model long-term. It must pair with a viable population health strategy in which the health system takes financial risk, commits to a digital engagement platform, and invests in the digital engagement of patients between episodes of telehealth care. Technology companies such as Amazon and Google have pioneered digital engagement over the past two decades, and the techniques for driving digital engagement are well known to them. Health systems must learn from technology companies about patient engagement, as they utilize consumer engagement learnings as they explore potential business opportunities as health care services providers. First, a health system should measure digital engagement. The most common metric is Monthly Active Users (MAU), which measures the number of unique users who visit a digital property in a given month. Second, a health system must build a digital engagement plan.

The fundamental challenge a health system faces in engagement is the lack of natural frequency of the use of their services. Americans, on average, see their physicians between two and four times a year as needed (McCarthy, 2014). This level of engagement is dwarfed by the consumer digital engagement platforms of large tech companies. Amazon's Prime program is one of the most successful engagement platforms in the industry. It serves more than 100 million members in the United States (Statista Research Department, 2020). Nearly 88% of Amazon Prime customers report shopping on the site at least once a month, with almost a third reporting that they shop there several times a week (Statista Research Department, 2020). Engagement matters because it reduces Customer (patient) Churn, another metric on which technology companies are focused. Customer Churn is the rate at which a patient switches to another source of care. It is a measure of patient loyalty. Patient churn is expensive for health systems (Providence estimates a 1% reduction in churn is worth $100M in economic benefit), and it is arguably bad for patients as switching between providers causes fragmentation of care. While this churn is sometimes unavoidable (patients switching plans, relocating, etc.), some of it is purely due to the lack of a compelling reason to stay with a given health care brand or provider.

Health systems need to build robust digital engagement programs that increase the relevance and frequency of digital interactions with patients between care episodes as they will be competing with technology companies who already have massive and loyal customer bases. These large and well-capitalized companies can leverage their customer base to experiment with disruptive health care delivery models, such as Amazon Care. The most relevant tactics many health systems are adopting are digitally engaging with patients about chronic conditions such as diabetes, fitness tracking, and other health-related content. Effective engagement, however, requires personalization so that only relevant content is shown to patients who will benefit. There are examples of personalized engagement platforms that serve specific, and very important segments of patient populations. For instance, Wildflower Health provides personalized content for women during their pregnancy journey. Women make 80% of health care decisions within a typical household (Matoff-Stepp, 2014). Building engagement and loyalty with women is a strategic imperative for most health systems. Wildflower's platform digitally engages women via an application that provides personalized content that is specific to each week of their pregnancy pre- and postpartum. Finally, health systems should try to move every offline instance of engagement and attempt to tie it to an opportunity to engage patients digitally. For example, Xealth allows physicians to prescribe any digital content, app, or video directly from the electronic medical record. It also allows the recommending physician to see if the patient has used the app, read the article, or viewed the video the clinician has recommended.

Once a patient is frequently visiting a digital engagement platform, the use of telehealth in the form of video visits, asynchronous communication, or bot-assisted care becomes more seamless and natural than one-off episodic visits. Marketing acquisition costs are also dramatically lower as the patient is continuously using the engagement platform and is aware of the telehealth services made available by the health system. In addition to brand loyalty and better continuity of care as benefits of digital engagement, population health is better achieved. Digitally engaged patients can be encouraged to commit to healthy behaviors and should be introduced to content, online coaching, and programs that may help them manage chronic conditions. When appropriate, these services can be accessed digitally, which will be more cost effective for the health system and more convenient for the patient.

ADMINISTRATION ENGAGEMENT

Administration engagement is what makes any telemedicine program transform from a project on paper to an active and running one. Interested patients and motivated clinicians are the key force to bring administration onboard. It is the sponsor's job to help champions grow administration engagement to meet needs from the following categories: strategic and logistical support, financial support, human resources support, and/or policy alignment (Sharma, 2019). The sponsor and the founding team, in collaboration with members of the administration, should formulate a strategic plan of what would benefit stakeholders and the institution in return for their support. An example is the plan implemented by the University of Virginia (UVA) telemedicine program, which achieved a smooth process (Wibberly, 2020).

In the "Top of Mind for Top Health Systems" report published by the Center for Connected Medicine and the Health Management Academy, executives of health institutions were surveyed about thoughts on the future of the field. They were optimistic regarding telehealth reimbursement, but they were worried about increased cyberattacks (Center for Connected Medicine and The Health Management, 2020). Many health organizations like the American Medical Association (AMA), the American College of Healthcare Executives (ACHE), the American Hospital Association (AHA), and the Healthcare Information and Management Systems Society (HIMSS) have participated, advised, developed, or published on the importance of telemedicine in the present and near future. The collection and citation of such articles or publications can strengthen the sponsor's team discussion with the administration and enhance their support. Additionally, the champion team needs an extensive review of the continually changing polices and regulations locally and nationally, given the fast pace of development in this area, particularly during a crisis such as the COVID-19 pandemic. Finally, it is important for administration and clinicians to establish metrics and to set goals, and on a reliable cadence (at least once monthly), to monitor progress in driving patient and clinical engagement (Table 4.3).

Table 4.3 WHAT C-SUITE LEADERS ARE THINKING ABOUT THE FUTURE OF TELEHEALTH (BASED ON THE TOP OF MIND FOR TOP HEALTH 2019 SYSTEMS RESEARCH PROJECT)

Subject	Opinions
Growth	Anticipate telehealth growth by 10% or more in the next three years.
Reimbursement	Optimistic about government and commercial telehealth reimbursement increasing in the next three years.
Funding	Expect the majority of funding for telehealth to come from commercial and government payers within the next three years.
Technology priorities	Integrate with the clinical workflow, ease of patient triage and virtual follow-up, and offer network of remote clinicians.
Value	Telehealth viewed as a cost-saving initiative; consider developing the patient connections and the associated potential downstream revenue as a proxy ROI.
Artificial intelligence	May help health systems implement more robust predictive risk modeling and preventative care.
Cybersecurity	Increasing concerns leading to increased spending.

STRATEGIC PLANNING AND MARKET PLACEMENT

Building a strategic plan for any telemedicine project should involve not only providers, but also members of the administration to increase their interest in the program and ensure fewer barriers as demonstrated in the UVA case (Wibberly, 2020). For better engagement from the executive level, the strategic plan should align with the institution's goals and vision. The AHA notes that medical institutions that don't address upcoming expectations in the telehealth market will be progressively confronted by new market entrants and other disruptors that encroach on existing patient–provider relationships (American Hospital Association, 2019). Extensive market analysis and the will to explore early entry to emerging markets is necessary, in addition to continuous work on the development and improvement of current services in competitive markets.

Human Resources

A well-developed Human Resources (HR) management plan aids in increasing administrator engagement of telehealth. The allocation of clinician availability to divide time between traditional care and telemedicine care can be achieved with the big picture view approach (PSJH, Patient Engagement Center, 2019). Telehealth skills can be integrated into organization learning management platforms and training requirements. HR leaders should consider centralization of licensure management, credentialing, and ancillary staffing. These concerns are addressed by extensive review of local and national polices, billing codes, principles for coverage and reimbursements, specific patients' needs, and types of telemedicine services. HR administrators can even use telemedicine programs as a retention and recruitment tool for new providers as the institution prepares for future staffing challenges.

FINANCIAL BENEFITS AND LOGISTICS

It is important to continually analyze the factors that prove the sustainability and stable financial benefits of a telemedicine program, such as improvement in readmission rates, cost savings, growing demand locally and nationally, improved reimbursement policies, and increased support and interest by the government (PSJH, Patient Engagement Center, 2019). The direct and indirect savings, costs, and benefits of the program should be conveyed in a manner that administrators can understand and thereby evaluate related benefits and risks. For example, showing how the use of telemedicine tools in their institutions would decrease penalties as a result of decreased readmission rates, coupled with improved general health outcomes, is very beneficial. Additionally, it is important to work with vendors and explore their present and future telemedicine solutions (Birk, 2020).

Data from AbilTo's Cardiac Health Program for the remote behavioral health intervention program showed 38% reduction in hospital admissions and 31% fewer hospital readmissions. Patients were 63% more likely to spend fewer days in the hospital and more engaged in their health care. These outcomes resulted in an overall reduction in the cost of care even after accounting for all collective program costs (Pande, 2015). Repurposing current capabilities and better management of available resources to expand care delivery to populations that are hard to reach and underserved will help administration understand the benefits of the program.

A broader example of the overall economics of patient engagement via telehealth and self-scheduling can be seen by studying Providence's experience. Engaging patients digitally not only brings more convenience for patients but also delivers lower costs to the health system. For example, self-service online scheduling delivers on average $4–6 in average cost savings versus phone scheduled appointments.

CONCLUSIONS

Engagement is the backbone for any successful telehealth program. Collaboration between clinicians, patients, and administrators cannot be achieved without a clear strategic plan. The experiences of many industry associations, government entities, and other organizations have provided guidance for health care institutions as they seek to drive their telehealth programs to success. Including digital engagement strategies will be important as other consumer-based industries look to move into the health care space. In this chapter we highlighted some of these experiences, including the most significant factors that are important for successful engagement in a telehealth program.

KEY TAKEAWAYS

- ➤ Establish a clear "why" to motivate providers to provide telehealth.
- ➤ Incorporate engagement strategies early in your telehealth initiatives to maximize utilization and benefit.
- ➤ Identify program sponsors among the clinician group you wish to engage.
- ➤ Formulate a multidisciplinary project team early in the process to develop the necessary plan.
- ➤ Build a realistic plan based on your institutional and population needs and resources.
- ➤ As part of a successful engagement strategy, adopt tactics to engage all key stakeholders, including clinicians, patients, and administration.
- ➤ Incorporate your informatics team early and resource required tools based on their recommendations.
- ➤ Study other institutions' best practices and lessons learned and stay up to date with local and national governmental policies and regulations.
- ➤ Keep measuring outcomes and iteratively modify the process to achieve better results.

REFERENCES

Alsher, P. (2019). Change leadership: The three actions needed by every sponsor. Accessed September 1, 2019, at https://www.imaworldwide.com/blog/change-leadership-the-three-actions-needed-by-every-sponsor.

American Hospital Association. (2019). Use of telehealth in hospitals and health systems—Members in action | AHA| AHA. Accessed September 6, 2019, at https://www.aha.org/bibliographylink-page/2017-12-11-use-telehealth-hospitals-and-health-systems-members-action.

American Hospital Association. (2020). Telehealth: A path to virtual integrated care report. Accessed January 17, 2020, at https://www.aha.org/system/files/media/file/2019/02/MarketInsights_TeleHealthReport.pdf.

ATA Accredited Telemedicine Training Programs—ATA Main. (2019). Accessed November 21, 2019, at http://legacy.americantelemed.org/main/ata-accreditation/training-programs.

Birk, S. (2020). Healthcare executive, telemedicine pearls from the experts. Accessed January 30, 2020, at https://healthcareexecutive.org/web-extras/telemedicine-pearls-from-the-experts.

Bryant, M. (2019). Telehealth fills void when weather emergencies disrupt normal provider-patient experience. Healthcare Dive. Accessed September 2019, at https://www.healthcaredive.com/news/telehealth-fills-void-when-weather-emergencies-disrupt-normal-provider-pati-1/508252.

CareAngel. (2019a). AI healthcare technology | Patient engagement at scale| Patient engagement at scale. Accessed September 8, 2019, at https://www.careangel.com/ai-and-voice-powered-virtual-nurse-assistant.

CareAngel. (2019b). Patient engagement solution | Care management. Accessed September 8, 2019, at https://www.careangel.com/care-angel-virtual-health-assistant.

CareAngel. (2019c). Outcomes | Care management success. Accessed September 8, 2019, at https://www.careangel.com/outcomes.

Center for Connected Medicine and the Health Management Academy. (2020). Top of Mind for Top Health Systems Research Report. Accessed January 17, 2020, at https://connectedmed.com/documents/tom2019/CCM_Top_of_Mind_2019_Research_Report_FINAL.pdf.

Comstock, J. (2019). For Providence St. Joseph, patient engagement begins with a call center. *MobiHealthNews*. Accessed September 8, 2019, at https://www.mobihealthnews.com/content/north-america/providence-st-joseph-patient-engagement-begins-call-center.

Ellimoottil, C., An, L., Moyer, M., Sossong, S., & Hollander, J. E. (2018). Challenges and opportunities faced by large health systems implementing telehealth. *Health Aff (Millwood)*, 37(12): 1955–1959.

Expert Program Management. (2019). Reinforcement theory of motivation. Accessed September 1, 2019, at https://expertprogrammanagement.com/2018/10/reinforcement-theory-of-motivation.

Folino, N. (2019). Personal Communication. November 4, 2019.

Freed Associates. (2019). Developing a successful physician engagement strategy. Accessed September 1, 2019, at https://www.beckershospitalreview.com/hospital-physician-relationships/developing-a-successful-physician-engagement-strategy.html.

Gillespie, S. M., Shah, M. N., Wasserman, E. B., et al. (2016). Reducing emergency department utilization through engagement in telemedicine by senior living communities. *Telemedicine J E-Health Off Journal of American Telemedicine Association*, 22(6): 489–496.

Ground, J. (2019). Jan Ground—Motivating providers to provide care virtually—Southwest Telehealth Resource Center. Accessed September 1, 2019, at https://swtrc.wistia.com/medias/cfwzd3lgth.

Hodge, R. (2020). Zoom security issues: Zoom Buys security company, aims for end-to-end encryption. [online] CNET. Accessed 19 May 2020, at <https://www.cnet.com/news/zoom-security-issues-zoom-buys-security-company-aims-for-end-to-end-encryption.

Kamins, C. (2019). What too many hospitals are overlooking. Gallup.com. Accessed September 2, 2019, at https://news.gallup.com/businessjournal/181658/hospitals-overlooking.aspx.

Mair, F. S., May, C., O'Donnell, C., Finch T., Sullivan, F., & Murray, E. (2012). Factors that promote or inhibit the implementation of e-health systems: An explanatory systematic review. *Bulletin of the World Health Organization, 90*(5), 357–364.

MDLIVE. (2018). Driving telehealth utilization to maximize value for organizations. Accessed February 1, 2020, at https://www.mdlive.com/wp-content/uploads/2018/03/MDLIVE_Telehealth-Utilization_Whitepaper.pdf.

MDLVE. (2019). Doctors on call 24 hours—Urgent care online doctor visits. Accessed November 21, 2019, at https://www.mdlive.com.

Ming Tai-Seale, N. Lance Downing, Veena Goel Jones, Richard V. Milani, Beiqun Zhao, Brian Clay, Christopher Demuth Sharp, Albert Solomon Chan, and Christopher A. Longhurst. Technology-Enabled Consumer Engagement: Promising Practices At Four Health Care Delivery Organizations. Health Affairs. March 2019 38(3) 10.1377/hlthaff.2018.05027

NewYork-Presbyterian. (2019). NYP OnDemand: A suite of online services | NewYork-Presbyterian| NewYork-Presbyterian. Accessed September 6, 2019, at https://www.nyp.org/ondemand.

O'Connor, S., Hanlon, P., O'Donnell, C. A., Garcia, S., Glanville, J., & Mair, F. S. (2016). Understanding factors affecting patient and public engagement and recruitment to digital health interventions: A systematic review of qualitative studies. *BMC Medical Informatics and Decision Making,* 16(1): 120.

Pande, R. L., Morris, M., Peters, A., Spettell, C. M., Feifer, R., & Gillis, W. (2015). Leveraging remote behavioral health interventions to improve medical outcomes and reduce costs. *American Journal of Managed Care,* 21(2): e141–151.

PatientEmanagementHIT. (2018). Telehealth closes patient care access gaps in rural Mississippi. Accessed September 6, 2019, at https://patientengagementhit.com/news/telehealth-closes-patient-care-access-gaps-in-rural-mississippi.

Pearl, R. M. (2019, July 10). Engaging physicians in telehealth. *NEJM Catalyst.* Accessed September 1, 2019, at https://catalyst.nejm.org/engaging-physicians-in-telehealth.

Providence St. Joseph Health. (2019a). Providence St. Joseph Health showcases one of U.S.'s largest telehealth systems at ATA18 | Providence and St Joseph. Accessed September 8, 2019, at https://www.psjhealth.org/news/2018/04/psjh-virtual-health-system.

Providence St. Joseph Health. (2019b). Patient Engagement Center | Providence Health and Services| Providence Health and Services. Accessed September 8, 2019, at https://www.providence.org/Clinical-Institutes/PEC.

PRWeb. (2019). A doctor in your stocking? DocChat offers telemedicine industry's first-ever gift certificates. Accessed September 6, 2019, at https://www.prweb.com/releases/2015/12/prweb13141905.htm.

Roga, A. (2019). Three tips for earning physicians' support for telehealth. Accessed September 2, 2019, at https://www.hhnmag.com/articles/8442-three-tips-for-earning-physicians-support-for-telehealth.

Sharma, R., Nachum, S., Davidson, K. W., & Nochomovitz, M. (2019). It's not just FaceTime: Core competencies for the medical virtualist. *International Journal of Emergency Medicine,* 12.

TeleHealth Services. (2019). iCare Navigator | TeleHealth Services. Accessed September 8, 2019, at https://www.telehealth.com/interactive-solutions/icare-navigator.

U.S. Telehealth Satisfaction Study | J.D. POWER. (2019). Accessed November 21, 2019, at https://www.jdpower.com/business/press-releases.| J.D. POWER. | J.D. POWER. 2019| J.D. POWER. | J.D. POWER. -us-telehealth-satisfaction-study.

Westerman, George; McAfee, Andrew. The digital advantage: How digital leaders outperfom their peers in every industry. (2012). Research Brief, MIT Center for Digital Business. MIT Sloan School of Management, Accessed Nov 15, 2020. http://sloan-ide.mit-dev.penzias.com/sites/default/files/publications/TheDigitalAdvantage.pdf

Wicklund, E. (2018). Using telehealth technology for care coordination during a disaster. mHealthIntelligence. Accessed September 7, 2019, at https://mhealthintelligence.com/features/using-telehealth-technology-for-care-coordination-during-a-disaster.

Wolverton, B. (2019). Finding (or developing) telehealth champions. *Northwest Regional Telehealth Resource Center.* Accessed November 21, 2019, at https://www.nrtrc.org/content/article-files/White%20Papers/Developing%20a%20Telehealth%20ChampionB.pdf.

Wootton, A. R., Legnitto, D. A., & Gruber, V. A., et al. (2019). Telehealth and texting intervention to improve HIV care engagement, mental health and substance use outcomes in youth living with HIV: A pilot feasibility and acceptability study protocol. *BMJ Open,* 9(7).

Wibberly, K. (2020, January 17). Personal communication (online interview).

Wicklund, E. (2015). A look ahead: Will 2016 be the year that telehealth gets creative? mHealthIntelligence. Accessed September 6, 2019, at https://mhealthintelligence.com/news/a-look-ahead-will-2016-be-the-year-that-telehealth-gets-creative.

5

Quality Assessment in Emergency Telehealth

JASON C. GOLDWATER AND JUDD E. HOLLANDER ■

INTRODUCTION

It is critical to remember that telehealth and telemedicine are a means to an end. Telemedicine is not about the technology; it is just a different form of health care delivery. Telemedicine does not change the type of care; rather, it is about access, utilizing another modality to connect with health care resources. It gives emergency medicine practitioners the ability to provide remote services in a variety of settings such as emergency departments (EDs), urgent care clinics, observation medicine units, and out-of-hospital settings such as emergency medical response and disaster sites.

Resources for both pre-hospital emergency medical services (EMS) services and ED services are becoming increasingly constrained as growing numbers of patients utilize these services for nonurgent complaints. In one report, it was estimated that approximately 13 to 16% of Medicare-covered 911 EMS transports involved conditions that were probably nonemergent or primary care treatable (Hauswald, Raynovich, & Brainard, 2005). Among those not admitted to the hospital, 34.5% had a low-acuity diagnosis that might have been managed outside the ED. This type of utilization results in high resource costs, as annual Medicare EMS and ED payments for low-acuity patients are approximately $1 billion per year (Knapp, Tsuchitani, Shelle, Prine, & Powers, 2009).

The use of telehealth as a model of providing care to these types of low-acuity patients is being increasingly examined as a method to provide needed services outside of the hospital setting. The types of technological modalities associated with telehealth are more patient-centered, reduce the burden on both the ED and EMS, enhance interactions with providers to improve patient care, and enable direct provider–patient interaction (Finn & Arendts, 2013). However, prior to the COVID pandemic telehealth had been typically used in rural areas or to provide care remotely for specialized diagnoses to patients who otherwise would not have access to needed medical services. The notion of utilizing telehealth for ED or EMS services has not been widely documented, and there are limited comparative effectiveness studies examining the use of telehealth versus traditional ED or EMS care (Patient Autonomy and Destination Factors, 2018). As a result, there are overarching concerns regarding the quality of telehealth services and whether their use provides the same level of care that patients receive onsite within the ED or EMS. Establishing metrics to track success for telemedicine programs is vital to promoting quality and influencing rational policy decisions.

Traditional Quality Paradigms in Telemedicine

New telemedicine programs have typically focused on measures of adoption. Depending on the particular use case, the metrics will vary. Depending on the type of service, some of the most assessed metrics include:

- Number of app downloads
- Number of patient registrations
- Patient experience (satisfaction) reports or scores
- Number or proportion of providers trained
- Provider utilization
- Provider experience/satisfaction, as assessed by formal surveys
- Platform performance (audio-video connectivity rates)
- Number of telemedicine encounters
- Number of repeat visits
- New customer acquisition

As telemedicine programs expand, metrics can often be tied to specific use cases and include items such as:

- Time from first contact to visit completion
- Number of repeat visits
- New customer acquisition
- Readmission avoidance
- Decreased cost of care

NATIONAL QUALITY FORUM TELEHEALTH QUALITY FRAMEWORK

More mature programs will align their metrics to national quality standards. In 2016, the United States Department of Health and Human Services (HHS) called upon the National Quality Forum (NQF) to develop a framework to create metrics to assess the use and effectiveness of telehealth services across multiple clinical settings, including both ED and EMS services. NQF convened a multi-stakeholder committee of 25 national experts in the field of telehealth to recommend various methods to measure the use of telehealth as a means of providing care. This committee was charged with developing a measurement framework that serves as a conceptual foundation for new quality measures, where needed, to assess the quality of care provided using telehealth modalities.

The NQF Committee began the project by conducting a comprehensive environmental scan to identify existing measures related to the use of telehealth in multiple clinical settings. Information was gathered through a multitude of sources, including documents published by operating divisions within HHS and other federal departments, such as the Department of Veterans Affairs (VA) and Department of Defense (DoD). These also included vendor-based white papers and reports issued by nonprofit organizations such as the American Telemedicine Association (ATA), the National Association for Community Health Centers (NACHC), the National Association of Rural Health Providers (NARHP), and the Health Information Management and Systems Society (HIMSS). Papers reviewed from various divisions of HHS—such as the Assistant Secretary for Planning and Evaluation (ASPE), AHRQ, and the Office of the National Coordinator for Health Information Technology (ONC)—included several published telehealth documents, such as ASPE's 2016 Report to Congress: E-health and Telemedicine and the 2016 Federal Telehealth Compendium.

The results of the environmental scan assisted the NQF Committee in developing a measure framework as a conceptual model for providing direction on telehealth measurement priorities and their impact on health care outcomes. The central organizing principle of the framework developed by the Committee was that the use of various telehealth modalities improves access to health care services. The use of telehealth does not represent a different type of health care within clinical settings, such as EDs, but rather a different method of health care delivery that provides services that are either similar or supplemental in scope or outcome to those provided during an in-person encounter.

Domains of the Telehealth Quality Framework

Encounters between a client and a provider or care team member through telehealth potentially enable the integration of telehealth services into a health care setting in a way that minimizes impact on workflow. Quality of care appears in each of the framework's domains and subdomains, as they all affect the quality of a health outcome or process. For example, an individual who is unable to receive health care services because of geographical constraints would have a poor-quality outcome. The Committee developed the framework around four major domains: access to care, financial impact, patient/provider experience, and effectiveness.

Access to Care

The first domain of the framework addresses access to care: specifically, whether the use of telehealth services allows remote individuals to obtain emergency clinical services effectively and whether remote hospitals can provide specialized services such as intensive care. With respect to emergency medicine, access is evaluated across five major areas:

1. Affordability—Are both patients and members of the care team willing to accept the potential costs of telehealth as opposed to the alternative of not receiving or delivering traditional emergency care at all, or receiving delayed care? What is the cost of providing telehealth services to those in need of emergency care, and what is its effect on hospitals and EDs?
2. Availability—Does a telehealth modality present access to an emergency medicine practitioner that can provide care when requested by the patient?
3. Accessibility—Is the technology necessary for an emergency telehealth consultation accessed and used by members of the care team?
4. Accommodation—Do the various modalities of telehealth accommodate the diverse needs of patients seeking emergency care?
5. Acceptability—Do both patients and clinicians accept the use of telehealth as a means of care delivery?

With these overarching guidelines, the Committee developed two subdomains under "access to care":

- Access for the patient, family, and/or caregiver refers to the ability of patients to receive emergency services from an emergency medicine specialist they could not access otherwise because of geographical barriers and other logistical difficulties (such as transportation and travel costs). These limitations lead to a potential lack of essential and critical services with patients who cannot initiate treatment at all.
- Access for emergency physicians and other clinical staff means they have appropriate access to the telehealth technologies needed to provide treatment when needed. For example, the access to a modality such as video-teleconferencing provides a method for clinicians and emergency medical technicians to provide specific guidance to patients with emergency conditions.

Financial Impact

The second domain of the framework addresses the financial impact/cost of telehealth services. This domain has four distinct subdomains: financial impact to patient, family, and/or caregiver; financial impact to care team; financial impact to health system or payer; and financial impact to society.

- The financial impact to a patient, family, and/or caregiver accounts for the potential cost savings and benefits of telehealth, such as less travel time to see a provider, reduction in ambulance-enabled ED utilization, and more appropriate levels of care for a patient seeking emergency services.
- The financial impact to emergency medical personnel and the patient includes the opportunity costs and both direct and indirect costs associated with providing care using a telehealth modality.
- The financial impact to payers and health systems is the net financial impact, including cost avoidance and opportunity costs.

- The financial impact to society includes the impact of telehealth on health care workforce shortages, the impact on hospitals of services provided at a distance, and the overall health status of a community, economic productivity, patient–provider convenience, and averted care.

Experience of Telehealth

The third domain focuses on the experience of telehealth, which represents the usability and effect of telehealth on patients, care team members, and the community at large, and whether the use of telehealth resulted in a level of care that individuals and providers expected. The Committee divided this domain into two separate subdomains: (1) patient, family, and/or caregiver experience and (2) care team member experience.

- For patients, family, and/or caregivers, experience refers to their ability to use the technology, the provision of a mechanism to connect with an emergency provider when needed, and the issue of whether the care delivered through various telehealth modalities is comparable to the quality of the care services they would receive during an in-person encounter.
- The care team subdomain reflects the utility of the technology to provide necessary information to assist in the provision of emergency care.
- For the community at large, the acceptance and consistent use of telehealth as provided to patients and their families, administrators, and executive leaders are critical to its ongoing use.

Effectiveness

The fourth domain focuses on effectiveness, which represents the health care system, clinical, operational, and technical aspects of telehealth.

- System effectiveness refers to the ability of a telehealth modality and the overall system to assist in the coordination of care across various health care settings; to assist in discerning between urgent and nonurgent care; and to facilitate the sharing of information between care teams in order to aid in decision making.
- Clinical effectiveness refers to the impact of telehealth on health outcomes as well as the comparative effectiveness of services provided in person or the alternative available to the patient at that time.
- Operational effectiveness revolves around how clinically integrated telehealth is within an emergency care setting.
- Technical effectiveness refers to the ability of the telehealth system to record and transmit images, data, and other information accurately to members of the emergency care team, as well as the system's ability to exchange information between stakeholders seamlessly.

Because of the complex interactions between the implementation and use of various telehealth modalities, multiple aspects of this framework likely apply to different telehealth issues. The assessment, evaluation, and effectiveness of telehealth are multidimensional; thus, quality measurement of telehealth requires varied and diverse approaches.

The Use of Telehealth for Emergency Medical Services

There are several examples of where the use of telehealth for emergency medical services demonstrated improvements in care that were eligible for assessment utilizing the NQF Framework. In 2014, the Houston Fire Department created a telehealth program designed to provide immediate treatment to primary care patients and avoid transport and admittance to an ED. The Emergency Telehealth and Navigation (ETHAN) program combined telehealth, social services, and alternative transportation that provide a model of care for low-acuity patients and those with nonemergent conditions (Langabeer et al., 2016). Using a case-control study design, the researchers divided patients who called 911 into an intervention group that incorporated ETHAN with community paramedicine and a control. They dispositioned patients to the appropriate level of care (local safety net clinical, referral to primary care, etc.), and the control group consisted of traditional ED patients. The intervention consisted of three components: telehealth capabilities between the paramedic, patient, and EMS physician; patient navigation and scheduling to safety net clinics; and taxi transportation and social service follow-up per incident. The results of the study, which included 5,570 patients in both cohorts, indicated that those in the intervention group had a significant decrease in transport to EDs for patients with nonemergent conditions. Additionally, the intervention group had a response time of 39 minutes (inclusive of EMS notification from 911 to unit back in-service time) as opposed to 83 minutes for the control group. This equates to approximately 2.1 times greater utilization from the EMS unit than the standard EMS control group, which results in significantly lower cost of care (Langabeer et al., 2016). Patient satisfaction with the ETHAN program was measured at 100% through surveys given to patients at the end of the encounter, and technical effectiveness was rated as high even with poor wireless signals at certain locations.

Another case study deals with the issues of ED overcrowding, which has led some EDs to use telemedicine to increase the number of providers during surges of patient visits and offer scheduled "home" face-to-face, on-screen encounters through telehealth providers (Rademacher, Cole, & Psoter, 2019). This cohort study compared the performance of real-time remote telescreening and in-person screening at a single urban academic ED over 22 weeks in the spring and summer of 2016. The study involved 337 standard screening hours and 315 telescreening hours. The primary process measure was patients screened per hour. Additional outcomes were rates of patients who left without being seen (operational effectiveness), rates of analgesia ordered by the screener (clinical effectiveness), and proportion of patients with chest pain receiving or prescribed a standard set of tests and medications (clinical effectiveness). The study demonstrated that compared to prior year-, date-, and time-matched data on weekdays from 1 a.m. to 3 a.m., a period previously void of provider screening, telescreening decreased the rate of patients who left without being seen from 25.1% to 4.5%. Analgesia was ordered more frequently by telescreeners than by in-person screeners (51.2% vs 31.6%), and there was no difference in standard care received by patients with chest pain between telescreening and in-person screening (29.4% vs 22.4%).

Effectively Using the NQF Framework for Emergency Telehealth Quality Measures

The continued advancement of telehealth to provide emergency care when needed and to appropriately identify nonemergent clinical situations or low-acuity patients, necessitate the development of a framework to appropriately assess outcomes provided by these services. The work of NQF provided a foundation to develop outcome-based measures that examine both the use and utility of telehealth across the four major domains. Prior studies demonstrated the value of telehealth within ED settings and how the NQF framework can be applied to develop a standard assessment method to evaluate telehealth outcomes.

The NQF report recommends measuring whether sufficient information was obtained during a telemedicine encounter to make clinical decisions regarding intervening or not intervening. The important concept is that obtaining the appropriate actionable information is more important than measuring diagnostic accuracy. The committee recognized that, just like in the ED, sometimes more information is needed to make a diagnosis. Thus, not knowing the diagnosis is not critical, but not referring to obtain the important information would be problematic.

> Obtaining the appropriate actionable information is more important than measuring diagnostic accuracy.

Outcome Measures

Outcome measures should depend on the specific application of telemedicine. Some examples are mortality, frequency of prescriptions such as antibiotics, and frequency of clinical worsening requiring an in-person visit or hospitalization.

Patient and provider experience (rather than just satisfaction) are important quality components and require special attention in telemedicine since direct in-person patient-to-provider contact is lacking. Satisfaction with the technological aspects of the interaction should be separated from that of the provider. Since interacting with a patient over telemedicine requires some differences in interaction, such as eye contact, environment, and audio-video quality, these aspects should be monitored.

CONCLUSIONS

The NQF measures are likely to be universally adopted, and therefore mature programs should be encouraged to measure and report quality outcomes in alignment with these recommendations. The four domains in the NQF report have already been incorporated into program metrics in primary care and internal medicine (Powell, Henstenburg, Cooper, Hollander, & Rising, 2017; Powell, Stone, & Hollander, 2018); urology (Glassman et al., 2018); general surgery (Nandra et al., 2018); otolaryngology (Rimer, Christopher, & Falck, 2018); preadmission testing (Mullen-Fortino et al., 2018); and oncology (Rising, Ward, Goldwater, Bhagianadh, & Hollander, 2018). We recommend the incorporation of telemedicine into emergency medicine in concert with program metrics capture and analysis. In this manner, we will be able to enhance the use and effectiveness of telehealth as a means of standard emergency care.

KEY TAKEAWAYS

- ➢ Studies over time have demonstrated the effectiveness of using telehealth for emergency care.
- ➢ The various modalities used for telehealth and emergency medicine have demonstrated utility for both patients and clinicians.
- ➢ There is a push to recognize telehealth not as an adjunct to care delivery, but as a specific means of care delivery—including emergency care.
- ➢ In order to accomplish this objective, it is essential to develop a set of quality measures that objectively assesses telehealth across specific domains: access to care, cost, effectiveness, and patient–provider experience.
- ➢ A framework was developed by the National Quality Forum in 2016 to help assist with the development of these measures.

REFERENCES

Finn, J., & Arendts, G. (2013). Evidence- based paramedic models of care to reduce unnecessary emergency department attendance—feasibility and safety. *BMC Emergency Medicine*, 13(1): 1–6.

Glassman, D., Puri, A. K., Weingarten, S., Hollander, J., Stepchin, A., Trabulsi, E., & Gomella, L. (2018). A single institution's initial experience with telemedicine. *Urology Practice*, 5(5): 367–371.

Hauswald, M., Raynovich, W., & Brainard, A. (2005). Expanded emergency medical services. *Prehospital Emergency Care*, 9(3): 250–253.

Knapp, B., Tsuchitani, S., Shelle, J., Prine, J., & Powers, J. (2009). Prospective evaluation of an emergency medical services administered alternative transport protocol. *Prehospital Emergency Care*, 13(4): 432–436.

Langabeer, J., Gonzalez, M., Alqusari, D., Langabeer- Champagne, T., Jakcson, A., Mikhail, J., & Persee, D. (2016). Telehealth- enabled emergency medical services program reduces ambulance transport to urban emergency departments. *Western Journal of Emergency Medicine*, 17(6): 713–720.

Mullen- Fortino, M., Rising, K., Duckworth, J., Gwynn, V., Sties, F., & Hollander, J. (2018). Presurgical assessment using telemedicine technology: Impact on efficiency, effectiveness, and patient experience of care. *Journal of Telemedicine and e-Health*. 25(2): 137–142.

Nandra, K., Koenig, G., DelMastro, A., Mishler, E., Hollander, J., & Yeo, C. (2018). Telehealth provides a comprehensive approach to the surgical patient. *American Journal of Surgery.* 218(3): 476–479.

Patient Autonomy and Destination Factors in Emergency Medical Services (EMS) and EMS- Affiliated Mobile Integrated Healthcare/ Community Paramedicine Programs. (2018). *Annals of Emergency Medicine,* 72(4): e57–58.

Powell, R., Henstenburg, J., Cooper, G., Hollander, J., & Rising, K. (2017). Patient Perceptions of Telehealth Primary Care Video Visits. *Annals of Family Medicine,* 15(3): 225–229.

Powell, R., Stone, D., & Hollander, J. (2018). Patient and health system experience with implementation of an enterprise-wide telehealth scheduled video visit program: Mixed methods study. *Journal of Medical Internet Research,* 6(1:e10): 1–7.

Rademacher, N., Cole, G., & Psoter, K. (2019, May 8). Use of telemedicine to screen patients in the emergency department: Matched cohort study evaluating efficiency and patient safety of telemedicine. *Journal of Medical Internet Research,* 7(2): e11233.

Rimer, R., Christopher, V., & Falck, A. (2018). Telemedicine in otolaryngology outpatient setting—Single center head and neck surgery experience. *Laryngoscope,* 128(9): 2072–2075.

Rising, K., Ward, M., Goldwater, J., Bhagianadh, D., & Hollander, J. (2018). Framework to advance oncology related telehealth. *Journal of Clinical Cancer Informatics.* (2): 1–11.

6

Legal, Regulatory, and Reimbursement Considerations

ALEXIS S. GILROY, KIMBERLY L. ROCKWELL,
ADAM RUTENBERG, CLAIRE MARBLESTONE,
AND KYLE Y. FAGET ■

INTRODUCTION

Health care services delivered through telehealth are impacted by numerous legal, regulatory, and reimbursement frameworks that apply at the local, state, and federal levels (Marcoux, 2016). Standard medical practices for consent, privacy, credentialing, and licensing have particular application to telehealth, depending on the practice setting, hospital by-laws, and state medical board. When one considers practice near state borders or those organizations with a multistate catchment area, cross-state practice complicates the need to share health information, multiple hospital credentialing processes, and, generally, the requirement for health care providers to be licensed in the state where the patient is located. Of particular interest to emergency care are the federal regulations related to emergency stabilization, so an examination of the Emergency Medical Treatment and Labor Act (EMTALA) must be considered through the lens of telehealth. Finally, reimbursements for services delivered by telehealth have been restricted and fragmented through a complicated web of rules that vary by service, payer, and location. It is important to understand the target population and payer mix to adequately determine which telehealth services may be reimbursable. Medicare, Medicaid, and private payer reimbursement vary by state, geography, and originating site of the patient. The COVID-19 pandemic accelerated telehealth adoption by waiver and alterations to regulatory barriers. As we emerge from the public health emergency, we find an urgency to make permanent regulations that promote broader access to telehealth. However, at this time significant regulatory uncertainty remains. Stakeholders that seek to advance telehealth locally or nationally must participate in advocacy for smart legislation that improves and simplifies access to equitable telehealth services.

COMPLIANCE TOPICS

Emergency Medical Treatment and Labor Act

EMTALA was enacted in 1986 to ensure that no individual seeking emergency department (ED) care in a Medicare-certified hospital has that care delayed or denied because of payer status or inability to pay. In other words, EMTALA was enacted to prevent patient dumping or the refusal to care for patients for financial reasons. Under EMTALA, all Medicare-certified hospitals with EDs must, with respect to any individual who "comes to the emergency department":

- Provide an appropriate medical screening examination within the capability of the emergency department, including ancillary services routinely available to the department, to determine whether an "emergency medical condition" exists; and
- If an emergency medical condition is determined to exist, provide any necessary stabilizing treatment, or an appropriate transfer.[1]

Some EMTALA requirements may be satisfied via telemedicine. The Centers for Medicare and Medicaid Services (CMS) has stated, "Telemedicine has great potential to expand availability of specialty care services, including emergency medicine services, to rural populations. However, misconceptions about. . . . EMTALA requirements may cause unnecessary concerns about, or create barriers to, using telemedicine."[2]

CMS has clarified, for example, that the use of audio, video, and other telehealth equipment by an onsite physician to perform medical screening examinations is not specifically prohibited under EMTALA.[3]

Under 42 CFR §489.24(a)(i), a medical screening examination must be performed by a qualified medical person (QMP), which requires the use of "adequate medical and nursing personnel qualified in emergency care." The QMP on-site conducting the required screening examination may be assisted or directed by a qualified telemedicine practitioner.[4] Additionally, when a physician is providing/directing diagnosis or treatment of individuals in a critical access hospital (CAH) ED via telemedicine, there is no requirement or expectation under EMTALA that the CAH must always require one of the local on-call physicians to come to the ED as well. However, if the QMP onsite and/or the physician providing care via telemedicine determine that hands-on treatment that is required to stabilize an individual's emergency medical condition is beyond the capability of the onsite QMP, then *a request for a local CAH physician to come to the ED could be required, depending on the circumstances.*

CMS's Survey and Certification Group has attempted to clarify how telemedicine may be used to satisfy EMTALA requirements. Therefore, practitioners and ED administrators interested in leveraging telemedicine to satisfy EMTALA requirements are advised to review their publications.

The QMP on-site conducting the required screening examination may be assisted or directed by a qualified telemedicine practitioner.[5] Additionally, when a physician is providing/directing diagnosis or treatment of individuals in a critical access hospital (CAH) ED via telemedicine, there is no requirement or expectation under EMTALA that the CAH must always require one of the local on-call physicians to come to the ED as well.

CONSENT FOR TELEHEALTH SERVICES

A majority of state telehealth laws and rules expressly require health care professionals using telemedicine technologies to obtain, in addition to consents typically required in a brick-and-mortar health care facility, a Telehealth Informed Consent (TIC) from patients before treatment. A TIC process ensures that patients understand the risks and benefits of using telehealth services. The best practice is to have an established patient affirmatively reacknowledge the TIC every time the patient has a new telehealth consultation. Alternatively, as a matter of course, the patient should affirmatively acknowledge the TIC at a minimum once per year.

Consenting Requirements

States have disparate laws and rules governing TIC requirements and may have multiple required disclosures. Components of an appropriate telehealth consent[6] used in Virginia, for example, are listed in Box 6.1.

Box 6.1

COMPONENTS OF A TELEHEALTH CONSENT IN VIRGINIA

- Identification of the patient, the practitioner, and the practitioner's credentials
- Types of activities permitted using telemedicine services (e.g., prescription refills, appointment scheduling, patient education)
- Agreement by the patient that it is the role of the practitioner to determine whether or not the condition being diagnosed and/or treated is appropriate for a telemedicine encounter
- Details on security measures taken with the use of telemedicine services, such as encrypting date of service, password protected screen savers, encrypting data files, or utilizing other reliable authentication techniques, as well as potential risks to privacy notwithstanding such measures
- Hold harmless clause for information lost due to technical failures
- Requirement for express patient consent to forward patient-identifiable information to a third party

---

Whereas some states like Virginia *encourage* practitioners to obtain informed consent, other states like California *require* it. Because the consent requirements vary across states, TIC should be conducted with careful attention for each state where telehealth services may be offered.

LICENSURE REQUIREMENTS

It is almost universally understood and accepted that practicing medicine requires a professional license, which is a state law issue subject to state medical board jurisdiction. In the context of telehealth, licensing and medical practice laws are based not on the physical location of the physician, but rather on the physical location of the patient at the time of the telehealth consult. In practice, this means that a physician licensed in Massachusetts and providing services to a patient located in Florida must have a license to practice medicine in Florida (or otherwise meet a state licensure exception). As telemedicine gains in popularity and acceptance across the United States, physicians looking to offer telehealth services in multiple states quickly encounter a licensure impediment due to cost and administrative burden.

Medical licensing is slowly becoming streamlined by efforts such as the Federation of State Medical Board's (FSMB) Interstate Medical Licensure Compact (IMLC), which offers a uniform, expedited pathway for physicians to obtain multiple licenses to practice in "Compact states."[7] The IMLCC is an agreement between multiple states and territories and the District of Columbia. Physicians who are licensed by different medical and osteopathic boards in one Compact state may go through a simplified licensing process in any other Compact state and can qualify to practice medicine across state lines, provided certain agreed upon eligibility requirements are met. The application process is expedited by the willingness of compact states to accept existing information from a physician's state of principal licensure. Once qualified, a physician may obtain a license in any number of Compact states in which they wish to practice.

The onset of COVID-19 led governors across the country to issue executive orders allowing for health care professionals (e.g., physicians, nurse practitioners, mental health providers, and physical therapists) to practice clinical care across state lines without the need for a permanent license. For example, Michigan authorized all "health care professionals" who are "licensed in good standing" in any U.S. state or territory to practice in Michigan. The authorization applies to health care professionals licensed under Article 15 of Michigan's Public Health Code, which specifically includes the categories of medicine, nursing, and physical therapy, and does not require individuals to apply for or be granted an exception. The Executive Order provides that "[a]ny and all provisions in Article 15 of the Public Health Code are temporarily suspended, in whole or part, to the extent necessary to allow health care professionals licensed and in good standing in any state or territory in the United States to practice in Michigan without criminal, civil, or administrative penalty related to lack of licensure. A license that has been suspended or revoked is not considered a license in good standing, and a licensee with pending disciplinary action is not considered to have a license in good standing. Any license that is subject to a limitation in another state is subject to the same limitation in this state."[8] Each state has approached emergency licensure exceptions differently, so health care professionals are advised to consult the applicable state emergency orders, medical board guidance, and the like before relying on a licensure waiver to practice in a state in which they are not licensed. The FSMB maintains a website with regular updates linking to state-by-state licensure exceptions during the pandemic. As the COVID-19 pandemic comes to a close, many states will be confronted with deciding whether and how to terminate the relaxed requirements.

Even outside the context of a public health emergency such as COVID-19, there exists a widely adopted licensure exception for providing medical services in response to emergency situations. Several states also offer a number of other exceptions to licensure that allow physicians licensed in one state to deliver care (typically on a limited basis) to patients located in the state where the physician is not located or licensed. For example, a number of states allow a licensure exemption for physician-to-physician (peer-to-peer) out-of-state consultations. In Minnesota, an out-of-state physician providing telemedicine services is exempt from licensure in the state if they are licensed in another state and (1) provide services less than once a month or to less than 10 patients per year or (2) provides services in consultation with a Minnesota-licensed physician who "retains ultimate authority over the diagnosis and care of the patient."[9] Another example includes the bordering or neighboring state exception. For example, the rendering of medical advice or information through telecommunications from a physician licensed to practice medicine in Virginia or an adjoining state, or from a licensed nurse practitioner, to emergency medical personnel acting in an emergency situation is not prohibited.[10] While certain exceptions exist in every state, they vary significantly, and providers should carefully understand the requirements or else risk unlicensed practice of medicine.

CREDENTIALING

Health care providers practicing telemedicine often seek privileges at multiple health care facilities. The federal government and hospital accrediting bodies, recognizing the problems caused by the increase in credentialing inquiries, have established credentialing by proxy (CBP) as a streamlined, efficient pathway to credentialing telemedicine health care providers. Implementing a CBP program can provide a broad range of improvements to the traditional credentialing process as it relates to telemedicine applicants, including expedited availability of new/augmented services, expanded access to health care providers, decreasing costs, and improved patient experience.

The Basics of Credentialing by Proxy

The traditional credentialing of health care providers is governed by the by-laws, policies, and procedures of each individual health care facility and includes a number of verifications, including employment verification, educational background verification, and human resource information collections, along with criminal background checks. Once the relevant information is collected from each applicant, medical staff reviews the information in relation to current licensure status, training, experience, current competence, and the ability to perform the requested privilege. When entities are confronted with the need to credential multiple telemedicine health care providers who may each have multiple current and past affiliations across multiple states, the traditional process becomes daunting, time consuming, and inefficient. This review process can quickly become unmanageable at a facility using telemedicine health care providers.

CBP can be an efficient and time-saving solution to the inefficiencies of the traditional credentialing process, but CBP requires paying careful attention to applicable legal and regulatory considerations. For example, hospitals must abide by the CBP requirements in the conditions of participation (CoPs), state regulations applicable to where the originating site is located, the standards required by their hospital accreditation program, and their own medical staff by-laws.

To utilize CBP, the originating site must enter into a written agreement with the distant site hospital or another entity providing telemedicine service, reflecting and confirming the following requirements:

1. The distant site hospital or telemedicine entity uses a credentialing or privileging program that meets or exceeds the Medicare standards that hospitals have traditionally been required to use.
2. The individual health care providers seeking to provide and/or are providing services via telemedicine to the originating site have been privileged at the distant site hospital or telemedicine entity.
3. The distant site hospital or telemedicine entity provides the originating site with a list of the current approved privileges for the telemedicine health care providers seeking and/or exercising privileges at the originating site.
4. The individual health care providers seeking and/or providing telemedicine services at the originating site are licensed or otherwise authorized to practice in the state where the originating site is located.
5. The originating site periodically reviews the services provided to its patients by the telemedicine health care providers and reports this information to the distant site hospital or telemedicine entity for use in performance evaluations. At a minimum, these reports must include all adverse events and all complaints related to each telemedicine practitioner's services provided at the originating site.
6. For contracts with distant site telemedicine entities only, the agreement must also state that the site is a contractor of services to the originating site that provides contracted telemedicine services in a manner that permits the originating site to comply with all CoPs.
   The CBP agreement requires the parties to share information regarding credentialing decisions and periodic reviews and assessments. Hospitals must remain cognizant of state laws regarding peer review decisions, confidentiality, health care provider disciplinary actions, and professional review actions under the federal Health Care Quality Improvement Act. Even if an agreement is entered into, the hospital is not required to use the CBP process for all telemedicine health care providers; traditional credentialing methods may be used to credential any and all health care providers.

Even when using CBP, the governing body of the originating site retains ultimate authority over privileging decisions regarding telemedicine health care providers. The originating site's medical staff by-laws should include provisions for CBP, and hospitals can consider creating a separate telemedicine staff category.

HOSPITAL ACCREDITATION STANDARDS

Many hospital accreditation bodies have amended their standards to align with CMS's requirements. Under the Healthcare Facilities Accreditation Program (HFAP), telemedicine health care providers must be licensed in both the state where they are located and the state where the patient is located. To allow for CBP, HFAP applies standards 3.00.02 and 3.00.03, which cover distant site hospital and telemedicine entity agreements. For distant site hospital agreements, HFAP allows the governing body of the originating site hospital to choose to have its medical staff rely on the credentialing and privileging decisions made by the distant site when making recommendations for privileges under certain conditions. Specifically, HFAP requires the following:

- That the distant site participate in Medicare.
- That the distant site provide the originating site with a list of all practitioners covered by the distant site hospital and telemedicine entity agreement, and outline each practitioner's privileges at the distant site.
- That the distant site ensure that all covered practitioners hold a license in the state where the originating site is located.
- That the originating site periodically review the telemedicine services provided and share feedback for the distant site's use in its own appraisals of the practitioners (at a minimum including all information on adverse events and complaints relating to the telemedicine services). *See standards 01.00.15; 01.00.16; 03.00.08; and 03.00.09.*

Similarly, DNV-GL Healthcare, an independent certification provider, accredits hospitals through its National Integrated Accreditation for Healthcare Organizations (NIAHO) program. In fact, the requirements applicable to DNV-GL are the same as those applicable to HFAP.

The Joint Commission (TJC) proposed revisions to its hospital accreditation standards regarding credentialing for telemedicine services because its original telemedicine standards required both the originating site and the distant site to be accredited by TJC, which was a limiting factor in the ability of TJC-accredited hospitals to utilize CBP. The proposed revisions, released in November 2017, would allow originating sites to use credentialing and privileging information provided by a distant site to grant their own hospital-specific privileges.

It is important to remember that utilizing CBP for credentialing telemedicine health care providers does not change the requirements for originating sites to query the National Practitioner Data Bank, and that each state has its own regulations regarding hospital based medical staff credentialing.

HEALTH INSURANCE PORTABILITY AND
ACCOUNTABILITY ACT

Health care providers delivering telehealth services in hospital EDs need to be aware of their obligations to ensure the privacy and confidentiality of protected health information (PHI) under the federal Health Insurance Portability and Accountability Act (HIPAA) and state law.

HIPAA applies to two types of entities—covered entities and business associates. A covered entity is defined as a health insurer, health care clearinghouse, or health care provider that engages in certain electronic transactions.[11] Business associates are third parties that contract with covered entities to provide services such as the receipt, creation, transmission, or maintenance of the covered entity's PHI.[12] In the context of emergency telehealth, the vast majority of physicians providing emergency telehealth services and the hospitals where such services are provided are considered covered entities. The telehealth software provider would most likely be considered a business associate of the hospital and/or the physician, depending on the structure of the telehealth arrangement.

As covered entities, the hospital and physician providing telehealth services need to comply with the HIPAA Privacy Rule. The obligations under this rule are extensive and accordingly cannot be sufficiently described here.[13] These obligations include providing a Notice of Privacy Practices to patients, which explains the patient's rights under HIPAA.[14] In addition, the hospital and physician must ensure that processes are in place to guarantee patient access to their PHI and that authorizations to use or disclose the patient's PHI are obtained when necessary.[15]

Covered entities and business associates must also comply with the HIPAA Security Rule and ensure that appropriate administrative, physical, and technical safeguards are in place to secure the confidentiality of patient's PHI.[16] The covered entity needs to enter into a business associate agreement (BAA) with all business associates who will receive or have access to PHI.[17] The BAA specifies each party's responsibilities with respect to PHI. Both the business associate and covered entity need to enact procedural and technical safeguards to protect patient data. The obligations include implementing a security management program, and conducting ongoing risk assessments.[18] The specific safeguards implemented by each covered entity or business associate should be tailored to their needs and capabilities, and may vary depending on the sophistication of the entity.[19] However, each covered entity and business associate must make sure that it has implemented some form of a safeguard to address all requirements under the HIPAA Security Rule (see Chapter 7).

HIPAA also requires covered entities and business associates to comply with the HIPAA Breach Notification Rule.[20] In the event there is a security incident or a breach of PHI, the business associate will need to notify the covered entity of the incident.[21] Covered entities may be required to notify the patient, the Office for Civil Rights, and/or the media of a breach of PHI.[22] Similarly, many state laws require health care providers, hospitals and physicians, or businesses that maintain medical information to notify state residents of a breach of security of their medical information. These state laws and HIPAA impose strict reporting timelines, so it is imperative to ensure that appropriate action is promptly taken after a security incident or breach.

The obligations to ensure privacy and security of PHI and medical information generated from an emergency telehealth encounter are complex and a critical component of compliance for hospitals, physicians, and their business associates. Proactive, compliance-focused preparation is essential to ensuring a meaningful relationship with telehealth patients, which balances the need for privacy of PHI, secure technology, and patient access to innovative digital health services.

REIMBURSEMENT REGULATORY OVERVIEW FOR TELEHEALTH SERVICES

Historically, a major barrier to telemedicine adoption has been lack of reimbursement by public and private payers. Medicare, Medicaid, and private insurers currently reimburse for telemedicine and related services based on idiosyncratic rules that do not apply to the provision of in-person clinical services. The following is a synopsis of reimbursement for telemedicine and related services by Medicare, Medicaid, and private commercial insurers, including as it relates to vendor agreements and clinical partnership considerations in the ED setting.

Medicare

While telemedicine reimbursement policy at the Centers for Medicare and Medicaid Services (CMS) appears to annually add new covered services to the Medicare program, CMS maintains several limitations on coverage that make reimbursement for these services difficult for many providers. As an initial matter, CMS only reimburses for telemedicine services that are provided via real-time audiovisual technologies, with rare exception.[23] Beyond that, outside the context of a public health emergency, CMS limits telemedicine reimbursement to patients receiving services in specific geographic locations, within specific types of facilities, and receiving specific types of services provided by specific types of practitioners.

In 2001 Congress passed the Benefits Improvement and Protection Act of 2000 (BIPA), which amended the Balanced Budget Act of 1997 to identify certain telemedicine services that CMS would cover if specific geographic, facility, technology, provider, and service-type qualities were present with the telemedicine encounter.[24] Currently, the greatest barrier to Medicare reimbursement for emergency telehealth services is CMS's ongoing requirement that the patient be located at a qualifying originating site when receiving the telemedicine services.[25] This requirement limits reimbursement to those cases where the patient is geographically located either in a county outside of a Metropolitan Statistical Area (MSA) or in a Health Professional Shortage Area (HPSA). The Health Resources and Services Administration (HRSA) advises CMS on HPSA classifications, while the U.S. Census Bureau determines the MSA and non-MSA areas. Note, however, that effective March 6, 2020, health care providers eligible to furnish Medicare telehealth services during the public health emergency, including physicians and certain nonphysician providers such as nurse practitioners, physician assistants and certified nurse midwives, may provide covered telehealth services to patients outside of rural areas, including treating patients in their homes.[26] As the public health emergency comes to an end, CMS will have to confront whether and how to continue the relaxed requirements for the provision of telehealth services.

Table 6.1 OTHER CMS COVERAGE LIMITATIONS ON MEDICARE REIMBURSEMENT
FOR TELEMEDICINE SERVICES

Originating Site Facility Types	Distant Site Practitioners	Services Relevant to Emergency Department
• Physician and practitioner offices • Hospitals • Critical access hospitals • Rural health clinics • Federally qualified health centers • Hospital-based or CAH-based renal dialysis centers • Skilled nursing facilities • Community mental health centers • Renal dialysis facilities • Homes of beneficiaries with end-stage renal disease getting home dialysis • Mobile stroke units	• Physicians • Nurse practitioners • Physician assistants • Nurse–midwives • Clinical nurse specialists • Certified registered nurse anesthetists • Clinical psychologists (with some limitations) • Clinical social workers (with some limitations) • Registered dieticians or other nutrition professional	• Telehealth consultations in the emergency department • Telehealth pharmacologic management • Psychiatric diagnostic interview examination • Neurobehavioral status examination • Telehealth consultation, critical care, initial and subsequent • Prolonged services in the in-patient or observational setting requiring unit/floor time beyond the usual service; first hour • Prolonged services in the in-patient or observational setting requiring unit/floor time beyond the usual service; each additional 30 minutes

Telehealth Services, MLN Booklet, Centers for Medicare and Medicaid Services, https://www. https://www.cms.gov/Outreach-and-Education/Medicare-Learning-Network-MLN/MLNProducts/Downloads/TelehealthSrvcsfctsht.pdf, March 2020 (last visited November 5, 2020).

Beyond this geographic limitation for originating sites, CMS places limits on originating-site facility type, the types of practitioners who may provide telemedicine services, and the types of services that may be reimbursed. (See Table 6.1.)

Ultimately, many emergency telehealth programs would likely qualify for Medicare reimbursement if not for the originating site geographic limitation. That said, CMS has implemented a host of other regulations more recently to expand coverage to specific types of services relevant to emergency telehealth to include services rendered to patients in all geographic locations. (See Table 6.2.)

Under these expansions, clinicians may now receive reimbursement for a range of emergency medicine services delivered via telecommunications technologies. Because telemedicine provides for efficiencies in services delivery and advancing outcomes with specialty engagement, telemedicine may be used as part of bundled payment initiatives without regard to the geographic limitation.[27] This is critical to EDs whose services are often bundled into chronic care management bundles for conditions such as chronic congestive heart failure and chronic obstructive

Table 6.2 SERVICES REIMBURSABLE BY MEDICARE REGARDLESS OF
PATIENT GEOGRAPHY

Service	Effective Date
Telemedicine services delivered as part of Bundled payment initiatives	January 2013
Telestroke services	January 2019
Interprofessional (peer-to-peer) internet consultations	January 2019
Telemedicine-based substance abuse treatment services	July 2019

pulmonary disease.[28] Furthermore, as of January 2019, CMS reimburses for telemedicine services "for purposes of diagnosis, evaluation, or treatment of symptoms of an acute stroke" for patients receiving these services from a qualifying facility (as detailed in Table 6.1) located in any geographic area.[29] CMS has similarly removed the geographic requirement (and added the patient's home as a permissible originating site) for telehealth services "furnished for purposes of treatment of substance use disorder or a co-occurring mental health disorder" as of July 2, 2019.[30] And finally, beginning January, 2019, CMS established reimbursement codes to cover "interprofessional internet communication" provided by a consulting health care professional.[31] These services do not require face-to-face patient contact but instead cover a consultation between health care professionals, resulting in verbal and written reports by the consultant to the patient's treating physician. This is relevant to a number of current emergency medicine outlays. Also notable are specific CMS requirements that influence utilization of telemedicine providers for certain workflows. For example, CMS typically requires that hospital admissions include an in-person "hands-on" exam by the admitting physician, although hospital admissions and ongoing care can often be supported by telemedicine services.[32]

Importantly, CMS also expanded the universe of available telemedicine services during the public health emergency by adding more covered services to the list of telehealth services.[33] In December of 2020, CMS issued its final 2021 Physician Fee Schedule Rule, which contains new telehealth services covered under Medicare.[34] CMS also included ongoing telehealth payment for a variety of services that will be covered until the end of the calendar year in which the PHE ends, including:

- Domiciliary, Rest Home, or Custodial Care services, Established Patients (99336, 99337)
- Home Visits, Established Patient (99349, 99350)
- Emergency Department Visits for Evaluation and Management of a Patient (99281–99283)
- Nursing Facilities Discharge Day Management (99315, 99316)
- Psychological and Neuropsychological Testing (96130–96133)

CMS, on a temporary and emergency basis under the 1135 waiver authority and Coronavirus Preparedness and Response Supplemental Appropriations Act, enabled Medicare to reimburse telehealth services under the Physician Fee Schedule at the same amount as in-person service.[35] Medicare reimbursement for telehealth services will continue to evolve, and the influence of the rule changes related to the PHE remains to be seen.

Medicare Advantage

While Medicare Advantage plans have historically had more leverage than traditional Medicare to provide coverage for telehealth services, CMS finalized policies in April 2019 to make it more likely that Medicare Advantage plans will, in fact, cover a broader range of telehealth services.[36] Pursuant to these policies, which became effective in January 2020, Medicare Advantage plans can now offer telehealth benefits as part of the standard benefits package and may reimburse for telehealth services even where the patient receives that care at home.

Medicaid

Almost all of the states now have legislation providing for some level of Medicaid coverage for telemedicine. Medicaid is a joint federal-state program and, in general, must follow federal requirements for reimbursing providers. For telemedicine specifically, however, state Medicaid programs can set unique payment policies and are encouraged to create innovative payment methodologies for telemedicine modalities. For example, states can determine, among other things, whether to cover telemedicine, the types of telemedicine services to cover, the types of technologies it will require, any originating site limitations, and the amount of reimbursement.

The Center for Connected Health Policy maintains a national survey that indicates that as of Fall 2020, 50 states and the District of Columbia provided some Medicaid coverage for telehealth services.[37] But while almost all of the state Medicaid programs cover telemedicine services, the method for delivering such service may limit the availability of coverage. According to the Fall 2020 report, for example, 16 states limit the type of facility that can serve as an eligible originating site; only 18 states provide reimbursement for store-and-forward technologies; and only 21 states reimburse for remote patient monitoring.[38] Thus, providers must evaluate state-specific Medicaid rules and coverage policies to determine reimbursement bounds for their particular state.

Private Commercial Payers

While some commercial payers voluntarily cover telemedicine services, many states require commercial payers to provide such reimbursement under what are known as "parity laws." According to the Fall 2020 report issued by the Center for Connected Health Policy, 43 states and the District of Columbia have adopted legislation governing the commercial payer's telehealth reimbursement.[39] While "parity" legislation appears to remove significant reimbursement barriers for telemedicine, the covered services and amount of reimbursement varies among the states with "parity" legislation. For example, some states require that telemedicine services be reimbursed at the same rates as in-person services, while other states only require "parity" in terms of *what* is covered rather than the level of reimbursement required.[40] And similar to public payers, there are differences among commercial payers regarding limitations related to originating site, technology requirements, and the like. That said, commercial payers are now increasingly developing programs to cover telemedicine services as a way to cut expenses for high-cost populations.

> While "parity" legislation appears to remove significant reimbursement barriers for telemedicine, the covered services and amount of reimbursement vary among the states with "parity" legislation. For example, some states require that telemedicine services be reimbursed at the same rates as in-person services, while other states only require "parity" in terms of *what* is covered rather than the level of reimbursement required.[41]

While "parity laws" are helpful in ensuring coverage for telemedicine services, commercial contract terms with providers (typically drafted for traditional bricks-and-mortar arrangements) may limit reimbursement for telemedicine services or provide mechanics for payers to deny claims. Simply stated, "parity laws" can be a helpful leverage in contractual negotiations, especially when paired with business justifications demonstrating the value basis for the telemedicine service. The COVID-19 pandemic spurred an onslaught of executive orders mandating that commercial payers cover telehealth services at the same rate as in-office visits for the duration of the public health emergency. State payment parity orders are limited to the timeframe contemplated by the specific order. However, a number of states have already begun legislative attempts to make payment parity permanent. For example, the Massachusetts senate unanimously passed a bill that addressed coverage offered by the commission to an active or retired employee of the commonwealth insured under the group insurance commission. The senate requires the commission to provide coverage for health care services via telehealth by a contracted health care provider and to cover services delivered via telehealth to the same extent as if they were provided via in-person consultation of delivery.[42]

BILLING AND CODING

Common Codes for Telehealth Services in the Emergency Setting

The process of evaluation and management (E/M) coding, which is often carried out by coding specialists and may be poorly understood by clinicians, gains a further level of complexity in telehealth because some requirements and codes are specific to telehealth services. As discussed in the preceding sections, reimbursement rules vary from payer to payer and from jurisdiction to jurisdiction, and additionally are not static over time. For example, in contract year (CY) 2017 a total of 89 Healthcare Common Procedure Coding System (HCPCS) codes were reimbursable by CMS for telehealth services. In CY 2018 this number rose to 96, and in CY 2019 it rose to 98.[43] While the core set of codes has remained relatively constant over this time, the number of reimbursable codes is likely to rise, and at the same time, codes can drop off the list as code definitions evolve. In CY 2019, services with the greatest number of telehealth-reimbursable codes under CMS rules included psychotherapy, end-stage renal disease management, and office or outpatient visits. Codes covering alcohol and tobacco cessation, certain types of health screening, nutrition management, and other areas were included as well. Notably absent from the list of reimbursable codes in 2019 were the primary CPT codes for ED visits (99281-99285).

The ED visit codes were made temporarily reimbursable after the public health emergency (PHE) was declared on January 31, 2020, in response to the developing SARS-CoV-2 pandemic. A total of 134 codes have been made temporarily reimbursable since the PHE declaration, including codes for in-patient care, in-patient observation care, critical care, ventilator management, home visits, physical and occupational therapy, speech therapy, and others. Per the 2021 Physician Fee Schedule that CMS issued in December 2020, some of these codes, including the ED visit codes, will remain reimbursable for telemedicine until the end of the calendar year in which the PHE ends.[44] It is not clear as of this writing what will become of these codes after this time.

Outside of the PHE, dedicated codes must be used in addition to the 9928x code when billing for telehealth consultations in the ED. These are G0425, G0426, and G0427. These codes are different from the typical "GC modifiers" and instead represent independent problem-focused, detailed, and comprehensive encounters, respectively (typically 30 minutes, 50 minutes, and 70 minutes spent communicating with the patient via telehealth). These same three codes are also used to bill for an initial *in-patient* consultation as well. In both cases, the codes must be appended with a POS 02 (Place of Service) or modifier (95 for Medicare and either 95 or GT for other payers) to represent teleconsultation. Under this system, the physician or provider at the distant site who provides the consultation must be distinct from the physician or provider at the originating site who has requested the consultation and who remains the local physician of record. Outside the public health emergency, ED telehealth consultations billed to Medicare are subject to the same set of eligibility rules around location and originating site previously discussed, though rules for consultations billed to Medicaid and private payers will vary by state and by payer.

When subsequent teleconsultation is required in the in-patient setting (including Skilled Nursing Facilities), the codes G0406, G0407, and G0408 are used and again refer to a problem-focused, expanded-focused, and detailed interval history, respectively (in this case, typically 15 minutes, 25 minutes, and 35 minutes spent communicating with the patient via telehealth). Initial hospital care (99221, 99222, and 99223) was temporarily covered under the PHE, but subsequent hospital care (99231, 99232, and 99233) was covered before the PHE.

Outpatient telehealth visits, such as those that take place at an urgent care center, are billed using the same codes as in-person visits (99201–99205 for new patients and 99211–99215 for established patients). These codes are appended with the GT or 95 modifier or POS 02 place of service to indicate that they are telehealth visits. The codes are selected based on the depth of required patient history, focus of the examination, time required for care, and complexity of the medical decision making as described in Box 6.2.

While standard E/M guidelines should be satisfied when billing for telehealth encounters, it is important to document findings accurately and appropriately within the limitation of the telehealth encounter. It is also best practice to include a

Box 6.2

DOCUMENTATION REQUIREMENTS FOR BILLING BASED ON EVALUATION AND MANAGEMENT GUIDELINES PUBLISHED BY CMS IN 1995 AND 1997

While a detailed discussion of general documentation requirements is beyond the scope of this chapter, for the most part, documentation requirements for telehealth visits mirror those of in-person encounters. Codes are built in sets, and multiple codes may represent the same basic service but at a different level of care. For example, the out-patient codes 99201–99205 all represent an office or out-patient visit for the evaluation and management of a new patient. However, these five codes are associated with different numbers of relative value unit (RVUs) and are selected based on the service provided. From a billing standpoint, the provided service is represented by the provider's documentation. The proper code is selected based on how narrow or broad the scope of the visit was, and it is assumed that this will be represented in the documentation. Each billable note must contain three components that should be familiar to any practitioner: a patient history, an examination, and a medical decision-making section. The patient history is subdivided into a chief complaint/HPI, a review of systems, and a history section (which includes past history, family history, and social history). A billing code is selected based on how comprehensive the documentation of the visit is. Specific definitions of history of present illness (HPI) components, review of systems requirements, physical exam requirements, and complexity of medical decision making are laid out in two sets of E/M guidelines published by CMS in 1995 and 1997.

telehealth disclaimer in the chart to document that specific telehealth reimbursement requirements have been met. The exact wording of the disclaimer should be based on the practice policies, local regulations, and payer requirements. For example, if payment is only provided for real-time two-way communication and not store-and-forward service, then the disclaimer should state the modality used. The patchwork nature of reimbursement rules may make certain services nonreimbursable, or only reimbursable in certain locations or for certain populations. Services provided outside of traditional third-party payer models, such as subscriptions, retainers, flat fees, and other arrangements, may offer more flexibility as long as they do not conflict with provider–payer contractual requirement or beneficiary coverages (Box 6.3).

Box 6.3

TELEMEDICINE DISCLAIMER EXAMPLE

"This encounter was provided via secure, real time two-way audio-video connection with the patient (telemedicine). The patient has provided informed consent to have an exam conducted via telemedicine, and I have addressed any questions or concerns. I have verified the location and identity of the patient to the best extent possible. The encounter was completed without any technical interruptions that would impact my provision of care."

RISK MANAGEMENT AND MALPRACTICE INSURANCE

The basic tests for malpractice claims—that a provider had a duty to care for a patient, that there was a breach of duty, that injury occurred, and that the breach caused the injury—are unchanged when care is delivered via telehealth. However, determining whether a breach occurred is dependent on whether the standard of care was violated. In 2014 the Federation of State Medical Boards adopted a policy position stating that "treatment and consultation recommendations made in an online setting, including issuing a prescription via electronic means, will be held to the same standards of appropriate practice as those in traditional (encounter in person) settings."[45]

However, not all states have adopted this standard, and some have not adopted any specific standard.[46] For example, the Hawaii statute states that "[t]reatment recommendations made via telehealth, including issuing a prescription via electronic means, shall be held to the same standards of appropriate practice as those in traditional physician-patient settings *that do not include a face-to-face visit* but in which prescribing is appropriate, including on-call telephone encounters and encounters for which a follow-up visit is arranged"[47](emphasis added). As with other aspects of telemedicine, standards of care may be inconsistent or incompletely defined, and there have been too few medical malpractice cases relating to telemedicine to characterize the standard of care.[48] Consequently, it is important that telemedicine providers be familiar with any expectations and laws around standard of care at both the distant site and the originating site. Providers should also know if their malpractice covers telemedicine or out-of-state care.

ADVOCACY

Variations in licensing laws, payment rules across geographic regions and payers, and accreditation and credentialing requirements limit one of the most substantial benefits of telemedicine: that it is fundamentally not limited by geographic borders or distances.[49] Easing barriers to practice across state lines and expanding payment for telehealth services have historically been goals for telehealth advocates. The temporary relaxation of federal and state laws governing licensure and payment during the COVID-19 Public Health Emergency has shown the potential for telehealth expansion under a more uniform and less restrictive set of telehealth regulations.

The Coronavirus Preparedness and Response Supplemental Appropriations (CARES) Act and subsequent CMS guidance temporarily lifted restrictions on originating site type and location for Medicare beneficiaries. Additionally, 46 states and 3 territories waived some requirements for in-state medical licensure for health professionals as long as they were licensed and in good standing in other states.[50] These federal and state changes were enacted to allow patients to receive medical care without risking exposure to SARS-CoV-2 and to permit states to increase medical staffing as necessary to confront the pandemic. These changes had a substantial immediate effect. For example, from February 2020 to April 2020, the number of primary care telemedicine appointments among Medicare fee for service beneficiaries increased from approximately 2,000 per week to 1.28 million per week.[51] The volume of telehealth claims increased 4,347% from March 2019 to March 2020.[52]

Many of the rules that were eased under the PHE will revert when the PHE is ended, and it is unclear what changes may become permanent and how they might impact telehealth availability and utilization. There are several coalitions and groups advocating for permanent changes to some of the rules that were adjusted under the PHE, or are tracking pending legislation. These are summarized in Table 6.3. In addition to those groups highlighted in the table, numerous other industry organizations that are not focused exclusively on telehealth track policy or put forth positions on telehealth expansion, including the American College of Emergency Physicians (ACEP), the Federation of State Medical Boards (FSMB), the Health Information Management Systems Society (HIMSS), the American Medical Association (AMA), and others. These organizations are an ongoing source of information on telehealth advocacy priorities and actions. There are telehealth advocacy priorities in addition to regulation and payment rule changes, such as the need to expand broadband access, provide telehealth education to students entering health professions, simplify patient information sharing while maintaining patient privacy, and expand research on telehealth outcomes and cost.

Table 6.3 INDUSTRY GROUPS AND OFFICES

Organization	About
Alliance for Connected Care	An organization made up of industry members "to create a legal and regulatory environment in which every provider in America is permitted to deliver safe, high quality care using telehealth technology at his or her discretion, and be compensated at a consistent rate regardless of care delivery location or technological delivery method."[53]
American Telemedicine Association	An industry group with a mission to "advance industry adoption of telehealth and virtual care, promote responsible policy, advocate for government and market normalization, and provide education and resources to help integrate virtual care into emerging value-based delivery models."[54]
Center for Connected Health Policy	The CCHP is "a nonprofit, non-partisan organization working to maximize telehealth's ability to improve health outcomes, care delivery, and cost effectiveness."[55] The CCHP monitors state and federal regulations, publishes regulation summaries, and engages in telehealth guidance and education projects.
National Consortium of Telehealth Resource Centers	A federally funded consortium of 12 regional and 2 national telehealth resource centers that aim to "lead the advancement and accessibility of telehealth with a focus in rural communities, Federally Qualified Health Centers (FQHCs), and Rural Health Clinics (RHCs)."[56]
Office for the Advancement of Telehealth	A federal office of the Health Resources and Services Administration (HRSA), it "promotes the use of telehealth technologies for health care delivery, education, and health information services," by "providing funds to promote and improve telehealth services in rural areas."[57]

CONCLUSION

Telehealth is governed by a complicated web of laws and rules issued by the federal government, states, medical boards, payers, provider organizations, and other stakeholders. These laws and rules touch on issues around privacy, licensing, credentialing, and reimbursement, and other regulatory topics. These rules and laws often differ from location to location and organization to organization. It is incumbent upon the administrators and practitioners in telehealth to understand the specific laws and rules that are applicable in the settings where they deliver care. Greater uniformity in regulation and payment will allow for the expansion of telehealth services, as demonstrated by temporary changes that occurred as a result of the public health emergency that was declared during the COVID-19 pandemic. There are a variety of additional legislative goals that will facilitate the expansion of telehealth, and there are organizations that focus on this work.

KEY TAKEAWAYS

- ➢ The provision of emergency care via telehealth is subject to the requirements of EMTALA.
- ➢ HIPAA Privacy Rules must be considered when selecting vendors and designing telehealth services.
- ➢ Patients must give consent for telehealth care and should understand the risks associated with telemedicine.
- ➢ Health care systems and clinicians providing telehealth services across jurisdictional lines must be familiar with licensing laws and credentialing rules at both the originating and distant sites, and must ensure that they are appropriately licensed and credentialed to provide care at the relevant site.
- ➢ Payment rules are not uniform from state to state and payer to payer.
- ➢ The COVID-19 public health emergency led to a rapid, temporary relaxation of licensing rules and expansion of reimbursement for telehealth services.
- ➢ Maintaining equitable access to telemedicine services after the expiration of the PHE will require advocacy, well thought out legislation, and interstate cooperation.

REFERENCES

1. 42 U.S.C. §1395dd.
2. Department of Health and Human Services, Centers for Medicare & Medicaid Services, Critical Access Hospital (CAH) Emergency Services and Telemedicine: Implications for Emergency Services Condition of Participation (CoPs) and Emergency Medical Treatment and Labor Act (EMTALA) On-Call Compliance, S&C: 13-38-CAH/EMTALA (June 7, 2013), available at: https://www.cms.gov/Medicare/Provider-Enrollment-and-Certification/SurveyCertificationGenInfo/Downloads/Survey-and-Cert-Letter-13-38.pdf.

3. Department of Health and Human Services, Centers for Medicare & Medicaid Services, Emergency Medical Treatment and Labor Act (EMTALA) and Ebola Virus Disease (EVD) – Questions and Answers (Q + A), S&C: 15-24-Hospitals (February 13, 2015), available at: https://www.cms.gov/Medicare/Provider-Enrollment-and-Certification/SurveyCertEmergPrep/Downloads/Survey-Cert-Letter-15-24-EMTALA-Ebola.pdf.

4. Department of Health and Human Services, Centers for Medicare & Medicaid Services, Critical Access Hospital (CAH) Emergency Services and Telemedicine: Implications for Emergency Services Condition of Participation (CoPs) and Emergency Medical Treatment and Labor Act (EMTALA) On-Call Compliance, S&C: 13-38-CAH/EMTALA (June 7, 2013), available at: https://www.cms.gov/Medicare/Provider-Enrollment-and-Certification/SurveyCertificationGenInfo/Downloads/Survey-and-Cert-Letter-13-38.pdf.

5. Department of Health and Human Services, Centers for Medicare & Medicaid Services, Critical Access Hospital (CAH) Emergency Services and Telemedicine: Implications for Emergency Services Condition of Participation (CoPs) and Emergency Medical Treatment and Labor Act (EMTALA) On-Call Compliance, S&C: 13-38-CAH/EMTALA (June 7, 2013), available at: https://www.cms.gov/Medicare/Provider-Enrollment-and-Certification/SurveyCertificationGenInfo/Downloads/Survey-and-Cert-Letter-13-38.pdf.

6. Virginia Board of Medicine Guidance Document 85-12, Section Two (Revised October 28, 2018).

7. Interstate Medical Licensure Compact, available at https://imlcc.org.

8. Executive Order 2020-30, https://www.michigan.gov/coronavirus/0,9753,7-406-98178_98455-521682--,00.html (last visited April 3, 2020); see also Michigan Licensing and Regulatory Affairs, Bureau of Professional Licensing, Clarification: Exemption of Michigan Licensure, Time of Disaster/State of Emergency (March 16, 2020).

9. Minn. Stat. §147.032.

10. Va. Code Ann. § 54.1-2901(A)(7).

11. 45 C.F.R. § 160.103.

12. *Id.*

13. *See* 45 C.F.R. § 164.500 *et seq.* Additional information regarding the HIPAA Privacy Rule can be found on the Office for Civil Rights website, available at: https://www.hhs.gov/hipaa/for-professionals/privacy/index.html.

14. 45 C.F.R. § 164.520.

15. 45 C.F.R. §§ 164.524, 164.508.

16. 45 C.F.R. § 164.302 *et seq.*

17. 45 C.F.R. § 164.308(b).

18. *See* 45 C.F.R. § 164.308(a).

19. 45 C.F.R. § 164.306(b).

20. 45 C.F.R. § 164.400 *et seq.*

21. 45 C.F.R. § 164.410.

22. 45 C.F.R. §§ 164.404, 164.406, 164.408.

23. Real-time audiovisual technologies are not required for services delivered as part of a federal telemedicine demonstration program conducted in Alaska or Hawaii. Moreover, certain other medical services delivered using telecommunications technology but not requiring the patient to be present—such as radiology and pathology services—are covered by Medicare much as are services delivered when a

patient is in-person at the medical facility and so are not considered telemedicine services. Further, recent CMS coverage of "telemedicine-like" services, referred to as virtual check-ins and interprofessional consultations do not require the patient to be present and thus are not subject to statutory telemedicine limitations.

24. U.S. Department of Health and Human Services, Program Memorandum Intermediaries/Carriers, Re: Revision of Medicare Reimbursement for Telehealth Services, Transmittal AB-01-69 (May 1, 2001), available at http://www.cms.gov/Regulations-and-Guidance/Guidance/Transmittals/downloads/AB0169.pdf.

25. *Telehealth Services*, MLN Booklet, Centers for Medicare and Medicaid Services, https://www.cms.gov/Outreach-and-Education/Medicare-Learning-Network-MLN/MLNProducts/downloads/TelehealthSrvcsfctsht.pdf, January 2019 (last visited September 9, 2019).

26. Medicare Telehealth Frequently Asked Questions (FAQs), *supra* note 14; *see also* Telehealth Services, MLN Booklet, Centers for Medicare and Medicaid Services, https://www. https://www.cms.gov/Outreach-and-Education/Medicare-Learning-Network-MLN/MLNProducts/Downloads/TelehealthSrvcsfctsht.pdf, March 2020 (last visited November 5, 2020)

27. *Bundled Payments for Care Improvement (BPCI) Initiative: General Information*, Centers for Medicare and Medicaid Services, http://innovation.cms.gov/initiatives/bundled-payments (last visited September 9, 2019).

28. Lewin Group, *CMS Bundled Payments for Care Improvement Initiative Models 2-4: Year 4 Evaluation Monitoring Annual Report*, June 2018. https://innovation.cms.gov/Files/reports/bpci-models2-4-yr4evalrpt.pdf. (last visited September 9, 2019).

29. *New Modifier for Expanding the Use of Telehealth for Individuals with Stroke.* MLN Matters. Centers for Medicare and Medicaid Services, https://www.cms.gov/Outreach-and-Education/Medicare-Learning-Network-MLN/MLNMattersArticles/Downloads/MM10883.pdf (last visited September 9, 2019).

30. *Final Policy, Payment, and Quality Provisions Changes to the Medicare Physician Fee Schedule for Calendar Year 2019.* Fact Sheet. Centers for Medicare and Medicaid Services, https://www.cms.gov/newsroom/fact-sheets/final-policy-payment-and-quality-provisions-changes-medicare-physician-fee-schedule-calendar-year (last visited September 9, 2019).

31. 83 Fed. Reg. 59,836 (November 23, 2018).

32. CMS has twice declined to include CPT codes for initial hospital care (CPT Codes 99221–99223) on the list of eligible telehealth service codes—first in 2010 (75 Fed. Reg. 73,860 (November 29, 2010)) and again in 2017 (82 Fed. Reg. 52,976 (November 15, 2017)). Most recently, CMS stated that "while initial inpatient consultation services [G0425-G0427] are currently on the list of approved telehealth services, there are no services on the current list of telehealth services that resemble initial hospital care for an acutely ill patient by the admitting practitioner who has ongoing responsibility for the patient's treatment during the course of the hospital stay." 82 Fed. Reg. 52,976 (November 15, 2017).

33. CMS, *List of Telehealth Services*, available at: https://www.cms.gov/Medicare/Medicare-General-Information/Telehealth/Telehealth-Codes.

34. https://www.cms.gov/newsroom/fact-sheets/final-policy-payment-and-quality-provisions-changes-medicare-physician-fee-schedule-calendar-year-1 (Last accessed December 20, 2020)

35. CMS, *Medicare Telehealth Frequently Asked Questions (FAQs)* (March 17, 2020), available at: https://www.cms.gov/files/document/medicare-telehealth-frequently-asked-questions-faqs-31720.pdf.

36. 84 Fed. Reg. 15,680 (April 16, 2019).

37. *Telehealth Medicaid and State Policy.* Center for Connected Health Policy. https://www.cchpca.org/telehealth-policy/telehealth-medicaid-and-state-policy (last visited November 15, 2020).

38. *Id.*

39. *Id.*

40. *Id.*

41. *Id.*

42. *See An Act Putting Patients First,* Bill S.2796 191st Sess. (Ma. 2020), available at: https://malegislature.gov/Bills/191/S2796.

43. https://www.cms.gov/Medicare/Medicare-General-Information/Telehealth/Telehealth-Codes.html (last accessed December 20, 2020)

44. https://www.cms.gov/medicaremedicare-fee-service-paymentphysicianfeeschedpfs-federal-regulation-notices/cms-1734-f (last accessed December 20, 2010)

45. Model Policy for the Appropriate use of Telemedicine Technologies in the Practice of Medicine: Report of the State Medical Boards' Appropriate Regulation (SMART) Workgroup. Federation of State Medical Board, 2014.

46. Russell, D; ed. (2018). *Telemedicine Risk Management Considerations* [White paper]. American Societ for Health Care Risk Management. https://www.ashrm.org/system/files/media/file/2020/01/TELEMEDICINE-WHITE-PAPER-Final.pdf

47. Hawaii Revised Statutes. §453-1.3(c) Practice of telehealth.

48. B. J. Kaspar, Legislating for a New Age in Medicine: Defining the Telemedicine Standard of Care to Improve Healthcare in Iowa, *Iowa Law Review*, (2014): 99, 839.

49. Thanks to Kathy Hsu Wibberly, PhD, Jeffery Davis, and Krista Drobac for perspective on this section.

50. U.S. States and Territories Modifying Requirements in Response to COVID-19. Federation of State Medical Boards. Available at https://www.fsmb.org/siteassets/advocacy/pdf/states-waiving-licensure-requirements-for-telehealth-in-response-to-covid-19.pdf.

51. Medicare Beneficiary Use of Telehealth Visits: Early Data from the Start of the COVID-19 Pandemic (Issue Brief). Office of the Assistant Secretary for Planning and Evaluation, Department of Health and Human Services. July 28, 2020.

52. Monthly Telehealth Regional Tracker, Data from Fair Health National Private Insurance Claims Database. https://www.fairhealth.org/states-by-the-numbers/telehealth

53. http://connectwithcare.org/overview/ (last accessed November 15, 2020).

54. https://www.americantelemed.org/about-us/ (last accessed November 15, 2020).

55. https://www.cchpca.org (last accessed November 15, 2020).

56. https://www.telehealthresourcecenter.org/about-us/ (last accessed November 15, 2020).

57. https://www.hrsa.gov/rural-health/telehealth (last accessed November 15, 2020).

7

Telehealth Cybersecurity

COLTON D. HOOD ■

INTRODUCTION

Complex interconnected clinical systems require the prioritization of cybersecurity strategies to ensure the privacy and security of health information. As telehealth expands in response to the COVID pandemic (Hoffman, 2020), health care providers and organizations need to increase their level of cybersecurity (NIST, 2020). Broadly speaking, telehealth consists of connecting two parties by the transmission of audio and/or visual information, ideally, combined with a way to document the encounter. Both patients and clinicians utilize a number of different interfaces and communications solutions to conduct telehealth visits. Given this variety, safeguarding protected health information (PHI) and earning the trust of patients are of utmost importance. Increasing the utilization of technology in the delivery of medical care makes the challenge of keeping information safe and confidential highly complex. There was a time when a patient's health information lived in a personal notebook. This evolved into the patient chart, which has physical security needs, and now information lives electronically, in local or cloud-based storage, making cybersecurity increasingly important. A thorough understanding of the interconnections and consequences of these systems is not practical for all users, but there are basic security concepts that impact all stakeholders.

People use and access dozens of secure computer systems daily to pay bills, listen to music, stream movies, check their email, and document in their patient's medical record. The first step in that process is to assign a username, the mechanism the computer system uses to identify a unique user and ultimately manage what information and procedures the user can access. User identities are secured by a credential such as a typed password (there may be additional credentials such as a fingerprint or a code generator resulting in two-factor authentication), used to authenticate with the system. The computer system is then responsible for authorizing access to a specific set of information. Information in the system may be encrypted during transmission or when it is at rest in storage; this process keeps the information secure from those who are not authorized to access it. Understanding the interplay between these

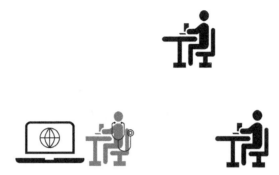

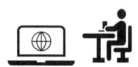

Figure 7.1 Telehealth providers must consider cybersecurity safeguards in public venues.

processes is just one step in understanding how health information is put at risk and how that risk can be mitigated.

Let's propose an exercise: You are taking your lunch break during a busy telemedicine shift. You are hungry and feel undercaffeinated, so you take your work-issued laptop to the local coffee shop, purchase a coffee and a sandwich, and decide to finish up the morning's charts while you enjoy your break. You connect to the coffee shop Wi-Fi and access your electronic health record (EHR) and while working on your charts, you get a call from your assistant that a patient is requesting a visit. The coffee shop is basically empty; you put in your headphones and connect to the patient through the patient portal video application (Figure 7.1). Is there anything wrong with this situation? Did we adhere to all the principles we discussed above, did we secure our identity, are we authenticated, is our information encrypted? Is there anything else we should consider?

CYBERATTACKS

Some of the most common types of cyberattacks include ransomware, denial of service, malware, phishing, advanced persistent threats, rogue software, and password attacks (Ponemon Institute LLC, 2016). Advanced persistent threats are stealthy long-term attacks designed to exfiltrate data over time (AO Kaspersky Lab, 2020b). These attacks can be categorized by how they affect the integrity, confidentiality, and availability of patient information as outlined in the Security Rule portion of the Health Insurance Portability and Accountability Act (HIPAA), but they also can have a direct impact on patient safety (Health Care Industry Cybersecurity Task Force, 2017). For example, a ransomware attack on a hospital system, such as those at Medstar Health (Reed, 2016) or Universal Health Services (Newman, 2020), could disable all vulnerable systems in the hospital. While there was no indication in these reports that patient information was at risk, such ransomware attacks could lead to the loss of confidentiality, if patient information were to be removed. Disabling computers could impact the availability of health information, and unplanned outages of clinical systems could impact patient safety. The integrity of records could also be at stake, if attackers attempted to modify health information.

A cyberattack, such as ransomware, is costly from the perspective of human resources, as well as damaged hardware and software. The impact to the company as a whole can include abnormal turnover of customers and diminished goodwill (Ponemon Institute LLC, 2012); 24% of companies reported that their reputation was diminished by the attack (Ponemon Institute LLC, 2017). These threats can be addressed by examining regulatory expectations which, when assessed, help to secure and protect telehealth programs.

HEALTH INSURANCE PORTABILITY AND ACCOUNTABILITY ACT AND LOCAL REGULATIONS

Typically, a telehealth- or technology-related care deployment will require support from an organizational information technology (IT) department, which generally includes security, compliance, and risk management assessments. In any health care organization, at least one person is assigned to be the HIPAA Compliance officer and a Security officer, but in larger organizations this assignment may require coordination between several different departments.

In the United States, security choices revolve around HIPAA, legislation that was enhanced by the Health Information Technology for Economic and Clinical Health Act (HITECH), itself a part of the American Recovery and Reinvestment Act of 2009. While the Privacy Rule has been covered extensively in Chapter 6, the Security Rule[1] will be discussed in the context of a telehealth solution that could include application-specific software and hardware.

After establishing that a company or person is a covered entity (CE) and that HIPAA applies, the aim of the Security Rule is to protect personal health information, or PHI. The HITECH act extends the Security Rule to electronic PHI (e-PHI). One of the first tasks is to perform a risk assessment and create a management plan, which is generally done by an IT professional who specializes in security or by a HIPAA Security specialist. Health and Human Services (HHS) and the Office of the National Coordinator (ONC) have provided guidance and assessment tools (such as the HIPAA Security Risk Assessment Tool (SRA)[2]), which provides a guided risk assessment. The SRA tool provides a threat and vulnerability rating, a summary of areas that need review, a detailed risk report, and an overall summary. Much of HIPAA compliance revolves around documenting policies, and CEs use it to assist and organize this endeavor. Additional detailed and easy-to-use guidance is available from the Office for Civil Rights (OCR) at https://www.hhs.gov/hipaa and the ONC at https://www.healthit.gov/topic/privacy-security-and-hipaa.

> Additional detailed and easy-to-use guidance is available from the Office for Civil Rights (OCR) at https://www.hhs.gov/hipaa and the ONC at https://www.healthit.gov/topic/privacy-security-and-hipaa.

The Security Rule has three overarching parts that can guide an assessment of security: physical safeguards, technical safeguards, and administrative safeguards. These categories all have aspects of the Security Rule that are required and addressable. The covered entity is responsible for addressing every specification; however, it may not be practical to implement every addressable specification, and so the Security Rule allows a covered entity to adopt an alternative plan, documented and measured when appropriate (45 C.F.R. § 164.306(d)).

Physical safeguards in a telehealth program will depend greatly on the details of the specific implementation. The two main topics in physical safeguards for facility access control are workstation and device security (45 C.F.R. § 164.310). This includes securing access to workstations and telehealth equipment. Some telehealth equipment may not be able to store any e-PHI, like most simple web cameras, but other devices, such as a laptop computer or tablet, will need to be secured to protect e-PHI (45 C.F.R. § 164.310). Once the physical equipment is secured, the next section to address is the technical safeguards.

Technical safeguards are controls that are more technology-driven in nature. Devices that store e-PHI must have access control, meaning only those who are authorized to access PHI can use them. Another factor is transmission security. Devices that use Wi-Fi need to do so in a secure manner. This is especially relevant to a telehealth solution where the audio and video that are transmitted are secured using encryption (45 C.F.R. § 164.312(e)). Other measures include the ability for activity on devices and software used to be logged so that they can be audited to ensure the integrity and security of e-PHI (45 C.F.R. § 164.312(b)).

Lastly, there are Administrative Safeguards that mainly revolve around creating and documenting security processes. There must be a designated Security Officer, and there must be a security management process, including a risk analysis. A risk analysis and review of policies should occur periodically (45 C.F.R. § 164.308(a)(8)). The technology needs to support the Privacy Rule such that the minimum necessary PHI is exposed by users. Organizations must supervise and train their workforce on their security policies and apply sanctions to those who violate them. To apply these safeguards to a telehealth solution, an organization needs to have robust training on the use of the telehealth system with its components. It is important to document not only processes, but also adherence to them, such as documenting completion of trainings.

State and local laws, such as the Massachusetts Data Protection Act (Massachusetts Court System Law Library, 2017) passed in 2010, has stipulations to protect customer information similar to those legislated in HIPAA. It is also important to be aware of any local regulations regarding PHI or Personally Identifiable Information (PII) that are usually, but not always, preempted by HIPAA (Office for Civil Rights, 2013). When handling the personal information of people located in the European Union (EU), the General Data Protection Regulation (GDPR) is in effect regardless of whether or not the company is located in the EU (European Parliament, 2016).

HARDWARE AND SOFTWARE ASSESSMENT

A vendor selection process for hardware or software should include an evaluation of how security is addressed. Beyond HIPAA, there are further security standards to consider with vendors such as System and Organization Controls (SOC) 2 (SOC for Service Organizations, n.d.). Organizations should look for a company that can provide automatic security updates for their software and ensure that basic functionality like password protection and encryption is present; the software should conform to the HIPAA regulations as outlined by their organization. If a software or hardware solution requires PHI, the vendor may need to become a business associate and enter into a business associate agreement (BAA). A BAA is an agreement between two organizations that delineates their responsibilities regarding the use of shared PHI and may be required to maintain compliance (Office for Civil Rights, 2017). If a vendor needs to handle organizational PHI, such as a vendor that hosts a real-time video solution or a specialized medical record, they will likely require a BAA to maintain HIPAA compliance.

Any hardware selected should be reviewed per written security policies. Understanding if telehealth devices store or hold e-PHI and how they transmit it is important for maintaining security and compliance. Organizations should consider the risk of permitting clinicians and staff to use personal devices to access telehealth or other secure information systems. A clear policy should be agreed upon with the understanding that there is risk of potentially unsafe hardware accessing the network and patients' health information. If the organization plans on allowing personal mobile devices to access the telehealth solution, HealthIT.gov has many suggestions on how to secure their use, include ensuring password use, device encryption, enabling remote wiping/disabling, installing firewalls or security software, keeping devices up to date, researching the mobile apps being utilized, ensuring security of patient data over public Wi-Fi networks, and making sure all health data is deleted before discarding the device (HealthIT.gov, 2019).

In addition to the security of personal devices, special attention should be made to USB telehealth peripheral devices. Studies have shown that malware-infected USB drives planted around hospitals can introduce malware to hospital networks. According to a report by Independent Security Evaluators, personnel are naturally curious to find out what the devices contain and plug them (Independent Security Evaluators, 2016). USB drives can also be used to remove ePHI from health care networks, with many organizations allowing read only access to all USB drives that are not securely encrypted. While USB drives provide a well-established risk to hospital networks, caution should be taken for any USB device, be it camera, stethoscope, or ultrasound probe. Understanding how these devices store data and interact with computer systems and the network is another important step in keeping data secure.

Secure Communication

Secure communication with patients is an essential component of high-quality care. Outside of ensuring a secure audiovisual connection, all other communications to patients needs to be secure and follow organizational guidelines. Caution should be taken with potentially insecure modalities such as email and short message service (SMS) messaging. It is good practice to keep patient communication within the patient portal of the EHR if the feature exists. The benefit of doing this practice is twofold: patient access is usually established and secure, and communications can be more easily documented.

Risk Assessment Tools

Zhou et al. took security one step further in 2019 with their report of a privacy and security questionnaire for telehealth providers (their complete questionnaire can be seen in Box 7.1). (Zhou, Thieret, Watzlaf, Dealmeida, & Parmanto, 2019). They assessed a total of 49 questions regarding a total of 31 programs and identified gaps in security and privacy in the domains of storage, transmission/accessibility, secure networks, encryption, consent, data backup plans, and authorization. They identified further problems, including: users not knowing if telehealth session information was stored on patients' computers or remote devices; users being unaware whether their telehealth vendor used encryption during transmission; failure to complete a thorough consent; and failure to have a system release PHI at patient request from the telehealth system. This paper highlights a more holistic evaluation of the program for both privacy and security. Ultimately, the effort taken to ensure robust privacy and security is essential in order to maintain patient and provider trust in the system (Hall & McGraw, 2014).

COFFEE SHOP REVISITED

Now let's return to the coffee shop where you were considering conducting a telehealth visit. Public Wi-Fi can be insecure due to the risk that data traffic can be intercepted and viewed between the access point and the connected computer (AO Kaspersky Lab, 2020a). Connected computers are vulnerable to malware from others accessing the Wi-Fi (AO Kaspersky Lab, 2020a). Every attempt should be made to secure traffic, such as encrypting it through a virtual private network (VPN) or using secure websites. Even with these protections. it is conceivably possible, though unlikely, that data could be put at risk. Public spaces are not always private, so it is also important to be mindful that your computer screen could be visible and that anyone could be listening (Figure 7.2).

Box 7.1

STATEMENTS OF THE TELEHEALTH SECURITY SELF-ASSESSMENT
QUESTIONNAIRE

D1: Policies
Q1. Does the telehealth system (vendor) have privacy policies in place?

Q2. Does the telehealth system (vendor) have security policies in place?

Q3. Are the privacy and security policies easy to understand?

Q4. Do the telehealth privacy and security policies include guidance on the best method to use to protect the security of patient information?

Q5. Are business associate agreements (BAAs) in place between the telehealth system (vendor) and other entities that do business with the telehealth system (vendor)?

Q6. If the vendor shares Protected Health Information (PHI) from the telehealth system (vendor) to other entities, are the privacy and security policies of those other entities checked before sharing?

Q7. Are the privacy and security policies and procedures kept current to meet federal and multi-state regulations?

Q8. Do the privacy and security features that are part of the telehealth system (vendor) meet federal and multistate regulations?

D2. Storage
Q9. Will PHI generated between the provider and patient be stored in any capacity by the telehealth system (vendor)?

Q10. Does the telehealth system (vendor) include guidance and information to clients on how best to store PHI which may include recordings of telehealth sessions?

Q11. When considering cloud service for data storage, is the telehealth system (vendor) compliant in keeping PHI highly secure?

Q12. Are clients discouraged from storing patient related information generated during the telehealth session offline on other storage devices?

Q13. Do you monitor whether any of the transmitted data during a telehealth session is stored on the patient's computer or other device's hard drive?

Q14. Is the telehealth system able to trigger remote erase of a mobile device used for telehealth sessions, if the mobile device is lost or stolen?

D3. Consent
Q15. Is the patient's or representative's informed consent obtained before the telehealth session begins?

Q16. Does the patient informed consent include the privacy and security features of the telehealth system?

Q17. Does the patient informed consent state that telehealth sessions may be recorded and pictures taken and stored?

Q18. Does the patient informed consent include recommendations that the environment and surroundings be secure?

Q19. Are patients provided the right to authorize a transfer of PHI outside of the existing system (e.g., to a biller, 3rd party payer, other entity)?

Q20. Are patients informed of the potential security risks when PHI is transferred between the health care provider and the telehealth system (vendor)?

D4. Transmission/Accessibility

Q21. Is PHI generated during the telehealth session accessible to others outside of the organization (such as law enforcement, government officials, etc.) as long as they have proper authorization?

D5. Encryption

Q22. Does the telehealth system (vendor) include details about encryption algorithms (such as the length of the key, for example, AES-256, the key management approach, and what specific data are encrypted)?

Q23. Do the encryption methods meet recognized standards from HIPAA, HITECH, the International Standards Organization (ISO) and the National Institute of Standards and Technology (NIST) as well as multistate regulations?

Q24. Are encryption keys periodically updated to meet the privacy and security policy?

D6. Data Backup Plan

Q25. If there was a technology breakdown, is there a data backup plan (e.g., be able to create and maintain exact copies of ePHI, establish what ePHI should be backed up, such as telehealth sessions/data) in place?

Q26. Is the data backup plan reviewed and updated on a regular basis (at least yearly)?

Q27. Are there appropriate redundant systems in place that ensure the availability of telehealth services even when one or a few components of the system are not working?

D7. Training

Q28. Is employee training provided on computer network privacy and security AND mobile device privacy and security?

Q29. Is HIPAA training, which includes instructional material tailored for telehealth privacy and security, provided at least on an annual basis, for all staff that use the telehealth system?

Q30. Are the risks of social media connections (e.g. risks of inadvertent linking of patients via social media as a result of using mobile devices with downloaded social media accounts on the device) discussed with all users of the telehealth system?

D8. Authentication/Access Control

Q31. Is proper user authentication (username, passwords, fingerprinting, PINs, and security questions) established before logging into the telehealth session?

Q32. Do you use strong passwords (uppercase, lowercase, minimum length, special symbols, digits, etc.) to access the telehealth system?

Q33. Is there an inactivity time out function available on the telehealth system that requires re-authentication to access the system after the timeout period has ended?

Q34. Is unauthorized viewing of patient information prevented by applying access controls (e.g., role-based, user-based, context-based access controls)?

Q35. Are all of the smart devices (smartphones, tablets, smartwatch etc.) that are used in telehealth sessions, password protected and encrypted?

D9. Authorization

Q36. Is prior written patient authorization required before any PHI content, developed as part of the telehealth session, is shared with other requestors?

Q37. Do qualified individuals with proper certification and backgrounds in privacy, security, and HIPAA regulations evaluate all requests for PHI?

Q38. Do patients receive an accounting of disclosures upon written request?

Q39. Will a patient's request for a restriction of uses and disclosures of PHI that is generated from the telehealth system be honored?

D10. Secure Networks

Q40. Do you connect only to secure networks (e.g., HTTPS, VPN, TLS, SSL) when using telehealth systems and avoid unsecure networks (e.g., public Wi-Fi)?

Q41. Do you use a Virtual Private Network (VPN) to access important websites?

Q42. Do you use Wi-Fi Protected Access-2 (WPA2) certification with AES-256 encryption for Wi-Fi?

Q43. Are privacy and security features of mobile apps used in telehealth practice carefully researched before being downloaded?

Q44. Is a disaster recovery plan (e.g., procedures in place to restore lost data, the types of data to be restored and copy of the disaster plan is readily available when needed) in place for the data collected during telehealth practice sessions?

Q45. Is an incident response plan in place for your telehealth practice?

Q46. Is there a security evaluation conducted by an independent party on the telehealth system to verify features such as Authentication, Encryption, Authorization, Wi-Fi settings, Data Management Plan, and all other proper privacy and security features?

Q47. Do you verify the source and integrity of the data when sending or receiving data during the telehealth session?

Q48. Are audit trails (a feature that records user activity in a telehealth system/vendor) used to track who has access to PHI that is collected during the telehealth session?

Q49. Are there up-to-date anti-virus, anti-malware programs installed on all devices used for telehealth sessions?

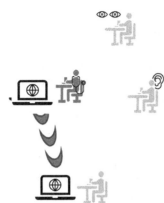

Physical Safeguards:
- Laptop screen could be visible
- Discussions can be overhead

Administrative:
- Organizational policies regarding clinical care in public spaces
- Using personal laptop for clinical care

Technical:
- Not securing clinical traffic, for example using a VPN
- Using insecure WIFI

The first coffee shop guest can see what is on the clinician's computer screen.
The second coffee shop guest can hear the discussion occurring during the telehealth visit.
The third guest is monitoring the clinician's network traffic through the insecure coffee shop WIFI.

Figure 7.2 How to apply physical, administrative and technical safeguards in public venues.

CONCLUSION

Health information systems are becoming increasingly complex, and telehealth is no exception. Whether launching a direct-to-consumer telehealth program or supporting emergency department staff with a telestroke program, security is paramount. Understanding the Security Rule is essential in order to provide telehealth services. Program evaluation tools can be helpful to assess risk as telehealth solutions become increasingly complex. Lastly, the effort made to keep the telehealth program secure should be explained to both the clinician and patient to help foster trust in the program.

KEY TAKEAWAYS

- Good security builds trust for both the patients and providers in telehealth.
- Risk assessments followed by thoughtful policies and good training will help keep telehealth deployments secure.
- Secure personal devices if they are to be used for telehealth.
- Be mindful of any PHI that could be stored on the patient's or distant site provider's device, or USB peripheral.
- Ensure all methods of communication are secure and encrypted.

NOTES

1. https://www.hhs.gov/hipaa/for-professionals/security
2. https://www.healthit.gov/topic/privacy-security-and-hipaa/security-risk-assessment-tool

REFERENCES

AO Kaspersky Lab. (2020a). *Public WiFi risk and what you can do about it.* Retrieved from kaspersky.com: https://usa.kaspersky.com/resource-center/preemptive-safety/public-wifi-risks.

AO Kaspersky Lab. (2020b). *What Is an advanced persistent threat (APT)?* Retrieved from kaspersky.com: https://www.kaspersky.com/resource-center/definitions/advanced-persistent-threats.

European Parliament. (2016). *Document 32016R0679.* Retrieved from EUR-Lex: https://eur-lex.europa.eu/eli/reg/2016/679/oj.

Hall, J. L., & McGraw, D. (2014). For telehealth to succeed, privacy and security risks must be identified and addressed. *HEALTH AFFAIRS,* 33(2): 216–221.

Health Care Industry Cybersecurity Task Force. (2017). *Health Care Industry Cybersecurity Task Force.* Retrieved from Public Health Emergency: https://www.phe.gov/Preparedness/planning/CyberTF/Documents/report2017.pdf.

HealthIT.gov. (2019, September 4). *How can you protect and secure health information when using a mobile device?* Retrieved from HealthIT.gov: https://www.healthit.gov/topic/privacy-security-and-hipaa/how-can-you-protect-and-secure-health-information-when-using-mobile-device.

Hoffman, D. A. (2020). Increasing access to care: Telehealth during COVID-19. *Journal of Law and the Biosciences,* 7 (Issue 1): lsaa043–lsaa043. https://doi.org/10.1093/jlb/lsaa043

Independent Security Evaluators. (2016). *Securing hospitals: A research study and blueprint.* Retrieved from https://www.ise.io/wp-content/uploads/2017/07/securing_hospitals.pdf.

Massachusetts Court System Law Library. (2017, October 2). *201 CMR 17.00: Standards for the protection of personal information of residents of the commonwealth.* Retrieved from https://www.mass.gov/doc/201-cmr-17-standards-for-the-protection-of-personal-information-of-residents-of-the/download.

Newman, L. H. (2020, September 28). *A ransomware attack has struck a major US hospital chain.* Retrieved from Wired: https://www.wired.com/story/universal-health-services-ransomware-attack.

NIST. (2020, February). *Telehealth remote patient monitoring system.* Retrieved from https://www.nccoe.nist.gov/sites/default/files/library/fact-sheets/hit-th-fact-sheet.pdf.

Office for Civil Rights. (2013, July 26). *399-Does the HIPAA Privacy Rule preempt state laws.* Retrieved from HHS.gov: https://www.hhs.gov/hipaa/for-professionals/faq/399/does-hipaa-preempt-state-laws/index.html#:~:text=In%20addition%2C%20the%20Department%20of,and%20which%20meets%20certain%20additional

Office for Civil Rights. (2017, June 16). *Covered entities and business associates.* Retrieved from HHS.gov: https://www.hhs.gov/hipaa/for-professionals/covered-entities/index.html.

Ponemon Institute LLC. (2012). *2011 cost of data breach study: United States.* Retrieved from Ponemon Institute: http://www.ponemon.org/local/upload/file/2011_US_CODB_FINAL_5.pdf.

Ponemon Institute LLC. (2016). *Sixth annual benchmark study on privacy & security of healthcare data.* Retrieved from Ponemon Institute: https://www.ponemon.org/

local/upload/file/Sixth%20Annual%20Patient%20Privacy%20%26%20Data%20 Security%20Report%20FINAL%206.pdf

Ponemon Institute LLC. (2017). *The rise of ransomware*. Retrieved from Ponemon Institute LLC: http://www.ponemon.org/local/upload/file/Ransomware%20Report%20Final%201. pdf.

Reed, T. (2016, March 29). *MedStar took 'extreme' measures to block cyber threat*. Retrieved from *Washington Business Journal*: https://www.bizjournals.com/washington/news/ 2016/03/29/medstar-took-extreme-approach-to-block-security.html

SOC for Service Organizations. (n.d.). Retrieved December 14, 2020, from AICPA. org: https:// www.aicpa.org/interestareas/frc/assuranceadvisoryservices/ socforserviceorganizations.html.

Zhou, L., Thieret, R., Watzlaf, V., Dealmeida, D., & Parmanto, B. (2019). A Telehealth Privacy and Security Self-Assessment Questionnaire for telehealth providers: Development and validation. *International Journal of Telerehabilitation*, 11(1): 3–14.

PART II

Originating Site Services

(Section Editor: Hartmut Gross)

8

Telestroke and Teleneurology

HARTMUT GROSS AND JEFFREY A. SWITZER ■

TELESTROKE

Introduction

With the institution in 1997 of alteplase, a tissue plasminogen activator (tPA), to treat acute strokes, it became apparent that new tools would be required to treat rural and distant patients quickly and safely. Helicopters were touted by some, but they were expensive and it took a long time to get patients transferred. Use of the internet to provide emergent live telemedicine was a completely new concept. Three large telestroke projects were independently established in 2003 and produced groundbreaking studies validating the concept, technology, safety, effectiveness, and applicability (Wang, 2003; Audebert, 2006; Meyer, 2005). Since then, telestroke has had the largest footprint in the telemedicine realm, especially within emergency telehealth. As emergency telehealth continues to expand, the construct of telestroke models and their metrics can be used to develop applications for other aspects of emergency care.

How Telestroke Works

Acute stroke patients presenting at rural, remote, and understaffed hospitals are disadvantaged because of their physical distance from stroke centers. These rural sites are often small centers staffed largely without board-certified emergency physicians, with limited or no neurology and radiology services besides a computerized tomography (CT) scanner. There are also a growing number of medium-sized community hospitals without 24/7 neurology availability where telestroke is filling in coverage gaps. These rural and community hospitals receiving telehealth consultations are referred to as "spokes" or "originating sites." Conversely, the consult is performed by the "hub" or "distant site." Consultants at the hub can provide urgent assessments and care, and facilitate transfer of patients, either inside or outside the network (Figure 8.1).

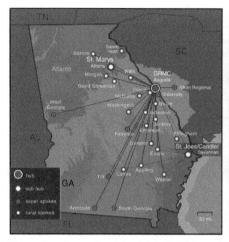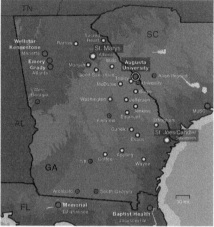

Figure 8.1 Example of the REACH Telestroke Network in Georgia and South Carolina. Hub (Comprehensive Stroke Center and regional location of consultants); Subhub (Primary Stroke Center and referral center for thrombolysis patients from affiliated rural spokes); Super spoke (medium-sized hospital lacking 24/7 neurology services); Rural spoke (small "stroke ready" hospital)
Grey circle: Mechanical thrombectomy-capable sites in and around Georgia.

With telestroke services, prompt acute stroke care can be provided, including (1) establishing if an acute stroke or a stroke mimic is present, (2) determining whether to treat with tPA, (3) managing blood pressure, (4) facilitating transfer to an appropriate next level center, (5) making recommendations for further diagnostic workup, (6) providing recommendations for secondary stroke prevention, and (7) providing rehabilitation. The provision of telestroke services has a number of associated benefits to patients, families, and the rural hospital (Box 8.1).

Spokes and hubs seeking Joint Commission Acute Stroke Ready Hospital Certification (ASRH; Joint, Quick Guide—Acute Stroke Ready Hospital Certification, 2018); Primary Stroke Center Certification (PSC; Joint, Quick Guide—Primary Stroke Center Certification, 2018); or Comprehensive Stroke Center Certification (CSC) must comply with the changing requirements to maintain their status. Hospitals can attain some level of stroke readiness, preventing EMS units from bypassing them with patients for whom they can safely provide care using telemedicine support. Care not only is timely, but also meets national metrics for acute stroke care. Small rural hospitals can work with the hub and acquire ASRH and PSC certification.

Telestroke Needs Assessment

A telemedicine program should never be started without first identifying what specific problems exist, determining if telemedicine may be a suitable solution, and deciding if those issues are a priority. An administratively mandated decision to use telemedicine without seeking input from spoke clinicians is likely doomed to failure.

Box 8.1

BENEFITS OF TELESTROKE

Initial stroke care provided at the distant site is equivalent to stroke center care.
Fill onsite neurology coverage gaps.
Each telestroke encounter is a learning and improvement opportunity for nurses and physicians.

- Bedside assistants become more efficient facilitating the hands-on examination.
- Originated site clinicians become more confident in their diagnoses and interventions.
- False alarms decrease

Originating sites retain more patients.

- Mild stroke patients not treated with tPA, kept in local facility and treated by hospitalists.
- Mild to moderate stroke patients receiving tPA, but not candidates for mechanical thrombectomy, are admitted at larger spokes with ICUs.

High patient satisfaction
Telestroke services are positive marketing messages to the community.
Excellent stroke care boosts originating site hospital reputation, restoring community and EMS confidence.
Restored patient volume may help prevent complete closure of the rural medical facility.

Buy-in is critical from the clinical staff that will actually use the equipment and interact with the virtual consultant. A number of important telestroke questions to ask are listed in Box 8.2.

An administratively mandated decision to use telemedicine without seeking input from spoke clinicians is likely doomed to failure.

VENDOR/PARTNER SELECTION
Once it has been concluded that telestroke services are needed or desired to fulfill mission-specific goals, the next step for stroke centers planning to provide telestroke services is deciding whether to build their own system or use an established vendor. For telestroke, a number of specific requirements must be considered (see Box 8.3).

Box 8.2

QUESTIONS TO ASK BEFORE STARTING ANY TELESTROKE PROGRAM

Why is telestroke being considered? Who wants it? Who are the stakeholders?
What are the coverage requirements? 24/7, overnights, or some other times?
Are the ED physicians already comfortable making a thrombolysis decision?
Is help needed with stroke mimics?
Is direction needed for mechanical thrombectomy consideration?
Is guidance requested by the admitting hospitalists for acute and subacute strokes?
Are emergent, urgent, and/or routine general neurology consults needed?
After evaluation of acute presentations, will follow-up be needed (in-patient and
    out-patient)?
Can the system support other specialty consultations if needed?
Can your hospital partner with other hospitals to bundle a group telestroke
    coverage deal?

Box 8.3

TELESTROKE-SPECIFIC HARDWARE AND SOFTWARE REQUIREMENTS

CMS and ATA have required video platform specifications that may include.

- Pan-tilt-zoom features are required to allow the telestroke clinician to
  adequately see the patient and detect subtle findings in particular body areas
  being examined.
- Bandwidth of at least 384 Kbps for upload and download with a minimum
  of 640 x 480 resolution at 30 frames per second are recommended
  (Krupinski, 2014).
- Evolving local and national requirements, for example, potential changes in
  the post-COVID era.

Radiology images must be easily accessible.

- Providers should be able to easily access each spoke's radiology PACS server
  and find CT stacks with their personal username and password.
- Optimal solutions push CT images to a separate secure server where the
  images are merged directly into the telestroke platform and the particular
  patient consult.

Documentation may be integrated into the consult platform or completed via a separate system.

- Availability of simultaneous charting by spoke and hub on a shared document.
- A shadow file may be archived on a secure server.
- Ultimately, notes must be included with the patient's hospital EMR.

CMS (Centers for Medicare and Medicaid); CT (computerized tomography); EMR (electronic medical record); Kbps (kilobytes per second); PACS (picture archiving and communication system)

Unless there are staff members who have considerable experience with telemedicine and software development, it may be reasonable to start with a telestroke vendor and then consider alternatives if the service proves unsatisfactory. For the hospitals looking to receive assistance via telestroke, choosing a vendor will be the next step and should be done very carefully. If services are already available some of the time and only intermittent fill-in is required, then a flexible provider with a customizable solution may be best. Some centers require 24/7 coverage and a turnkey, full-service contract. Stroke consultants may be general or vascular neurologists or, rarely, emergency medicine physicians, who rotate call. As a result, the term *strokologist* has been coined to reflect this diverse pool of specialists. The virtual telestrokologists may be a stable local group of physicians who provide all consults, or a regional, even national, pool of physicians who rotate call. Smaller sites prefer having a consistent group of consultants whom they get to know and with whom they become comfortable. This group will also know more about the region and available resources, building more rapport with patients and families. Whatever arrangement is selected may affect patient and staff satisfaction to some degree.

TELESTROKE OPERATIONS

Telestroke involves far more than putting a telemedicine cart into an ED; it should be integrated into existing resources. Those services start with prehospital care. EMS communications, training, and notifications must dovetail with ED processes, notably by allowing early activation of the stroke team, including the telestroke system. Some hospitals have neurologists onsite during certain hours on certain days and use telestroke to fill in the gaps. Patient flow must be worked out and refined to streamline throughput, and standardized order-sets must be developed. Memorandums of understanding (MOUs) and contracts must be in place between the hospital and the telestroke service. Protocols must be set up describing when and how to activate a "stroke alert" and how to initiate the telestroke consult. The issue of documentation and how notes merge into the patient record must be addressed. For patients needing transfer, processes must be developed with agreements that referral sites will readily accept patients, whether it is the stroke hub, a closer stroke center, or an endovascular capable facility. Usually, the telestroke physician makes the determination and facilitates the transfer. Telestroke services may also be extended from the ED to in-house strokes where similar processes should be in place.

Recent advances now permit telemedicine oversight in mobile stroke units. In this unique situation, the EMS vehicle has an onboard CT scanner. The crew operates under standing EMS medical protocols, augmented by a hub telestrokologist, to initiate tPA administration before arrival to the hospital. Other onboard ED-directed telemedicine applications are likely to follow, improving the accuracy of traditional radio or telephonic online medical control.

Usually, the telestroke physician makes the determination and facilitates the transfer.

LOCAL HUMAN RESOURCES NEEDED

Any telestroke service requires a wide variety of human resources from both the originating and distant site. Without buy-in from both sides, the network will fail. Overly inconvenienced or underpaid strokologists have been known to simply stop answering consult requests, threatening collapse of the entire network. Similarly, clinicians at the spoke may baulk at initiating consult requests if they do not perceive a need for the service or are not involved or are sidelined during the development stages. A cohesive guiding force is required at each end. At the hub, it is essential to have a telestroke medical director and a clinical director who maintain close contact with all spokes to help set up, instruct, update, give feedback, provide additional training for staff turnover, and troubleshoot. These critical persons must also monitor the volume and timing of calls, decide if the staffing is adequate or needs backup, and keep track of physician satisfaction with the clinical load and equipment. An originating site stroke champion and ED medical director who keep up momentum, address concerns, and liaise with the hub directors are vital to the spoke site success.

On-call schedules must be made each month and must be kept updated. While spokes could be sent schedules and contact the telestrokologist directly, it is often simpler to have a central call center that is contacted by the spoke. The center in turn contacts the scheduled physician, can capture "face sheets" for billing, and can help facilitate transfers. Alternative models may have the calls first go to an RN screener. Some sites have the case discussed between ED physician and telestrokologist to determine if direct visualization is needed or if recommendations by phone are sufficient.

Stroke protocols to be used by the spoke must be developed or may be offered by the hub. They can then be modified and implemented by the spoke. Items to address include doorway assessment, expedited CT imaging, initiation of the telemedicine consult, bedside presenter/assistant (who may be an APP, RN, and/or MD), and handling of documentation. With repetition, the spokes become progressively more confident and facile in their care of stroke patients. Regular practice sessions, refreshers, and drills put on by the stroke champion keep a telestroke spoke "at the ready."

LOCAL INFORMATION TECHNOLOGY RESOURCES NEEDED

There are a number of information technology (IT) considerations particular to telestroke. To perform consults both *from* a center as well as *into* another center requires penetration of firewalls and circumventing security protocols; IT services are required to implement this. Internet bandwidth requirements are relatively small but must be present and stable. Without dedicated bandwidth, surge internet and intranet activity may slow and cripple video and audio streams, especially when there is high internet traffic by hospital patients and staff. It is also needed to ensure that wireless connections are seamless wherever the telemedicine services are to be provided (ED, floor, ICU) and to address hardware issues such as network upgrades that may cause connectivity loss. Equipment (cameras, speakers, bridges, computers, battery backups) that wears out or fails must be monitored and repaired or replaced by IT promptly. Contingencies for failures must be planned before they occur. A telestroke turnkey service should provide continuous monitoring (pinging equipment even when it is not in use) and prompt 24/7 service in the event of technology problems.

EVIDENCE FOR THE EFFICACY OF TELESTROKE
Existing benchmarks compare processes before and after telestroke implementation and have validated the shorter treatment times, efficacy, and safety of telestroke (Box 8.4; Johansson, 2010).

Telestroke Metrics

The time-sensitive nature of acute stroke has prompted the meticulous dissection of the telestroke workflow into many discrete pieces (Box 8.5). Many metrics parallel the in-person management of stroke patients. They serve as benchmarks for both spokes and telestroke providers (Wechsler, 2017; Demaerschalk, 2017; Johansson, 2010).

MONITORING FOR EFFECTIVENESS OF A TELESTROKE PROGRAM
Ongoing continuous quality improvement (CQI) processes through regular chart reviews will ensure optimal performance by both the spoke and telestroke consultants. Telestroke metrics to monitor the effectiveness of telehealth versus bedside services can be grouped into four broad categories (Johansson, 2010; Wechsler, 2017).

1. General information about the spoke, patients, distances, training and education, consult numbers
2. Process indicators for patient treatment
   a. Time from onset to thrombolysis (onset-to-needle)
   b. Time from admission to thrombolysis (door-to-needle)
3. Immediate quality, utilization, and process reports that should include tPA use, intracerebral hemorrhage (ICH) rate, length of stay, mortality, transfer rates, and technical failures.
4. Patient health outcomes that include immediate, delayed, and follow-up indicators. These include pre- and poststroke scales and patient level of function, discharge location, ongoing required supportive care, and interval mortality.

Monitoring for low use of a telestroke system is essential. Reasons include unfamiliarity or treatment delay perceptions, technical problems (sound or image quality, connectivity, or difficulties/delays in getting access to equipment) and lack of 24/7 IT staff, lack of staff confidence, or fear of clinical hemorrhagic or other complications. Low case volumes and staff turnover may exacerbate unfamiliarity. Periodic mock cases and use of the system for other (nonstroke) clinical presentations may be helpful to maintain staff confidence.

Box 8.4

PROVEN CLINICAL METRICS FOR TELESTROKE

Telestroke is superior to telephone consults for correct diagnosis, management decisions, and documentation.

Radiologist and telestroke physician agreement over the presence or absence of radiological contraindications to tPA is excellent. Interrater reliability for ASPECTS score is equally high.

IV tPA use via telestroke is as safe as treatment at a stroke center, with equal long-term outcomes.

Telestroke systems are highly accurate in identifying patients with large vessel occlusions.

Telestroke use significantly increases alteplase delivery for acute ischemic stroke patients.

Telestroke increases number of drip and keep/admit patients.

Admission of telestroke managed patients increases staff efficiency and improves stroke outcomes.

Using telestroke, rural hospitals were able to reduce in-patient LOS an average of 3 days.

Occupational or physical therapy to stroke patients via telemedicine is effective.

Hemorrhagic stroke patients may be screened and treated at outlying hospitals using telemedicine.

Telestroke may increase recruitment of rural patients into acute stroke studies.

LOS-length of stay

Box 8.5

TELESTROKE WORKFLOW METRICS

Door to telestroke registration

Door to consult initiation

Time to head CT scan retrieval and read

Time of consult initiation to tPA decision

Door to needle (alteplase administration)

Consult initiation to consult completion (discern between recommendations given vs chart completion as paperwork may need to wait if there are simultaneous consultations)

Consult duration depending on whether or not tPA is given

Door-in to door-out (transfer) time for endovascular intervention candidates

PUBLISHED GUIDELINES

In 2017, the American Telemedicine Association released its telestroke guidelines (Demaerschalk, 2017). Similar guidelines were published by the American Heart Association (Wechsler, 2017) and the Canadian Heart and Stroke Foundation. (Blacquiere, 2017). Telestroke consultations must meet all the requirements of an in-person encounter: obtaining an appropriate history and physical examination; reviewing available test results and assessments and recommendations with the patient and/or family; discussing diagnosis and plan with the consult-requesting health care provider; and finally documenting the encounter in the patient's medical record. At all times, patient privacy and confidentiality must be maintained.

FINANCIAL BENEFITS OF TELESTROKE

Many states offer start-up grants to fund various telehealth projects, including telestroke. Charges for ED stroke services, as well as the rare acute in-house stroke care, may be billed, including administration of alteplase, regardless of whether the patient will remain at the spoke or be transferred. The mixing and administration of the medication is simple; the difficult step is having someone "pull the trigger" to recommend/order the tPA. It is well established that patients treated early fare better than those treated late in the therapeutic window or those who miss the treatment window altogether. Improved outcomes and shorter hospitalizations result in better reimbursement for the hospital, especially the tertiary hospital if patients are transferred. Telestroke networks are cost-effective from the hospital perspective (Switzer, 2013). These cost savings are maximized by spokes if the transfer rates are low.

COMMON BUSINESS MODELS

Depending on the flexibility of the program and the vendor as well as available finances, any number of business models or combinations thereof are possible (Box 8.6).

CODING AND BILLING

In 2020, billing for initial telemedicine Medicare patient consultations used G0 (G-zero, not the letter O) codes. For acute stroke, these codes are used for telehealth, ED, or initial in-patient consultation. The differences in the three codes are based on the amount of time spent communicating with the patient and complexity (Table 8.1).

The Furthering Access to Stroke Telemedicine (FAST) Act of 2017 (U.S. Senate, 2017) specifies that, under Medicare, telehealth services include telehealth-eligible stroke services provided to an individual soon after the onset of acute-stroke symptoms. The law states that "[c]ertain originating-site requirements applicable to telehealth services under Medicare shall not apply with respect to such" stroke services. FAST, then, effectively removes the rural restrictions for originating sites for Medicare beneficiaries.

The 2020 CARES Act (Congress, 2020) temporarily reimburses a wide use of non-face-to-face encounters, including interactive telephonic patient consultations. In response, CMS has released many guidelines for waivers and flexibility for clinicians to provide patient care (Centers for Medicare and Medicaid, 2020). After the COVID emergency declaration expires, telemedicine is projected to continue to expand, and financial support must follow.

Box 8.6

BUSINESS MODEL EXAMPLES

Federal and state telehealth grants

- Often available to start up a telehealth program and should not be overlooked.
- May significantly defray equipment and installation costs.

Spokes should have some minimal monthly fixed charge.

- May be a nominal charge for small spoke hospitals.
- Several spokes may each chip in to cover an on-call stipend for a strokologist.
- "Pump-priming" by the hub may be required to get financially stressed spokes on board.
- Even if the hub picks up most of the cost for a spoke, there needs to be "skin in the game" to encourage use of the system. Telestroke experience demonstrates that when it is free, it is underutilized.

There may be a charge for larger spokes based on the estimated number of stroke patients.

- National ED volumes demonstrate approximately 0.5% of encounters are acute stroke presentations.*
- The national average does not take into account that some communities have an older population or a higher incidence of stroke (e.g. in the Southeastern stroke belt).
- An audit of strokes seen at the site over the previous few years would be good for all negotiating parties to be aware of as they discuss contracts.
- After a predetermined time, the spoke stroke numbers can be reviewed and charges adjusted based on the actual number of consults.

There may be a system that begins with a rough estimate of cases per month.

- There may be an added "per click" or "per activation" charge for any overage.
- There may be charges for nonacute strokes for which an emergent consult is initiated, although no emergency exists (e.g. the patient will be admitted, but the hospitalist is requesting guidance for working up and treating the patient).

Charges may be based on specific spoke needs.

- Neurology coverage exists 8 a.m.–5 p.m. weekdays, but backfilling for nights and weekends is required.
- Coverage is needed for the vacationing onsite neurologist.
- If a 24/7/365 telestroke system is already in place for a network, then having the hub add randomly needed coverage at another site is simple; it doesn't

matter where consults originate from, since the on-call consultant is going to be near a computer anyway.

For the telestroke system to be sustainable, consults must be billed.

- Hub-and-spoke negotiations and contracts will ensure this is a transparent, mutually acceptable, fluid process.
- The hub may need to archive spoke site notes (essentially shadow charts) for coding and billing purposes.

---

* Based on annual incidence of strokes in the United States and total ED volumes.

RETURN ON INVESTMENT AND OTHER INDIRECT BENEFITS OF TELESTROKE

The return on investment (ROI) by the spoke will be both direct and indirect. If properly announced and marketed, patients will see the benefit of timely, excellent care via telemedicine at their nearby hospital. They will start going to their community hospital for stroke and other care as confidence is restored. Because of excellent networks and relationships, if a patient is transferred, the spoke hospital with telehealth oversight can comfortably use swing beds to return patients for rehabilitation, skilled nursing facility, or even long-term nursing home care in their beds. Initially, this can be done with stroke patients, and later for other conditions as the programs expand. Patients and families are far happier being returned to their community rather than driving long distances back and forth for ongoing care at the tertiary referral center. The successes will continue to build on themselves. The revenue infusions into the spoke hospitals will help struggling centers keep their doors open.

The return on investment by the hub will also be both a direct and indirect one. Patients can be screened for appropriateness of transfer. Acute stroke patients can be treated earlier and, when transferred, will have better outcomes and shorter hospitalization stays. Patients can be screened for possible mechanical thrombectomy candidacy, and the endovascular team can be mobilized ahead of arrival. A well-run telestroke program will leave a positive impression with the spoke hospital, which is then likely to work with the hub on other projects and patient transfers for other medical conditions. Large hospitals progressively need larger networks to refer and pass patients back and forth for appropriate level of care and keep beds turned

Table 8.1 TELEHEALTH BILLING CODES

G0425	*Typically about 30 minutes with the patient, including problem-focused history and problem-focused examination via telehealth and straightforward medical decision making.*
G0426	*Typically, about 50 minutes communicating with the patient, including detailed history and detailed examination via telehealth and moderate complexity medical decision making.*
G0247	*Typically, about 70 or more minutes communicating with the patient, including comprehensive history and comprehensive examination and high complexity medical decision making.*

over for the correct acuity. Telehealth systems are critical for facilitating this, and telestroke models are leading the way on both the front and the back ends.

TELENEUROLOGY

As with acute stroke decision making, telemedicine may be a useful tool to facilitate diagnosis and treatment for patients presenting with emergent nonstroke neurologic conditions, including stroke mimics. Most neurologic disorders, including epilepsy, multiple sclerosis, headache, Parkinson's disease, dementia, and neuromuscular conditions, can be assessed via telemedicine. However, the originating site for nonstroke diagnoses has most commonly been the home or clinic as opposed to the ED or in-patient hospital setting, and these evaluations are often done for follow-up care as opposed to an initial diagnostic evaluation. Further, when compared with telestroke, the evidence base for nonstroke teleneurology is limited.

In the ED or in-patient setting, when a neurologist is not available at the bedside, consultation with a remote expert for nonstroke conditions may be useful for diagnosis, transfer decisions, and, in some cases, urgent treatment. In many EDs, consultations for confusion, coma, seizures/status epilepticus, dizziness, and generalized weakness are not uncommon. It is important to recognize the limitations of emergency nonstroke teleneurology, which may have a bearing on diagnostic accuracy. Whereas the National Institutes of Health (NIH) stroke scale score can typically be performed remotely with a high degree of reproducibility compared with bedside assessment, numerous elements of the neurologic exam that are needed for nonstroke diagnosis require direct physical contact with the patient and cannot be performed remotely or require significant bedside assistance from an experienced practitioner (Table 8.2). As a result, there are certain clinical scenarios, such as evaluation of brain death and prognostication following cardiac arrest, that may not be optimally evaluated by teleneurology. Nevertheless, in some situations, recognizing the limitations of the exam, consultation with a neurologist may still add value to the decision-making process and clarify the need for further imaging and transfer to a center with onsite neurologic expertise.

Table 8.2 NEUROLOGIC EXAM FOR NONSTROKE DIAGNOSIS REQUIRING IN-PERSON EVALUATION

Clinical context	Neurologic exam elements limited by teleneurology (requiring bedside assessment)
Coma	Vestibulo-ocular reflex, cold calorics, corneal reflex, pupillary light response, and response to noxious tactile stimulation
Acute dizziness	HINTS exam (head impulse test, pattern of nystagmus, and test of skew)
Generalized weakness (neuromuscular failure)	Muscle tone, effort against resistance, deep tendon reflexes, and plantar reflex
Functional limb weakness	Hoover's sign, Hip Abductor sign, and co-contraction of opposing muscle groups

One small study from 2004 (Craig, 2004) demonstrated that in-patient teleneurology consultations at two small, rural hospitals in Northern Ireland shortened length of stay without increase in mortality or hospital resources. No patients underwent MRI scans. The applicability of this data to the current U.S. health care system is unclear. Future research is needed on nonstroke in-patient and emergency teleneurology to better clarify the feasibility, safety and diagnostic accuracy of remote consultations, and to determine the impact on interhospital transfer rates and length of stay, as well as the cost-effectiveness of these systems from societal and hospital perspectives (Craig, 1999).

CONCLUSION

Telestroke now has over 15 years of experience and a track record of safety, speed, and excellence, comparable to an in-person encounter. Many stroke mimics or simply nonstroke neurologic conditions are similarly assessed and managed via teleneurology. The acute and time-sensitive nature of telestroke provision has mandated many benchmarks for improved care delivery. The most recent changes are narrowing the door to needle time and looking at shortened door-in to door-out times for endovascular transfers. Telestroke has set a high mark that other timely patient care telehealth consult systems can use as a roadmap and set comparable goals to achieve. Less critical consults can eliminate unneeded benchmarks and substitute their own. As new treatments are developed and implemented, telestroke and teleneurology have demonstrated that they are well positioned to deliver them in an efficient manner.

KEY TAKEAWAYS

➤ Provide acute stroke consultations 24/7/365. Flexible providers can deliver a full-service line or fill in schedule gaps as needed.
➤ To lower costs, bundle telestroke services with other nearby rural facilities with same needs.
➤ When initiating telestroke services, be sure to work with EMS, local providers, and news media.
➤ Have a telestroke medical director, network coordinator, and spoke stroke champion.
➤ Provide 24/7 IT support services. Have alternate contingencies thought out *before* a failure occurs. Monitor for and correct problems promptly.
➤ Have treatment and transfer protocols thought out well ahead of time.
➤ Provide a regular newsletter and launch a periodic telestroke conference inviting spoke staff to the comprehensive stroke center to bolster the unity of the network.

REFERENCES

Audebert, H. J. (2006). Telemedic pilot project for Integrative Stroke Care Group. Effects of the implementation of a telemedical stroke network: The Telemedic Pilot Project for Integrative Stroke Care (TEMPiS) in Bavaria, Germany. *The Lancet Neurology*, 5(9): 742–748.

Blacquiere, D. (2017). *Canadian stroke best practice recommendations: Telestroke*, Sixth Edition. Retrieved from Canadian Stroke Best Practice Recommendations: https://www.strokebestpractices.ca/-/media/1-stroke-best-practices/telestroke/csbpr-telestroke-module-final-april2017-1.ashx?la=en&hash=A4CEA397731F3B6365154CF443FF676B2622FABC.

Centers for Medicare and Medicaid. (2020). *Physicians and other clinicians: CMS flexibilities to fight COVID-19*. Retrieved from https://www.cms.gov/files/document/covid-19-physicians-and-practitioners.pdf.

Craig, J. (2004). A cohort study of early neurological consultation by telemedicine on the care of neurological inpatients. *Journal of Neurological Neurosurgery and Psychiatry*, 75: 1031–1035.

Craig, J. J. (1999). Neurological examination is possible using telemedicine. *Journal of Telemedicine and Telecare*, 5: 177–181.

Demaerschalk, B. M. (2017). American Telemedicine Association: Telestroke Guidelines. *Telemedicine and e-Health*, 23(5): 376–389.

Demaerschalk, B. M. (2017). American Telemedicine Association: Telestroke Guidelines. *Telemedicine and e-Health*, 23(5): 376–389.

Johansson, T. (2010). Telemedicine in acute stroke management: systematic review. *International Journal of Technology Assessment inHealth Care*, 26(2): 149–155. Retrieved from https://www.acep.org/globalassets/sites/acep/blocks/section-blocks/telemd/final-whitepaper---sans-definition-8-7-19.pdf.

The Joint Commission. (2018). *Quick guide—Acute Stroke Ready Hospital (ASRH) certification*. Retrieved from https://www.jointcommission.org/-/media/tjc/documents/accred-and-cert/certification/certification-by-setting/disease-specific-care-certification/03---dsc-quick-guide---asrh-4-9-digital.pdf.

The Joint Commission. (2018). *Quick Guide—Primary Stroke Center (PSC) certification*. Retrieved from https://www.jointcommission.org/-/media/tjc/documents/accred-and-cert/certification/certification-by-setting/stroke/psc-quick-guide---psc-4-9-digital.pdf.

Krupinski, E. A. (2014). *Core operational guidelines for telehealth services involving provider-patient interactions*. Retrieved from American Telemedicine Association Guideline: http://www.medicalinfo.ch/images/articles/ATA-Core-Operational-Guidelines-for-Telehealth-Services.pdf.

Meyer, B. C. (2005). Prospective reliability of the STRokE DOC wireless/site independent telemedicine system. *Neurology*, 64: 1058–1060.

Switzer, J. A. (2013). Cost-effectiveness of hub-and-spoke telestroke networks for the management of acute ischemic stroke from the hospitals' perspectives. *Circulation: Cardiovascular Quality and Outcomes*, 6(1): 18–26.

U.S. Congress. (2020). *S.3548—CARES Act*. Retrieved from S.3548—116th Congress (2019–2020): https://www.congress.gov/bill/116th-congress/senate-bill/3548/text?q=product+actualizaci%C3%B3n.

U.S. Senate. (2017). *Furthering access to Stroke Telemedicine Act*. Retrieved from Congress.gov: https://www.congress.gov/bill/115th-congress/house-bill/1148.

Wang, S. (2003). Remote evaluation of acute ischemic stroke: Reliability of National Institutes of Health Stroke Scale via telestroke. *Stroke*, 34(10): e188–191. Epub 20.

Wechsler, L. R. (2017). Telemedicine quality and outcomes in stroke: A scientific statement for healthcare professionals from the American Heart Association/American Stroke Association. *Stroke* (48): e3–e25.

9

Emergency Telepsychiatry

EWALD HORWATH, THOMAS E. DELL, AND ZEINA SALIBA ■

INTRODUCTION

According to the National Alliance on Mental Illness (NAMI), 4.6% (11.4 million) of adults in the United States experienced serious mental illness in 2018. Suicide is the tenth leading cause of death in the United States, and NAMI further reports that among those between the ages of 10 and 34, suicide is the second leading cause of death (Mental Health by the Numbers, 2019). About 16% (23.1 million) of all emergency department (ED) visits in 2017 were for mental and substance use disorders, accounting for over $5.6 billion in costs (Karaca, 2020). Further, in children and adolescents, there was a 28% increase in psychiatric ED visits from 2011 to 2015, and a 2.5-fold increase in adolescent suicide-related visits (Kalb, 2019). The number of ED patients with behavioral health conditions is growing, and providing timely evaluation is a major challenge for both rural and urban EDs, where access to psychiatrists and other behavioral health professionals is limited or unavailable.

The use of telehealth to provide virtual care for mental health disorders is often referred to as *telepsychiatry* (often shortened to telepsych), or the broader term *telemental health*. It is a subset of *telemedicine*, providing psychiatric evaluation and treatment using telecommunications technology. In this chapter, we will use these three terms interchangeably. Telepsychiatry, with its beginnings at the Nebraska Psychiatric Institute in 1959, has expanded as telecommunications technology has improved, and it is now used to connect psychiatrists, psychotherapists, and other behavioral health clinicians with patients in a wide variety of settings. It has primarily grown in response to the national shortage of psychiatrists, especially in rural areas. Limited access to mental health specialist care and services can lead to increased ED visits, extended ED consultation wait times, increased ED involuntary holds, and negatively impacted overall ED care (Nesper, 2016). Downstream effects may include unnecessary hospital admissions and transfers to other facilities, both of which incur high costs, inconvenience to patients, causing them additional stress, and lower quality of care. By making mental health resources and specialists more easily accessible to patients, telemental health can lead to quicker service, lower health care and transportation costs, and often provide better outcomes for those who struggle with access to psychiatric care. The American Psychiatric Association

(APA) endorses telepsychiatry as a validated and effective modality of care, a component of the mental health delivery system that must be used ethically and within all applicable regulations, with appropriate safeguards that protect patients (APA Policy on Telepsychiatry, 2018).

The APA's Telepsychiatry Toolkit (https://www.psychiatry.org/psychiatrists/practice/telepsychiatry/toolkit) is a helpful reference for those practicing telepsychiatry and for those considering the implementation of a new telepsychiatry program.

EMERGENCY TELEPSYCHIATRY

Emergency telepsychiatry, according to one definition, is "psychiatric care delivered over live interactive videoconferencing to assess and treat patients experiencing potential imminent dangerousness to themselves (suicidal or grossly disturbed behavior) or dangerousness to others (homicidal or other violent behaviors)" (Shore, 2007, p. 200). However, in the ED setting, emergency telepsychiatry services are often used for a broader subset of patients; they are used to support patients with depressive symptoms, anxiety attacks, stress, psychosis, obsessive-compulsive disorder, and other new and exacerbations of mental or behavioral health conditions that require urgent evaluation and treatment. Typically, emergency telepsychiatry occurs when the patient is in a hospital ED. Less commonly, emergency telepsych services may be part of a public health response to a disaster situation. EDs around the country are overcrowded and almost half of U.S. hospitals struggle to maintain psychiatric coverage to meet the needs of ED patients (Yellowlees, 2008).

Telepsychiatric services to support the ED can come from within the hospital or health system, from a statewide network, or from a telepsychiatry vendor. The first model distributes resources and makes them available when and where needed. For example, during the COVID-19 pandemic, psychiatric hospitalists were able to use telepsychiatry to evaluate patients with psychiatric concerns in the ED, limiting exposure of both clinician and patient to infection and reducing use of personal protective equipment (PPE). In a multihospital system, mental health clinicians (such as psychiatrists, psychologists, social workers, psychiatric nurse specialists, and counselors or therapists) at one site can evaluate a patient in an ED at another network hospital. This allows for improved resource management by distributing limited personnel to sites without trained clinicians. If there is no capacity in the system, a health care organization can contract with a state network or private company with mental health clinicians available for on-demand consultation. One model to describe the distribution of specialists, including in telepsychiatric care, is that of the "hub and spoke," in which psychiatrists are at a central location, or the "hub," and patients are at any number of understaffed EDs in more remote locations, or the "spokes." Often a hybrid model is used in which requests come from a spoke, while connectivity and governance are centralized at the hub, but clinicians operate out of their clinics or personal workspaces. Common among all models of telepsychiatry for ED patients is a promising technology to reduce wait times for psychiatric evaluation, avoid unnecessary admissions, and decrease costs (Seidel, 2014).

EVIDENCE BASE FOR TELEPSYCHIATRY

Telepsychiatry is a well-established practice with a strong evidence base. Sam Hubley's 2016 systematic review of 134 articles provides a guide to understanding the efficacy of telepsychiatry by focusing on the following domains: (1) satisfaction, (2) reliability, (3) treatment outcomes, (4) implementation outcomes, (5) cost-effectiveness, and (6) legal issues.

Patient satisfaction for telemental health services is generally high, with 23 of 31 studies demonstrating ratings of telepsych from good to excellent, with major benefits attributed to convenience, reduced time, and lower cost associated with transportation. Those studies demonstrating lower ratings commonly cite concerns related to technology-related issues, assuring privacy, and establishing a rapport with the clinician. A commonly used patient instrument to assess patient satisfaction in these studies is the six-item Client Satisfaction Questionnaire (CSQ-6; see Table 9.1) (Larsen, 1979). While some clinicians have reservations regarding establishing a therapeutic relationship over a video visit, most psychiatrists, primary care providers, and emergency practitioners report adequate to high satisfaction with telepsych. Prior reviews of telepsych have not found statistically significant

Table 9.1 Six questions from the Client Satisfaction Questionnaire

1. How would you rate the quality of service you received?

4	3	2	1
Excellent	Good	Fair	Poor

2. Did you get the kind of service you wanted?

1	2	3	4
No, definitely not	No, not really	Yes, generally	Yes, definitely

3. To what extent has our program met your needs?

4	3	2	1
Almost all my needs have been met	Most of my needs have been met	Only a few of my needs have been met	None of my needs have been met

4. If a friend were in need of similar help, would you recommend our program to him/her?

1	2	3	4
No, definitely not	No, I don't think so	Yes, I think so	Yes, definitely

5. How satisfied are you with the amount of help you received?

1	2	3	4
Quite dissatisfied	Indifferent or mildly dissatisfied	Mostly satisfied	Very satisfied

6. Have the services you received helped you to deal more effectively with your problems?

4	3	2	1
Yes, they have helped a great deal	Yes, they helped somewhat	No, they really didn't help	No, they seemed to make things worse

See reference for correlates and variations (Larsen, 1979).

differences in symptoms, quality of life, or patient satisfaction, as compared to face-to-face assessments (Garcia-Lizana, 2010).

Telepsychiatric assessments are generally comparable to face-to-face (FTF) assessments, according to Hubley's review. It is unclear how bandwidth and video quality may impact these evaluations. In one study, comparison of two different levels of bandwidth affecting image quality showed high reliability (Matsuura, 2001), while another showed lower interrater reliability in lower bandwidth cohort members as compared to controls (Yoshino, 2001). Fortunately, in the setting of ED telepsychiatry, systems are typically in place to manage bandwidth access and ensure adequate video quality.

The next domain examined whether telepsych interventions are as effective as FTF interventions; they have indeed been shown to deliver similar treatment outcomes, and some patients are more likely to engage in ongoing therapy using telemental health, due to convenience and lack of need to travel. The primary focus of psychiatric consultation in the ED is patient assessment, treatment, and safe disposition planning. A 2014 study of ED patients who required psychiatric assessment demonstrated very high concordance when comparing telepsych with FTF evaluation for suicide risk and appropriate disposition decisions (Seidel, 2014).

The fourth domain in the review is implementation outcomes. The general acceptance of telepysch by care team members and patients is high. With broad engagement from all stakeholders and proper training, ED telepsych programs have been shown to be well accepted and quickly adopted (Bhandari, 2011).

Cost-effectiveness is an important domain for those considering new implementation of ED telepsychiatry programs. Many cost analyses related to telehealth focus on reduced patient wait times and decreased transportation costs. Emergency telepysch often reduces time to consult, in turn improving throughput and ED revenue (Paavola, 2018). In the setting of ED telepsych, a major contributor to cost-effectiveness is reducing ED boarding and its downstream impact on throughput and patient care. Telepsych may offer an alternative to the high cost of hiring locum tenens psychiatrists. It may also help reduce the costs of adding sitters, creating larger security teams, and expanding boarding areas (Paavola, 2018). In low-volume EDs, a distributed model of on-demand telepsych coverage would result in a significant return on investment and expanded coverage hours, when compared with the cost and availability of having full-time in-person mental health coverage.

The final domain in the Hubley review involves legal issues. Telepsychiatry is not different from the larger domain of telemedicine from a licensing and credentialing perspective. The remote psychiatrist must be licensed where the patient is located, and in some cases a state may require the clinician to also be licensed in the distant site. Consideration for the licensing of additional care team members should be consistent with their regulatory boards. There may be privacy considerations that are elevated for psychiatric care as compared to general medical treatment, especially around the sharing of medical information and access to medical records. Additionally, in multistate implementations, it is important for clinicians to know that mental health legislation, processes, patient rights, and standards may vary by state, and they must be aware of state and jurisdiction-specific regulations that impact their patients' care.

PROGRAMMATIC CONSIDERATIONS

Implementation

Strong and supportive leadership is important in implementing telehealth services for emergency psychiatric care. As with other telehealth services, a needs assessment that includes all stakeholders is an important step in developing the program. Stakeholders in emergency telemental health include psychiatrists, behavioral health care team members (such as nurses, social workers, crisis counselors, and case managers), ED clinicians, stepdown programs and local psychiatric facilities, administration, information technology (IT), and patients. An important step in the process is to reach consensus regarding the type of clinical scenarios for which telepsychiatry is appropriate, and to develop a simple flowchart for ED clinicians to follow to access the services. Shared protocols must address defining a psychiatric emergency, accessing the covering virtual psychiatric team, transfer procedures, admission procedures, and the management of patient consent (Shore, 2007). The treatment of time-sensitive conditions like stroke and ST-elevation myocardial infarction may offer a framework when implementing programs for improving the care of ED behavioral health patients. This treatment can also help to ensure that timely evaluation and treatment (acute and ongoing pharmacological interventions) are prioritized (MacKenzie, n.d.).

Resources

Like other telehealth programs, emergency telepsychiatry programs have basic human and IT resource needs. In some cases, the telepsychiatry coverage may be a comprehensive solution (i.e., 24/7 service), and in others it may extend the hours of in-person coverage. Outside vendors may need to be credentialed at the hospital or emergency facility and may need access to the electronic health record. ED clinicians complete initial evaluations (which should consist of history and physical exam) and order appropriate testing (vitals, labs, and possible imaging) to aid in differential diagnosis as well as determine level of medical stability to identify the most appropriate level of care needed.

In most cases, ED patients who are considered a danger to themselves or others are placed with a sitter. Sitters may assist with initiation of videoconferencing and sometimes serve as telepresenters, but in most cases they remain at observation distance so that the patient can have a confidential one-on-one interaction with the clinician. ED security should be aware when consultations are occurring in case the patient escalates and the clinician providing virtual evaluation needs a mechanism to notify security personnel about acute situations or behaviors. Additionally, there needs to be a clearly identified plan in the event that the patient warrants an in-person response.

Emergency telepsychiatry does not require expensive or complicated technology infrastructure and can typically piggyback onto the existing infrastructure (e.g., computers/tablets, carts, and connectivity). A simple model consists of a tablet on a stand that can be wheeled from one patient to a nurse or doctor to another patient, with cleaning in between uses. A more sophisticated setup might include a computer on wheels with a pan-tilt-zoom camera and a larger screen. These can be mobile to the patient's bedside or fixed in a dedicated telemedicine space. Dedicated bandwidth is also useful to improve the audio and visual quality of telepsychiatry visits. In addition to the proper audiovisual equipment, software programs that support HIPPA-compliant communication are needed.

Policy and Regulations

It is necessary to follow both federal and state regulations when practicing emergency telepsychiatry. Where they differ, the more restrictive takes precedence. Federal telehealth policy is addressed in Chapter 6, and state policies vary regarding telepresenters, consent, and reimbursement, depending on telemedicine originating sites. State regulations for both the originating and distant sites must be reviewed and followed (Shore, 2007).

Each state (and sometimes a locality) has unique laws governing legal holds and commitment procedures, including specific regulations regarding the credentials required to sign documents, the number of individuals needed to initiate commitments, and the duration of legal involuntary holds, as well as procedures for due process. In some areas, judges will hold proceedings in hospitals or psychiatric facilities, or virtually, while in others, patients and petitioners must physically travel to a courthouse. Telemedicine requires the clinician to be licensed in the state where the patient is located (and in some states, the clinician must also be licensed in the state where they are physically located when practicing); specific local licensing or credentialing may also be required for involuntary certifications. Standards regarding the duty to warn and interactions with law enforcement may vary by state and local jurisdiction (Shore, 2007). There is also variance regarding medical liability laws, which has implications for assignment of legal responsibility. When there is disagreement in disposition decision between the in-person ED clinician and the virtual mental health provider, a psychiatrist should be involved in direct discussion with the emergency physician to determine a safe disposition.

Guidelines

To ensure the safety of both patients and physicians, it is important that telepsychiatry programs adhere to standard operating procedures. Shore et al. outlined a set of standard competencies that should be addressed before beginning to practice emergency telepsychiatry (see Box 9.1) (Shore, 2007).

Box 9.1

EMERGENCY TELEPSYCHIATRY GUIDELINES AND
MANAGEMENT CONSIDERATIONS

1. Administrative Issues
   a. Perform a remote site assessment.
      i. Obtain information about local regulations.
      ii. Identify local mental health facilities (voluntary and involuntary) and outpatient resources.
   b. Create emergency protocols with clear delineations of roles and responsibilities of the ED physicians and APPs, support staff, and the psychiatry consultants.
   c. Establish guidelines to trigger a telepsychiatry consult.
   d. Decide telepsychiatry coverage hours (should be 24/7/365).
2. Legal/Ethical Issues
   a. Know local civil commitment and duty-to-warn regulations.
   b. Provide access to appropriate civil commitment forms and criteria (e.g., dangerousness to self or others, grave disability) and appropriate forms needed to reverse an involuntary commitment.
3. General Clinical Issues
   a. Be aware of the impact of telepsychiatry on the ED physician's perception of control over the clinical interaction, and how this might impact the ED physician's management.
   b. Be aware of safety issues with patients displaying strong affective or behavioral states upon conclusion of a session, and how patients may then interact with remote site staff.
   c. Discuss firearm ownership and safety. Be prepared to negotiate with patients over firearm disposition, and consider involvement of patients' families as appropriate.
   d. Be sensitive to impact of disclosures made during emergency management on patient confidentiality and relationships.
   e. Include families in emergency treatment situations where possible, but assess and be attentive to exacerbation of family tensions.
   f. Assess therapeutic medication use and administration as well as substance use issues. Be familiar with local resources for substance use assessment and treatment, and be prepared to play a role in recommending substance use treatment.

Adapted from Shore 2007.

Business Models

Hospitals may finance their start-up telemedicine programs at both the hub and spoke sites through federal and state legislative appropriations, grants, insurance reimbursement, philanthropic donations, and funds allocated by a hospital system. In order to be sustainable, the program must generate enough revenue and cost savings to the hospital to cover the operating costs of the telepsychiatry service, including information technology and operational support, subscription fees, training, consultant and staff salaries, and program management. Some hubs with a large number of spoke sites will bill the spoke sites on an hourly or per-visit basis in order to support the hub site (third-party services may also bill this way). Smaller hospitals may elect to collectively provide an on-call stipend for a telepsychiatry provider.

Legislatures, national organizations, and other prospective sources of funding for telepsychiatry programs are interested in the clinical outcomes of telepsychiatry as well as its profitability. Return on investment (ROI), which compares net revenue to amounts invested, is a measure used by investors to determine the "cost" of spending money on a program. Some existing data indicate that a telepsychiatry program can produce a favorable ROI. For example, North Carolina's NC-STeP program reported a 75% ROI in 2018.

CASE STUDIES

Case studies of existing emergency telepsychiatry programs can be instructive. However, it is important to note the context in which each case is designed. The South Carolina Department of Mental Health (SCDMH) ED Telepyschiatry program was developed in the setting of an integrated public mental health system. The South Carolina Department of Mental Health (DMH) operates all of the state's in-patient psychiatric hospitals, outpatient centers, and clinics connected by a common electronic health record (EHR). The ED program targets the rural areas of the state where ED psychiatric evaluations can be delayed for days (Telepsychiatry Program History, 2018), and only 32% of South Carolina's EDs were found to have emergency psychiatric services (Narasimhan, 2015). All participating telepsychiatrists were from the DMH. The program had significant impact during its first four years, as demonstrated by analysis using matched controls compared to those receiving emergency telepsychiatric consults through live video. Patients with telepsychiatric access had significantly higher 30-day and 90-day out-patient follow-up rates, were less likely to be admitted, and had decreased 30-day inpatient costs and overall health care charges (Narasimhan, 2015).

The North Carolina Statewide Telepsychiatry Program (NC-STeP), like the SCDMH Program, was launched in response to North Carolina's inadequate staffing for management of psychiatric emergencies in the ED. At the time of NC-STeP's introduction in 2013, nearly 10% of all North Carolina EDs were assigned at least one mental health disorder diagnostic code, and the admission rate for these patients was double that of nonbehavioral health patients (Hakenewerth, 2013; Saeed, 2018). NC-STeP connects 80 spoke hospital EDs throughout North Carolina to 6 hub hospitals, but unlike the SCDMH, there is not a single EHR. The network links psychiatric care through a NC-STeP portal that facilitates documentation, scheduling, tracking, and reporting of telepsychiatry encounters across the network (Saeed, 2018). Saeed et al. (2011) proposed that access to a telepsychiatric network could provide law enforcement with information regarding patient condition or history when they respond to calls for residents in crisis (Saeed, 2011). From 2013 to 2018, the program saved $21 million by preventing unnecessary hospitalizations (North

Table 9.2 NC-STeP 2014 Emergency Telepsychiatry Diagnosis, *N* > 6000

Diagnosis	Percent of Patients
Mood Disorders—Bipolar	31.1%
Mood Disorders—Depression	26.5%
Psychotic Disorders	24.9%
Mood Disorders—other	7.2%
Trauma and Stressor Related	3.4%
Neurocognitive Disorders	2.4%
Substance Use Disorders	1.7%

Carolina Telepsychiatry Program, 2018). NC-STeP has overturned 43% of involuntary commitments, a statistic that has nationwide relevance since all states have some form of involuntary commitment laws, and these patients often are detained in EDs due to the insufficient availability of psychiatric consultation or in-patient psychiatric beds for a variety of diagnoses (see Table 9.2). More recent data from the program found a statistically significant increase in patients discharged home and a decrease in those transferred to a psychiatric facility (Kothadia, 2020). Interestingly, these outcomes were more significant in patients with longer ED lengths of stay.

The emergency telepsychiatry program at CaroMont Regional Medical Center ED in Gastonia, North Carolina, was established in 2016 in collaboration with a private telepsychiatry vendor, Specialists On-Call (SOC). This program targeted long ED wait times for psychiatric assessment and subsequent ED crowding and boarding. The program was able to leverage the technology already in place for an SOC telestroke program to launch emergency telepsychiatry. The emergency telepsychiatry program supplements the availability of local psychiatrists and resulted in 70% decrease in length of stay for behavioral health patients in the ED as well as improvement in bed availability for nonbehavioral health patients and reduced crowding (Case Study: CaroMont Regional Medical Center).

CONCLUSION

Emergency telepsychiatry offers great promise for improving access to psychiatric care in hospital EDs. This is especially true in rural and other underresourced communities where few behavioral health resources are available but demand for ED psychiatric consultation is high. The best and safest disposition and treatment plans require the availability of psychiatrists for evaluation and treatment recommendations and social work support to identify social issues impacting health and to connect patients to resources guides. It is clear that ED staff are more comfortable with patient treatment and care when telemental health is available (Yellowlees, 2008). Emergency telepsychiatry addresses problems of prolonged lengths of stay and delayed treatment. Although there are regulatory and logistic challenges to implementing emergency telepsychiatry, the experiences of existing services suggest that emergency telepsychiatry can provide high-quality, accessible, and financially sustainable psychiatric consultation.

KEY TAKEAWAYS

➤ Telepsychiatry improves access to psychiatrists and mental health services, especially in rural and other underresourced communities.

➤ The efficacy of telepsychiatry has been shown to be equivalent to face-to-face psychiatric care.

➤ Emergency telepsychiatry shortens prolonged lengths of stay and delayed treatment that patients with psychiatric disorders often experience in hospital EDs.

➤ Emergency telepsychiatry provides more timely treatment and disposition decisions, which can lead to cost savings for hospitals and health systems.

➤ Understanding federal and state regulations is essential to creating successful emergency telepsychiatry programs.

➤ Protocols to be used in conjunction with telepsych must be developed jointly with hospital administration, ED leadership, as well as the telepsychiatry service.

➤ The increased acceptance of telehealth during the COVID-19 pandemic provides an opportunity to further expand emergency telepsychiatry services.

REFERENCES

APA Policy on Telepsychiatry. (2018). Retrieved December 15, 2020, from American Psychiatric Association: https://www.psychiatry.org/psychiatrists/practice/telepsychiatry.

Bhandari, G. (2011). Meeting community needs through leadership and innovation: A case of virtual psychiatric emergency department (ED). *Behaviour and Information Technology*, 30(4): 517–523.

Garcia-Lizana, F. (2010). What about telepsychiatry? A systematic review. *Primary Care Companion Journal of Clinical Psychiatry*, 12(2).

Hakenewerth, A. M. (2013). Emergency department visits by patients with mental health disorders—North Carolina, 2008–2010. *Morbidity and Mortality Weekly Report*, 62(23): 469–472.

Hubley, S. (2016). Review of key telepsychiatry outcomes. *World Journal of Psychiatry*, 6(2): 269–282.

Kalb, L. G. (2019). Trends in Psychiatric Emergency Department visits among youth and young adults in the US. *Pediatrics*, 143(4): 1269–1276.

Karaca, Z. (2020). *Costs of Emergency Department visits for mental and substance use disorders in the United States, 2017.* Retrieved from Agency for Healthcare Research and Quality: https://www.hcup-us.ahrq.gov/reports/statbriefs/sb257-ED-Costs-Mental-Substance-Use-Disorders-2017.jsp.

Kothadia, R. J. (2020). The impact of the North Carolina Statewide Telepsychiatry Program (NC-STeP) on patients' dispositions from emergency departments. *Psychiatric Services*, 71(12): 1239–1244.

Larsen, D. L. (1979). Assessment of client/patient satisfaction: Development of a general scale. *Evaluation and Program Planning*, 2: 197–207.

MacKenzie, J. (n.d.). Create parity and equity using telebehavioral health. *Telehealth Innovation Forum*. Retrieved December 16, 2020, from https://teladochealth.com/resources/video/create-parity-and-equity-using-telebehavioral-health.

Matsuura, S. H. (2001). Application of telepsychiatry: A preliminary study. *Psychiatry and Clinical Neurosciences*, 54: 55–58.

Mental health by the numbers. (2019). Retrieved December 14, 2020, from National Alliance on Mental Illness: https://www.nami.org/mhstats

Narasimhan, M. (2015). Impact of a telepsychiatry program at emergency departments statewide on quality, utlization, and cost of mental health services. *Psychiatric Services*, 66(11): 1167–1172.

Nesper, A. C. (2016). Effect of decreasing county mental health services on the emergency department. *Annals of Emergency Medicine*, 67(4): 525–530.

North Carolina Telepsychiatry Program. (2018). Office of Rural Health. North Carolina Department of Health and Human Services. Retrieved December 17, 2020, from https://files.nc.gov/ncdhhs/2018%20NC%20DHHS%20ORH%20 Telepsychiatry%20Program%20One%20Pager_0.pdf.

Paavola, A. (2018). *Top 5 benefits of telepsychiatry in the ED*. Retrieved December 16, 2020, from Becker's Hospital Review at https://www.beckershospitalreview.com/telehealth/top-5-benefits-of-telepsychiatry-in-the-ed.html.

Saeed, S. A. (2011). Use of telepsychiatry to improve care for people with mental illness in rural north Carolina. *North Carolina Medical Journal*, 72(3): 219–222. Retrieved from https://www.researchgate.net/profile/Richard_Bloch2/publication/51627771_Use_of_telepsychiatry_to_improve_care_for_people_with_ mental_illness_in_rural_North_Carolina/links/09e4150d0974f376a0000000/ Use-of-telepsychiatry-to-improve-care-for-people-with-ment.

Saeed, S. A. (2018). Successfully navigating multiple electronic health records when using telepsychiatry: The NC-STeP experience. *Psychiatric Services*, 69(9): 948–951.

Seidel, R. W. (2014). Agreement between telepsychiatry assessment and face-to-face assessment for emergency department psychiatry patients. *Journal of Telemedicine and Telecare*, *20*(2): 59–62.

Shore, J. H. (2007). Emergency management guidelines for telepsychiatry. *General Hospital Psychiatry*, 29(3): 199–206.

Telepsych highlites 2015. (2015). East Carolina University, Center for Telepsychiatry. Retrieved December 17, 2020, from https://www.ecu.edu/cs-dhs/ncstep/upload/ TelepsychHighlites2015.pdf.

TelePsychiatry improving outcomes and metrics at CaroMont Regional Medical Center ED. (n.d.). Retrieved December 17, 2020, from https://www.soctelemed.com/: https:// files.nc.gov/ncdhhs/2018%20NC%20DHHS%20ORH%20Telepsychiatry%20 Program%20One%20Pager_0.pdf.

Telepsychiatry program history. (2018). Retrieved December 17, 2020, from South Carolina Department of Mental Health: https://scdmh.net/dmhtelepsychiatry/ telepsychiatry-and-telehealth-program-history.

Yellowlees, P. (2008). Emergency telepsychiatry. *Journal of Telemedicine and Telecare*, 14(6): 277–281.

Yoshino, A. S. (2001). Telepsychiatry: Assessment of televideo psychiatric interview reliability with present- and next-generation internet infrastructures. *Acta Psychiatrica Scandinavica*, 104: 223–226.

10

Role of Telemedicine in Guiding Rural Emergent Neurosurgical Care

M . OMAR CHOHAN, MARTINA STIPPLER,
SUSY SALVO WENDT, AND HOWARD YONAS ∎

INTRODUCTION

Neurosurgical and neurovascular emergencies are time sensitive, with outcomes linked to interventions that occur during the initial hours post-onset of injury (Matsushima & Inaba, 2015; Rosenfeld, 2012). They require rapid assessment and disposition, especially for those who need emergent intervention (Esposito, 2005). Historically, tertiary centers have accepted the transfer of all patients with neurosurgical complaints without assessment of the true risk of a significant brain and spine condition. In more than 70% of emergent air transfers however, patients are discharged within hours or a few days without any intervention. (Carlson, 2010; Stippler, n.d.). The availability of a virtual neurosurgeon, via real time audio and video, to emergency departments (EDs) without bedside neurosurgery coverage can improve this triage process.

The following case study describes a teleneurology and teleneurosurgery program. Later sections of this chapter will intermittently refer to this model to demonstrate various aspects of effectiveness.

CASE STUDY

The University of New Mexico (UNM) neurology and neurosurgery departments recognized that a high volume of patient transfers was received from the Gallop Indian Health Hospital. Over half of the patients did not require admission after arrival at UNM. By creating a mechanism for a timely transfer of images (Net Medical, Albuquerque), UNM neurosurgeons were able to combine a phone consultation with simultaneous review of radiologic images. Over approximately five years, the program reduced transfers by 50% and saved the Indian Health Service (IHS) over one million dollars (Holquin, 2011). The program observed no harm to patients retained at Gallop Hospital.

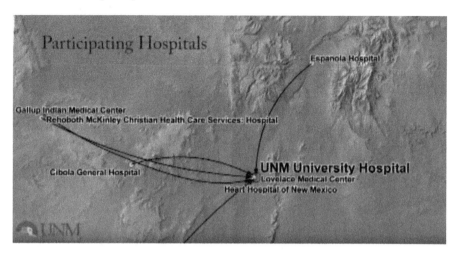

University of New Mexico Neurovascular Network (Yonas, 2009)

Based on the IHS experience, together with later integration of video consultations, funding from the Centers for Medicare and Medicaid Services (CMS) was obtained in 2014 to develop a New Mexico rural telemedicine neuro emergent program, ACCESS (Access to Critical Cerebral Emergency Support Services). Over the next two years, the teleneurosurgery team was able to reduce the neurosurgical consult transfers from 12 rural New Mexico hospitals to 13%, with 50% of those transferred patients requiring neurosurgical intervention. Of the 87% of retained in local hospital or discharged "neurosurgical" patients in rural hospitals, there were no late transfers due to neurological deterioration. The program has been very successful, continues to grow, and has doubled in size.

RESOURCE MANAGEMENT

Limited neurosurgical staff and intensive care unit (ICU) bed capacity in tertiary neurosurgical centers restricts the ability to accept transfer of patients who may need a higher level of care. Many patients resolve the neurosurgical question within a few hours, but an ED clinician often does not have the neurosurgical backup available to support decision making regarding the admission, transfer, or discharge of these patients. The ED clinician is also under intense pressure to disposition patients as quickly as possible to avoid long length of stays and boarding. Consultations by a teleneurosurgeon can help differentiate high-risk patients with a spectrum of neurosurgical diagnoses. The high-risk patients are appropriately transferred to a center capable of providing the needed care. The patient determined to be low risk, such as one who has a chronic or minimal subdural hematoma, having completed a teleneurosurgical consultation, can be admitted and monitored at the spoke hospital. The ACCESS program demonstrated that the collaborative consultation of the patients, their family, and the ED staff with a virtual neurosurgeon dramatically increased the willingness to keep patients at rural hospitals (Whetten, 2018).

There is a diminishing number of neurosurgeons providing ED on-call services. This is due to age attrition as well as reduced interest in providing emergency care, especially trauma (Rosman, 2013). Nonetheless, access to neurosurgical consultation is necessary for ED clinician support in rural and community hospitals to determine more focused diagnoses, facilitate rapid disposition, and provide families with clear and confident treatment plans. Because one neurosurgeon can provide a virtual neurosurgical presence at many rural hospitals while maintaining an active clinical practice, teleneurosurgery is the ideal means for provision and management of this critical resource.

PROGRAMMATIC CONSIDERATIONS

Like every hospital-based telemedicine program, a teleneurosurgical consult service requires (1) technology to be able to provide an optimal video consultation enhanced by rapid image transfer and integration; (2) state licensure and hospital credentials; and (3) a viable business model for all stakeholders.

Technology

The necessary telemedicine technology that is now widely available for telestroke programs meets many of the needs of a teleneurosurgery program (see Chapter 8, this volume, for more detail). A real-time two-way audio and video capability that allows the neurosurgeon to examine a patient and discuss recommendations with the patient, their family, as well as the ED staff, has been essential for acceptance of teleneurosurigcal recommendations. The virtual neurosurgical consultation does require the aid of the clinical staff at the originating site hospital to serve as a telepresenter, helping perform the neurological exam with the neurosurgeon's guidance.

The advent of cloud-based communication for telemedicine has greatly improved the ability to provide rural specialty care. These systems have significantly lessened the cost of acquisition and operation of the technology. The teleneurosurgery system utilized for the UNM program included a mechanism to acquire and transfer image data simultaneously with establishing the consultation. The Net Medical (Albuquerque, New Mexico) program contacted the appropriate specialist (neurosurgeon vs neurologist) as triaged by a Net Medical operator who identified consultants from on-call lists. ACCESS neurosurgical consultants were members of the full-time faculty at UNM, while stroke neurology consultants included neurologists in practice elsewhere in the United States. Within 30 minutes of consult completion, Net Medical sent a clinical report documenting clinical data and recommendations to the spoke ED.

The ease of access for the consultant via a portable computer has also made providing consults more consistent with clinical practice and a normal work-life balance.

Reimbursement

Appropriate compensation for consulting physicians is important for program buy-in and program longevity. A fair market value assessment of a teleneurosurgical consultation was determined to be $1,200, based on local standard community salaries in 2014 combined with the expected volume of emergent consultations. Both New Mexico Medicaid and local insurance companies have accepted this number. While this represents a significant investment by a hospital or an insurance company, reducing the transfer rate from 90 to 13% has many positive implications. Originating site hospitals are able to keep additional patients and the associated diagnosis-related group (DRG), which has had a major financial impact for rural hospitals (Podbielski, 2015; Friedman, 2016). The avoidance of air transport has an even greater impact on the health care system. Because most patients in large and significantly rural states like New Mexico are transported by emergency air ambulance, the cost of moving patients is significant. A recent analysis reported an average air ambulance cost of nearly $46,000 per transfer (Air Ambulance Memorial, 2017). The avoidance of >80% of neurosurgical transfers from 2016 to 2018 of 350 consults under the UNM ACCESS program has reduced air transport costs by over 10 million dollars. The result explains the willingness of insurance companies to cover the costs of neurosurgical telemedicine consultations. Rural hospitals and New Mexico Medicaid have approved a bundle payment model, and Medicare is currently assessing a possible wider national application.

EDUCATION AND TRAINING

Many rural and urban physicians are uncomfortable with the management of cranial or spine trauma, as well as a spectrum of tumors and hemorrhagic processes. This often places ED clinicians in the middle of negotiating admission to the hospitalist service or finding a neurosurgeon to accept the patient in transfer. The ACCESS program addressed this issue by providing the originating site ED clinicians and allied staff with over 8 hours of education (Box 10.1). The training, combined with teleneurosurgery consultation, led to a major shift in the willingness of local clinicians to keep patients in their hospitals. Because of the relatively high rate of new physicians entering practices in rural communities, education needs to be ongoing. Another aspect of developing a sustainable and successful program is the development of relationships between consulting neurosurgeons and local providers. While a trust relationship can be built with multiple consults over time, the best way to build rapport is for the neurosurgical provider to be part of the offered training to local physicians. In the case of the ACCESS program, this was accomplished with monthly teleconferences and inclusion to UNM Neurological weekly Grand Rounds presentations and education.

Box 10.1

ACCESS EDUCATION PROGRAM (ADAPTED FROM UNM EDUCATION AND
TRAINING WEBSITE, 2020)

Onsite in-person training and education workshop
- Stroke
- Trauma
- Spectrum of other neurological disorders

Neuroscience Distance Learning Series
- Acute spinal cord injury
- Brain death
- Brain injury, including traumatic brain injury and acute brain injury case
  studies
- Neurological assessment
- Status epilepticus
- Stroke, including acute ischemic stroke, hemorrhagic stroke, stroke recovery
  and rehabilitation, and tPA for review and competency

Annual ACCESS Conference
- Annual 2-day conference focused on a specific neurology education theme

HUMAN RESOURCES

An essential ingredient in the success of a neurosurgical telemedicine program is
having a cohort of dedicated neurosurgeons. Various strategies are available for
obtaining the involvement of actively practicing neurosurgeons, but the most effective ones include appropriate staffing and support to ensure a manageable workload.
The telemedicine system needs to be easy to use, reliable, and accessible on multiple
devices. Referral of appropriate patients into the neurosurgeon's practice should be
possible, and teleneurosurgery coverage should be adequately compensated. Because
of availability limitations related to surgery schedules at the distant site, the neurosurgery practice needs a backup surgeon who can respond to a consult when the
primary person on-call is not available.

The field of telestroke has evolved very rapidly. A variety of organizations leverage
the capacity of neurologists to provide stroke-focused consultation for many small
and moderate-size hospitals. Program costs related to acquiring and maintaining telemedicine technologies, on-call fees, consultation fees, and subscription fees are beyond the means of most low-volume rural hospitals. An alternative model initiated
at the UNM is a bundled charge built around the consult. This means that if a hospital sees one neurology or neurosurgery emergent patient in a month, they would
only be charged for the one consult. Low-cost access to expert guidance and added
rural hospital revenue gained by retaining more patients have more than paid for the
consult. Physician retention improved as one-third of ED physicians reported that

having the ability to consult with ACCESS neurospecialists provided them the support they needed to want to continue to practice in rural New Mexico.

DIAGNOSES: SPECTRUM OF NEUROSURGICAL DIAGNOSES AND MANAGEMENT

Table 10.1 lists the first 252 neurosurgical diagnoses for which ACCESS consultations were requested by rural ED physicians.

The following examples illustrate how a teleneurosurgeon can assist with the management and disposition of several diagnoses.

Subdural hematomas: Acute subdural hematomas are associated with significant brain injury and require neurosurgical consultation. The virtual neurosurgeon can evaluate imaging to determine if a subdural hematoma requires transfer to a tertiary center versus observation at the local site. In some cases, consultation may clarify that the subdural is actually chronic and is with little risk for progression. These cases can be managed with outpatient in-person follow-up or potentially by utilizing telemedicine.

Skull and spine fractures: Fractures of the skull that are not associated with significant depression of the level of consciousness or intracerebral hemorrhage rarely warrant emergency transport. It is the role of the consulting teleneurosurgeon to identify the uncommon fracture, such as when it involves the frontal sinus, where the risk

Table 10.1 Neurosurgical Consultation Diagnoses ($N = 252$)

Abscess	
Brain	2
Spine	4
Aneurysm	3
CSF leak, posttraumatic	5
Epidural hematoma	3
Intracranial Hemorrhage	
Spontaneous	14
Traumatic	5
Subarachnoid hemorrhage	
Spontaneous	5
Traumatic	8
Shunt malfunction	3
Spine, degenerative	51
Spine, trauma	35
Subdural hematoma	
Acute	8
Chronic	49
TBI, moderate	35
Tumor, brain	22

of a CSF leak exists. In addition, most spine fractures do not alter the stability of the spinal axis and can be managed acutely with an external support and elective referral to a spine specialist. It is the role of the teleneurosurgeon to identify if an unstable fracture exists, for which emergent transport is indicated.

Subarachnoid hemorrhage: Subarachnoid hemorrhage (SAH) is a common ED diagnosis, with only a small percentage being due to a ruptured aneurysm. Ruptured aneurysms are emergencies that need transfer to a specialty team. Unruptured aneurysms are far more common as incidental findings on a CT scan and require elective referral. Traumatic SAH is an even more common finding in an ED, but fortunately the vast majority of them are self- resolving without the need for neurosurgical intervention. The role of a virtual neurosurgeon in an ED is to help define the type of SAH, its risk for worsening, and a follow-up plan.

Malignancies: The spectrum of intracranial or spine tumors can present in many ways including as seizures or as a progressive deficit. While an occasional patient presents with a life-threatening clinical picture, most lesions, including malignant brain tumors, can appropriately be managed with high-dose corticosteroids and an anticonvulsant. The teleneurosurgeon can help determine when and where the patient should be referred.

Futile Care: The unfortunate reality is that some patients suffer lethal neurologic catastrophes. Massive intracerebral hemorrhage with mass effect and midline shift may present no chance of survival, regardless of procedural or surgical intervention. The teleneurosurgeon can identify these cases and provide families with realistic expectations and discuss the futility of further interventions. These patients will not benefit from transfer and are best admitted near family for comfort care at the originating site.

OUTCOMES, QUALITY, AND METRICS

Some quality and outcome metrics for teleneurosurgery programs should include the number of consults, time to begin consultation after request, transfer rates, and patient satisfaction. As mentioned in Chapter 4, a comprehensive quality program could be built around the four domains of the National Quality Forum (NQF) quality framework. The teleneuro-emergent program at UNM received start-up funding by CMS, with the goal of developing a clinical platform for caring for the full breadth of neurological and neurosurgical disorders. As part of measuring the impact of the program on patients, families, nurses, and physicians, three-day and three-month assessments were made after discharge from the ED. Patients provided positive feedback regarding the teleneurosurgery consultation process and their interactions with the teleneurosurgeon. They particularly felt that the teleneurosurgeon listened to them and understood their concerns. Patients were also appreciative of avoiding travel and receiving care in their own community. Both nurses and physicians gave a >85% satisfaction rating to the consultation process. They reported the process as convenient and simple, and emphasized that the telehealth consultation enabled them to provide better care than without the consult.

Developing standard consult forms and tracking treatment and transfer recommendations are useful tools to facilitate review for quality purposes. These tools also help improve consistency of service and assure that teleneurosurgery services are providing high-level care. Reviewing the data concerning duration of time from placement of consultation to final report allows response times to be monitored. The quality of the technology is monitored with an assessment by the consulting physician who reports any technical difficulty with the audio, video, or radiographic image transfer during the consultation. A 97% technically successful consultation rate was recorded in the last two years of the current UNM program. In instances where the internet connection failed to support audio, video, or image transfer, a phone conversation supplemented by a smart phone image was sufficient for decision making.

While acute stroke consultations require a rapid expert response, the majority of neurosurgical consultations are less emergent. ACCESS requests for consultation were classified as emergent or routine, with response standards ranging from 10 minutes to 60 minutes. The average neurosurgery response time has been 30 minutes. The majority of neurosurgical consultations have served to reaffirm the ED clinician's plan of care or to reexamine an X-ray that was read by a radiologist as "cannot rule out" an injury. As of 2019, 50 of 350 neurosurgical consultations in which the major concern was addressing this type of radiological read demonstrated no emergent pathology. Without neurosurgical involvement these patients would have been transferred from rural hospitals.

ENGAGEMENT AND UTILIZATION

There is a major unmet need for both expert neurology and neurosurgery consultation in rural and underserved EDs. To date, however, teleneurosurgery has not been as widely adopted as telestroke. During the four years of the ACCESS grant (three primary years and one additional year), the acceptance of this mode of consultation has steadily increased. The number of neurosurgery consults has remained about 7% of all of the 5,515 ACCESS consults processed as of March 2019. The strategies of ongoing training and relationship building are effective at maintaining rural ED provider engagement with a teleneurosurgery program. Further evidence of the benefit of ACCESS was the progressive enrollment of new hospitals, with 17 engaged in the program by the end of CMS funding and 7 additional hospitals in the process of joining at that time.

Rural providers and hospitals may benefit from some reduction in medicolegal risk by utilizing a teleneursurgery program. The ACCESS team initially believed that ED physicians would learn how to confidently triage head trauma cases, resulting in a decline of neurosurgical consultations over time. However, in many situations, the ED physicians developed reasonable treatment plans based on clinical experience and the literature, but still activated the virtual neurosurgical consultant to gain agreement and patient confidence. In other cases, the ED physician's decision to admit the patient and observe them locally received pushback from the hospitalist. They might refuse the admission unless a virtual neurosurgical consult was completed. Each stakeholder in the chain of care can benefit from expert consultation; therefore, those benefits must be highlighted, measured, and routinely reported to administrators to help sustain the program.

CONCLUSION

A severe shortage of neurosurgical expertise in rural hospitals has resulted in a pattern of emergent transfers to a tertiary center; a high percentage of these neurosurgical diagnoses did not require transfer for optimal care. The significant waste of time, resources, and increased risk from helicopter transfer could be avoided. A virtual neurosurgical consult in a rural ED is possible today, resulting in fewer unnecessary transfers and the opportunity for the rural hospital to retain patients in their own community. Improved education for rural hospital doctors and nurses, combined with modern telemedicine can help resolve the current unmet need. Teleneurosurgeon support to less resourced hospitals can serve as a model to improve access to care while supporting local communities. While challenges to widespread adoption continue, the evolving technology and regulatory environments, in addition to greater awareness of the impact of telehealth interventions such as teleneurosurgery, offer innovative emergency physicians and departments mechanisms to improve care.

KEY TAKEAWAYS

➤ Teleneurosurgery has a significant role to meet the current unmet need for delivering tertiary care to rural and underserved hospitals.

➤ A significant infrastructure for maintaining and accessing a network of consulting specialists, timely transfer of images, creation of reporting, as well as an extensive educational effort are needed to deliver this type of care.

➤ Coupling teleneurosurgery with an existing telestroke service may be a simple solution.

➤ Teleneurosurgery is effective in selecting which patients require and which can be safely admitted at a rural site or even be discharged home with follow-up.

➤ Quality Reviews and Education are critical pieces in the success of a teleneurosurgery program.

REFERENCES

Air Ambulance Memorial. (2017). Study Report, State of New Mexico, Office of the Superintendent of Insurance (HM78/SM62). Retrieved October 12, 2020, from https://www.nmlegis.gov/handouts/ERDT%20083117%20Item%208%20NM%20 Superintendent%20of%20Insurance%20Air%20Ambulance%20Memorial%20 Study%20Report.pdf.

Carlson, A. P. (2010). Low rate of delayed deterioration requiring surgical treatment in patients transferred to a tertiary care center for mild traumatic brain injury. *Journal of Neurosurgery, Neurosurgical Focus* 2, 29(5): E3.

Esposito, T. J. (2005). Neurosurgical coverage: Essential, desired or irrelevant for good patient care and trauma center status. *Annals of Surgery*, 242(3): 364–370.

Friedman, A. B. (2016). Trends in hospital ED closures nationwide and across Medicaid expansion, 2006–2013. *American Journal of Emergency Medicine*, 24(7): 1262–1264.

Holquin, E. (2011, May). Management of acute head trauma in rural locations; University of New Mexico Teleradiology Initiative for Mild Traumatic Brain Injury. *The HIS Primary Care Provider*, 26(5): 99–104. https://hsc.unm.edu/health/for-medical-professionals/access/how-access-works/education.html. (n.d.).

Matsushima, K., & Inaba, S. S. (2015). Emergent operation for isolated severe traumatic brain injury: Does time matter? *Journal of Trauma and Acute Care Surgery*, 79(5): 838–842.

Podbielski, C. (2015). *Share the wealth: Extending valuable neurosurgical care and the legal considerations thereof*. From *AANS Neurosurgeon* 24 (4). https://aansneurosurgeon.org/departments/share-the-wealth-extending-valuable-neurosurgical-care-and-the-legal-considerations-thereof/#

Rosenfeld, J. V. (2012). Early management of severe head traumatic brain injury. *Lancet*, 380: 1088.

Rosman, J. (2013). Is there a shortage of neurosurgeons in the United States? *Neurosurgery*, 73(2): 356–365.

Stippler, M. (n.d.). Utility of routine follow-up head CT scanning after mild traumatic brain injury: A systematic review of the literature. *Emergency Medicine Journal*, 29(7): 528–532.

UNM Education and Training website. (2020). Adapted from https://hsc.unm.edu/health/for-medical-professionals/access/how-access-works/education.html.

Whetten, J. (2018). Cost-effectiveness of Access to Critical Cerebral Emergency Support Services (ACCESS): A neuro-emergent telemedicine consultation program. *Journal of Medical Economics*, 21(4), 398–405.

Yonas, H. (2009). *Neurosurgery telehealth system*. From https://www.youtube.com/watch?v=emyNuGQySSs&feature=youtu.be.

11

Emergency Ocular
Telehealth Services

ANIKA GOODWIN AND CHLOE T. L. KHOO ■

INTRODUCTION

Emergency medicine practitioners manage common ophthalmic issues directly, with outpatient follow up performed by an ophthalmologist. However, there remain certain ocular conditions where an ophthalmologists' evaluation is essential in optimizing patients' final visual outcome. Visual disorders among adult Americans pose substantial costs for the U.S. economy (Rein et al., 2006; Vision Health Data, 2019, 2020); the estimated annual burden reaches approximately $35.4 billion, with $16.2 billion in direct medical costs.[1] More concerning is that an estimated 61 million adults at high risk for serious vision loss have disparate access to eye care (Zhang et al., 2007). Ocular telehealth can reduce the financial burden of ocular conditions and increase access of care to the U.S. population. In addition, with increasing risk for medical litigation (Jena, Seabury, Lakdawalla, & Chandra, 2011; Thompson, Parikh, & Lad, 2018), emergency departments (EDs), urgent care centers (UCCs), and hospital systems should consider implementation of ocular telehealth systems.

Programmatic Considerations

Some EDs and hospitals require 24/7 access to ophthalmology coverage in order to maintain their designation or status, including level 1 trauma centers and burn centers. The real conundrum lies with EDs and UCCs in smaller cities and rural areas where there may not be an ophthalmologist within 50 miles. A study looking at the geographic distribution of eye care providers in the United States reported that 24% of U.S. counties had no ophthalmologists or optometrists, and 60.7% of counties were in one of the lower two quartiles of both ophthalmologist and optometrist availability (Gibson, 2015). The EDs and UCCs in rural areas are also more likely to be staffed by nonemergency-medicine-trained physicians or advance practice providers (APPs) who may lack experience or confidence in handling certain ophthalmologic emergencies. Facilities with these staffing models will benefit from a remote option to access an ophthalmologist. The alternative is transferring a patient to a larger facility with specialty coverage, which can add to the total costs of care and increase patient inconvenience (Kindermann, Mutter, Houchens, Barrett, & Pines, 2015).

Technology

Equipment needs are a hallmark of the specialty of ophthalmology, so start-up costs must be considered. Many EDs and UCCs already have certain items within their inventory, including a slit lamp for anterior segment evaluation and a tonometer for intraocular pressure measurement. However, a lack of training and equipment familiarity has led to the underutilization of ophthalmic equipment. The advancement in telehealth has brought about innovation with ophthalmic devices. There are now smaller, simpler devices that are more portable and user-friendly, allowing trained ancillary staff members (i.e., nurses, medical assistants, or technicians), in addition to emergency medicine practitioners, to care for patients with more acute ophthalmic issues. These same ancillary staff members can be trained to obtain additional ophthalmic exam elements and act as facilitators when presenting the patient to the tele-ophthalmologist, allowing the ED workflow to move forward efficiently. In addition to ophthalmic equipment, image communication devices (i.e., computers, servers, and network devices) that are FDA-approved and HIPAA-compliant are available for data transfer (Telemedicine for Ophthalmology Information Statement, 2018).

Utilizing ophthalmic equipment may seem daunting and costly but is essential in the ophthalmic examination due to the nature of the exam and the anatomy of the eye. Next, each piece of equipment will be addressed in detail (Table 11.1).

The ophthalmic equipment described above is essential in performing an eight-point eye examination (Table 11.2) (Rupp, 2016; Bowe et al., 2020). The Fundus photography vs. Ophthalmoscopy Trial Outcomes in the Emergency Department (FOTO-ED) study performed at Emory University demonstrated in its first two phases that ED clinicians perform significantly better with fundus photography than with direct ophthalmoscopy (Bruce et al., 2020). Hence, EDs considering ocular telehealth support should ensure that all necessary equipment is available for the comprehensive eye examination.

An exam room in the ED, UCC, or hospital fully equipped with ophthalmic equipment can be turned into an examination space for patients with ocular issues. Ocular information obtained from the eight-point eye examination can be documented in the EMR to be assessed by a remote ophthalmologist. The eight-point eye exam may also be conducted by the technician under video supervision of the tele-ophthalmologist.

Any digital images or recordings can be transferred via a secured HIPAA-compliant software (e.g., RetinaVue® Network Software) for further interpretation. Bandwidth capable of supporting synchronous audio and video communication between the remote ophthalmologist, facilitator, provider, and patient will allow for a real-time encounter interviewing the patient for additional history, performing an external exam, interpreting captured images, suggesting any required additional

Table 11.1 REQUIRED EQUIPMENT AND EXAMPLES

Ophthalmic Equipment	Description	Price per unit
Tonometry, e.g., Tono-Pen™, iCare®	A hand-held instrument used to provide intraocular pressure readings in mmHg.	~$3,000–4,000
Slit lamp, e.g., Haag-Streit BM 900 Table LED slit lamp	A microscope with bright light that allows the examiner to view the structures of the eye with greater magnification.	~$15,000–19,000
Hand-held slit lamp, e.g., Horus Hand-held digital slit lamp (Figure 11.1)	A portable version of the slit lamp microscope with the ability to capture images or recordings of the anterior segment for disease screening and diagnosis. Images or video clips can be transferred via an SD card or USB cable to be uploaded to electronic medical records (EMR).	~$4,000–6,000
Retinal or fundus camera, e.g., Topcon NW400 (Figure 11.2)	A device that captures nonmydriatic full-color 45° images of the posterior segment, which are transferred via a secure HIPAA-compliant software and then made available to interface with EMR or picture archiving and communication systems (PACS).	~$16,000–18,000
B-scan ultrasonography, e.g., Keeler B-scan plus	A device that offers two-dimensional cross-sectional view of the eye to evaluate for retinal detachments and vitreous hemorrhage.	~8,000–9,000

testing or imaging, diagnosing, recommending treatment plans, providing patient education, and scheduling follow-up by the remote ophthalmologist.

More recently, artificial intelligence (AI) has been increasingly implemented in the field of ophthalmology and may play a role in ocular telehealth, once its limitations and challenges are overcome. AI based on deep learning has been applied to imaging devices such as fundus cameras and may be incorporated with telehealth to screen, diagnose, and monitor ocular pathology (Ting et al., 2019).

Reimbursement Models

The cost profile of beginning an ocular telehealth program should be directly compared to the cost of either employing multiple ophthalmologists who take on-call coverage as a requirement of their contract versus paying local ophthalmologists

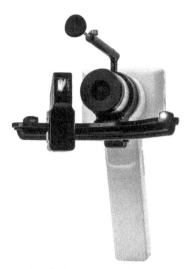

Figure 11.1 Example of a portable slit lamp: Horus hand-held digital slit lamp. Image courtesy of Medimaging Integrated Solution, Inc. (Miis).

to provide coverage (recent rates average approximately $1,200 per 24-hour period). As ophthalmic surgical services transition from hospital settings to outpatient surgical centers, fewer ophthalmologists are hospital staff members. Hospitals with few or no staff ophthalmologists are having a hard time obtaining on-call coverage, despite compensation from hospitals and payment from patients and their insurance (Telemedicine for Ophthalmology Information Statement, 2018; On Call Compensation for Ophthalmologists, 2014). Ocular telehealth can be a solution to provide patients with on demand care. However, one of the challenges of telehealth is the absence of widespread payment coverage for telehealth by federal, state, and private payers Telemedicine for Ophthalmology Information Statement, 2018). With the advent of COVID-19 and increasing transition to telehealth, Medicare policies have been amended to include approximately 180 different service codes for reimbursement if provided via telehealth, including eye exams for new and established patients (Telehealth Coverage Policies in the Time of COVID-19, 2020). While billing requirements are in a constant state of flux and should be referenced with Centers for Medicare and Medicaid Services and the Academy of Ophthalmology, there are three main types of reimbursable visits in ophthalmology: telehealth visits, virtual check-ins, and digital encounters (Center for Medicaid and Medicare Services, 2020; Saleem, Pasquale, Sidoti, & Tsai, 2020).

Outcomes, Quality, and Metrics

One of the most valuable aspects of ocular telehealth services is the ability to provide a definitive diagnosis in cases of diagnostic uncertainty. This is comforting to both the patient who may need reassurance on vision potential, and the ED clinician who can provide a sound plan of care. In addition, the availability of on-demand ocular telehealth services can prevent gaps in on-call coverage. Having access to board

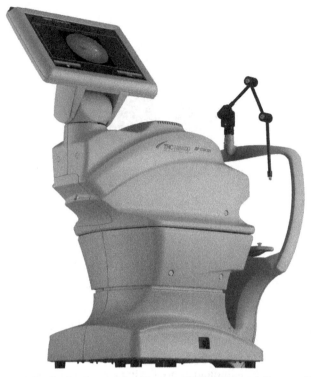

Figure 11.2 Example of a fundus camera: Topcon NW400 Retinal Camera. Image courtesy of Topcon Healthcare.

certified ophthalmologists to assist in the diagnosis and treatment plan can lead to overall economic savings for the patient and health care system and may also help mitigate medical liability risk.

According to another study looking at eye-related ED visits from 961 hospitals in the United States, the majority of ophthalmic issues were nonemergent (Vaziri, Schwartz, Flynn, Kishor, & Moshfeghi, 2016). The most common ICD-9 diagnoses include conjunctivitis (33.8%), corneal injury without foreign body (13.1%), corneal foreign body (7.8%) and eye pain (4.2%). Of all patients, 97.2% did not require hospital admission or transfer (Vaziri et al., 2016). Despite these statistics, hospitals that hire ophthalmology on-call services are contracted to pay for 24 hours of coverage, regardless of whether the covering physician's services are rendered. These nonemergent/urgent ocular complaints could have been effectively managed via ocular telehealth provided by board-certified ophthalmologists. Guidance from a remote ophthalmologist can facilitate transfer of patients requiring a procedure (outside the scope of the ED clinician) or surgery to a facility with an in-house ophthalmologist. The ability to consult a remote ophthalmologist via telehealth will ease the ED clinician's decision to transfer a patient, knowing that the time and cost involved were necessary in ensuring the highest quality of care and the best final visual outcome for the patient.

Table 11.2 EIGHT-POINT EYE EXAMINATION

Eight Points	Description
Visual acuity	• In the clinic setting, visual acuity is typically measured at 20-foot distance with the Snellen visual acuity chart. • In a consult setting in the hospital, visual acuity at near can be measured at bedside using a hand-held near card. • If patient is unable to see the largest letter on the card, visual acuity can be measured (from better to worse) with counting fingers (CF), hand motion (HM), light perception (LP), and no light perception (NLP).
Pupils	• Check if the pupils are equal, round, and reactive to light. • If anisocoria is present, carefully check the pupil size in both well-lit and dark conditions.
Intraocular pressure	• Intraocular pressure measurements can be performed with Tono-pen™ or iCare®. • If there is a suspicion for a ruptured globe, skip this part of the exam, as applying pressure with tonometry could cause extrusion of intraocular contents.
Extraocular motility and alignment	• Check for motility by having the patient look in six cardinal positions of gaze.
Confrontation visual fields	• Examining one eye at a time, assess each quadrant by having the patient count the number of fingers that the examiner has up.
External examination	• Evaluate the eye and periorbital region externally for any gross deformities, injuries, swelling, or lacerations especially involving the eyelids. • Perform a cranial nerve exam for patients with diplopia or neurologic symptoms.
Slit lamp examination	• With the standard or hand-held slit lamp, examine the anterior segment of the eye, including the eyelids for any deformity or lacerations involving the eyelid margin, conjunctiva for redness or hemorrhage, cornea for abrasions or ulcers, iris for irregularities, and lens for cataracts or dislocated lens.
Fundoscopic examination	• With the direct ophthalmoscope, examine the optic nerve for edema and the macula for any gross hemorrhages or retinal detachments. • Using a retinal camera will allow capture of retinal images, which can then be sent electronically to a remote ophthalmologist.

Having ocular telehealth services may also be a useful tool in recruiting ophthalmologists to a hospital or to an area. As patients can be effectively triaged by on-call ocular telehealth providers, call responsibility for ophthalmologists will be limited to surgical or procedural ocular issues, which is an attractive option.

Increased patient satisfaction, better clinical outcomes, less cost for the hospital, and improved hospital/physician relationships are all compelling reasons to consider adding ocular telehealth services to the ED or UCCs. The availability of ocular telehealth could also lead to increased ED physician recruitment and retention.

Receiving care in the setting of a UCC or ED is only a small part of the equation. The true measure of excellent care is in the follow-up. The paucity of eye surgeons overall, especially in small towns or rural areas, makes this a much more difficult task. In addition, the fact that not all specialists participate in all insurance plans, particularly government-run plans, makes this an even more challenging task. Ocular telehealth is extending the reach of the limited number of practicing ophthalmologists, as shown by the Technology-Based Eye Care Services (TECS) study (Maa et al., 2017). This study, conducted in five primary care clinics in Georgia surrounding the Atlanta Veterans Affairs hospital, demonstrated patient and physician time savings of 25% and 50%, respectively. In addition, the access to ophthalmology care improved, with 99% of patients seen within 14 days of contacting the eye clinic having a no-show rate of 5.2% (Maa et al., 2017). The findings from this study were encouraging and prove that ocular telehealth has the potential to reduce cost, improve efficiency, and significantly improve access to care on a larger scale.

While access to eye care is improving with ocular telehealth, it is still not readily available in all states, leaving patients who need to be seen as outpatients after an ED visit with a conundrum. While local optometrists may play a role in following patients with ocular issues that do not require additional procedures or surgeries, certain patients may need follow-up with an ophthalmologist for further management. Despite this fact, ocular telehealth can still assist making a diagnosis in the emergency setting and beginning a potentially sight saving treatment.

Emergency Department and Urgent Care Center Settings

The use cases for ocular telehealth within a hospital system are quite diverse and span both outpatient and inpatient service offerings. Within the ED setting, ocular telehealth services are often useful, especially with ocular emergencies and urgencies (Table 11.3). Ophthalmic exam findings utilizing slit lamp video recordings and fundus photography can help guide what can often be more difficult diagnoses (Telemedicine for Ophthalmology, 2018; Center for Medicai and Medicare Services, 2020; Woodward et al., 2017; Cao & Fecarotta, 2015; Ting et al., 2017). In this setting, the remote ophthalmologist would be able to recommend and review radiographic and sonographic imaging and help guide the examination. In cases where procedures or surgical intervention are necessary, having this remote access can make this decision-making process much more efficient and less doubtful, all while preparing the patient for the next level of care with confidence.

UCCs will also find ocular telehealth services particularly useful. Patients who desire a cheaper, faster, and more convenient care option to ED visits often look to UCCs as the solution, particularly for perceived low-acuity complaints. UCCs run on thin financial margins and often employ APPs in order to meet these budgeting constraints. Many of these providers have little hands-on experience with ocular

Table 11.3 LIST OF COMMON EMERGENT/URGENT OCULAR CONDITIONS AMENABLE
TO OCULAR TELEHEALTH EVALUATION, DIAGNOSIS, AND DISPOSITION

Diagnoses that can be discharged home or admitted locally with follow-up	Diagnoses that require transfer
• Acute or chronic conjunctivitis (viral or bacterial etiology) • Central retinal vein occlusion • Chalazion • Chemical injury, depending on severity • Corneal abrasion • Corneal foreign body, depending on severity • Dry eye syndrome • Herpes zoster without ocular involvement • Hordeolum or stye • Idiopathic intracranial hypertension, aka Pseudotumor cerebri • Orbital fracture with no evidence of extraocular muscle entrapment and no evidence of globe injury or rupture • Preseptal cellulitis • Subconjunctival hemorrhage	• Acute angle closure glaucoma • Corneal ulcer • Central retinal artery occlusion • Endophthalmitis • Eyelid laceration involving the eyelid margin • Globe rupture • Intraocular foreign body • Orbital fracture with evidence of extraocular muscle entrapment or evidence of globe rupture • Orbital cellulitis • Retinal detachment • Vitreous hemorrhage

complaints. Similar to teleradiology services (e.g., NightHawk Radiology®), ocular telehealth offers the same concept for on-demand, accurate ophthalmic diagnoses in this setting. APPs could elect to consult with a board-certified ophthalmologist whenever needed for ready assistance with diagnosis and treatment planning. In this way, patients gain access to the highest level of care in the most convenient way, while potentially saving significant costs in the process.

Extending Use of the ED-Based Ocular Telehealth Program

An ED-based ocular telehealth program may benefit the local health system. Hospitals with level 3 neonatal intensive care units are very familiar with the utility and necessity of having ocular telehealth options for diagnosing and managing retinopathy of prematurity in at-risk neonates (Cao & Fecarotta, 2015). The number of ophthalmic specialists who perform such exams is limited; hence, remote options will allow these few specialists to reach many. Early diagnosis, close observation, and timely intervention allows these infants the opportunity to live full and productive lives by providing the benefit of good eyesight.

Affiliated primary care clinics and critical access hospitals may benefit as well. Offering these services locally help keep revenues, retain patients in the community, and could dramatically improve compliance in patients with chronic disease who require annual eye examinations.

Special Considerations for Training Telepresenters in Ocular Telehealth

Long-standing screening programs for diabetic retinopathy and retinopathy of prematurity have led to well-accepted standard protocols and procedures that ensure interpretation accuracy. Since ocular telehealth for acute care is a newer use case, these protocols are rapidly evolving and are certain to further elevate the quality of care provided.

Easy-to-use equipment and a manual of best practices have simplified training medical and ancillary staff to help facilitate the eye exam and gather data to be sent to the remote ophthalmologist. Telepresenters are the remote ophthalmologist's hands and feet on the ground. These facilitators are not expected to perform at the level of a certified ophthalmic technician. A half-day training session should be planned at the onset of the program to help these telepresenters master the components of the basic eye exam—specifically, vision check, pupil examination, and assessment of extraocular motility. The skills necessary to obtain pieces of information utilizing the eight-point eye exam are easily learned. The reliability of the diagnoses and treatment plans are heavily dependent on the quality and consistency of the information shared with the remote ophthalmologist. As these are essential components of an ocular telehealth program, recertification and skill testing should be offered to ensure intertelepresenter reliability. Digital procedure manuals with high-quality images and online videos can act as a reference in training new hires. The availability of a hands-on training protocol, with user-friendly equipment and secured HIPAA-compliant software for information transfer, will facilitate enthusiastic adoption by staff and commitment to making ocular telehealth a success.

Infection Control

The care, cleaning, and maintenance of the equipment are also essential considerations. Staff members should be trained on these aspects of the program to ensure equipment longevity and problem-free function. If renting, the equipment, service and maintenance are typically covered; if purchasing, equipment malfunction within the warranty period is solved through contacting the manufacturer. These items have a long history of use within ophthalmology and are often able to be serviced by outside technicians. To ensure cleanliness and prevention of disease transmission, ophthalmic equipment should be disinfected with sodium hypochlorite (dilute bleach) disinfectant wipes or 70% isopropyl alcohol wipes after each use. Sodium hypochlorite is effective against adenovirus (the cause of epidemic keratoconjunctivitis) and herpes simplex virus, which are commonly associated with nosocomial outbreaks in eye care (Junk et al., 2017).

The advent of the COVID-19 pandemic has brought about new recommendations to help prevent disease transmission. In keeping with recommendations to promote social distancing by limiting unnecessary patient–physician interaction, ocular telehealth visits, especially in the primary care setting, have gained increasing relevance. Due to the nature of the ophthalmic examination where patient–examiner interaction is often less than 6 feet apart, various modifications to ophthalmic equipment have been tried and tested to limit further exposure of COVID-19 to both patient and examiner. Face shields made of materials such as polycarbonate, acetate, and clear plastic have been redesigned with specific dimensions to fit slit lamps to act as a barrier between patient and examiner. Recently, it has been noted that slit lamp shields made of hydrophilic material with antiviral properties such as gold or silver nanoparticles and graphene oxide may act as an improved barrier for infectious droplets, thus reducing transmission risks (Ong et al., 2020).

CONCLUSION

Ocular telehealth services in the ED and UCC setting can aid in the diagnosis and management of ocular complaints, especially in small cities and rural areas with no access to ophthalmologists. The benefits of ocular telehealth services far outweigh the cost of obtaining ophthalmic equipment and training telepresenters. Ocular telehealth has shown that it can improve patient satisfaction and overall clinical outcome, mitigate medicolegal implications, increase eye care access to the U.S. population, and reduce overall economic burden to the health care system.

KEY TAKEAWAYS

> The availability of ocular telehealth can facilitate the diagnosis and management of ocular diagnoses.
> Essential ophthalmic equipment includes the visual acuity chart, tonometry, slit lamp, direct ophthalmoscope, and a retinal or fundus camera. Information obtained can be conveyed via documentation in EMR systems, and images can be transferred via Food and Drug Administration-approved and secured HIPAA-compliant software.
> Valuable aspects of ocular telehealth include the ability to provide patients with definite diagnoses and plan of care, leading to increased patient satisfaction and improved outcomes.
> In the long run, it is cost-effective to invest in ocular telehealth services to mitigate medicolegal risk, reduce the overall financial burden, and improve eye care access.
> Ophthalmology telepresenters can become skilled via training sessions conducted by certified ophthalmic technicians.

REFERENCES

Bowe, T., Hunter, D., Mantagos, I., et al. (2020). Virtual visits in ophthalmology: Timely advice for implementation during the COVID-19 public health crisis. *Telemedicine Journal and E-Health*, 26(9): 1113–1117.
Bruce, B. B., Thulasi, P., Fraser, C. L., et al. (2013). Diagnostic accuracy and use of nonmydriatic ocular fundus photography by emergency physicians: Phase II of the FOTO-ED study. *Annals of Emergency Medicine*, 62(1): 28–33.e1.

Cao, F. X., & Fecarotta, C. M. (2015, May). Telemedicine for ROP screening. Review of ophthalmology. Accessed August 20, 2020, at https://www.reviewofophthalmology.com/article/telemedicine-for-rop-screening.

Center for Medicaid and Medicare Services Medicare Telemedicine Health Care Provider Fact Sheet. (2020, March). cms.gov. Accessed at https://www.cms.gov/newsroom/fact-sheets/medicare-telemedicine-health-care-provider-fact-sheet.

Gibson, D. M. (2015). The geographic distribution of eye care providers in the united states: Implications for a national strategy to improve vision health. *Preventive Medicine*, 73: 30–36.

Jena, A. B., Seabury, S., Lakdawalla, D., & Chandra, A. (2011). Malpractice risk according to physician specialty. *New England Journal of Medicine,* 365(7): 629–636.

Junk, A. K., Chen, P. P., Lin, S. C., et al. (2017). Disinfection of tonometers: A report by the American Academy of Ophthalmology. *Ophthalmology*, 124(12): 1867–1875.

Kindermann, D. R., Mutter, R. L., Houchens, R. L., Barrett, M. L., & Pines, J. M. (2015). Emergency department transfers and transfer relationships in United States Hospitals. *Academic Emergency Medicine*, 22(2): 157–165.

Maa, A. Y., Wojciechowski, B., Hunt, K. J., et al. (2017). Early experience with technology-based eye care services (TECS): A novel ophthalmologic telemedicine initiative. *Ophthalmology,* 124(4): 539–546.

On-call Compensation for Ophthalmologists–2014. (2014, February). aao.org. Accessed August 20, 2020, at https://www.aao.org/clinical-statement/oncall-compensation-ophthalmologists.

Ong, S. C., Yap, J. X., Tay, T. Y. F., Mo, Y., Loon S. C., & Koh, V. (2020). Considerations in the use of slit lamp shields to reduce the risk of respiratory virus transmission in coronavirus disease 2019. *Current Opinion in Ophthalmology,* 31(5): 374–379.

Rein, D. B., Zhang, P., Wirth, K. E., et al. (2006). The economic burden of major adult visual disorders in the United States. *Archives of Ophthalmology*, 124(12): 1754–1760.

Rupp, J. (2016, May 24). The 8-point eye exam. aao.org. Accessed August 20, 2020, at https://www.aao.org/young-ophthalmologists/yo-info/article/how-to-conduct-eight-point-ophthalmology-exam.

Saleem, S. M., Pasquale, L. R., Sidoti, P. A., & Tsai, J. C. (2020, August). Virtual ophthalmology: Telemedicine in a COVID-19 era. *American Journal of Ophthalmology*, 216: 237–242.

Telehealth Coverage Policies in the Time of COVID-19. (2020, April). cchpca.org. Accessed September 1, 2020, at https://www.cchpca.org/resources/covid-19-telehealth-coverage-policies.

Telemedicine for Ophthalmology Information Statement–2018. (2018, February). Accessed August 20, 2020, at aao.org. https://www.aao.org/clinical-statement/telemedicine-ophthalmology-information-statement.

Thompson, A. C., Parikh, P. D., & Lad, E. M. (2018). Review of ophthalmology medical professional liability claims in the United States from 2006 through 2015. *Ophthalmology*, 125(5): 631–641.

Ting, D. S. W., Cheung, C. Y., Lim, G., et al. (2017). Development and validation of a deep learning system for diabetic retinopathy and related eye diseases using retinal images from multiethnic populations with diabetes. The *Journal of the American Medical Association*, 318(22): 2211–2223.

Ting, D. S. W., Pasquale, L. R., Peng, L., et al. (2019). Artificial intelligence and deep learning in ophthalmology. *British Journal of Ophthalmology*, 103(2): 167–175.

Vaziri, K., Schwartz, S. G., Flynn, H. W., Kishor, K. S., & Moshfeghi, A. A. (2016). Eye-related emergency department visits in the United States, 2010. *Ophthalmology.* 123(4): 917–919.

Vision Health Data and Surveillance System. (2019). cdc.gov. Accessed August 22, 2020, at https://www.cdc.gov/visionhealth/data/index.html. Updated April 2, 2019.

Vision Health Initiative (VHI) Resources and Publications. (2020). cdc.gov. Accessed August 20, 2020, at https://www.cdc.gov/visionhealth/resources/publications/index.htm. Reviewed March 12, 2020.

Woodward, M. A., Bavinger, J. C., Amin, S., et al. (2017). Telemedicine for ophthalmic consultation services: Use of a portable device and layering information for graders. *Journal of Telemedicine and Telecare,* 23(2): 365–370.

Zhang, X., Saaddine, J. B., Lee, P. P., et al. (2007). Eye care in the United States: Do we deliver to high-risk people who can benefit most from it? *Archives of Ophthalmology,* 125(3): 411–418.

12

Medical Subspecialty Telehealth Consults

SUSIE Q. LEW, SHAILENDRA SHARMA, MARC O. SIEGEL, HANA AKSELROD, SIMRANJIT KAUR, ANITA KUMAR, MARIE L. BORUM, AND HARTMUT GROSS ■

INTRODUCTION

Emergency medicine practice consists of the rapid evaluation and stabilization of acute, unscheduled care. The current payment structure is primarily fee for service; however, health care reforms are advancing new care models that emphasize population-based outcomes. Emergency clinicians are being challenged to provide more coordinated care. Emerging value-based models are creating the impetus for increased collaboration in order to provide high-quality care at lower cost by reducing admissions when possible and increasing access to specialists (for further detail, see Chapter 22). Additionally, in rural and community-based settings alike, advanced practice providers are a growing part of the emergency medicine workforce. Emergency telehealth can be used to provide supervision of emergency department (ED) care and procedures (see Chapter 17), but there are times when it may be valuable to include a specialist or primary care provider as part of delivering comprehensive and coordinated care.

As care paradigms evolve, there is a need to explore the indications and roles of a telehealth medical subspecialty consult request from the ED. In some instances, medical subspecialists from cardiology, endocrinology, gastroenterology, hematology, infectious disease, nephrology, pulmonology, or rheumatology could add value to an individual's ED care. However, few instances have been reported in the literature evaluating their benefit or describing their operation.

ED clinicians frequently request medical subspecialty consultation for complex cases and follow-up care consults for established patients. Traditionally, these consults have been in-person or via the telephone. In some settings, secure messaging is used to improve communication between the ED and the subspecialty or primary care physician, especially in integrated delivery network or academic settings. These consults have value in directing a known patient's evaluation and disposition, in addition to transition of care.

Depending on location and local resources, a medical subspecialty consult may be obtained from (1) a central remote service in areas that do not support a subspecialist, (2) a local network with an organized call schedule for new consults, or (3) the patient's specialty physician with whom an established relationship already exists. In the last-named situation, a phone call between the ED clinician and subspecialist generally addresses care and follow-up arrangements. An urgent subspecialty condition (i.e., gastroenterologist to manage an acute GI bleed) generally will result in the patient being admitted or transferred to a tertiary hospital. For nonurgent matters, a patient may be recommended to follow up with their primary care physician or referred for subspecialist outpatient consultation. Presently, the need for an audio-video conference between the patient in the ED and the subspecialist remains underexplored and underutilized.

Telemedicine has been used by clinicians to circumvent subspecialty physician shortages in communities that cannot attract or support a subspecialist (Rheuban, 2006). This application improves patient access to specialty care and may impact outcome. It allows patients to be seen promptly and without requiring either clinician or patient to travel.

An example of a successful specialty telemedicine consult from the ED is the telestroke system, which permits urgent remote evaluation of the patient by a specialized neurologist or strokeologist, who can expedite and supervise thrombolytic treatment or make a decision for urgent transfer to a stroke center (Demaerschalk et al., 2009). Telestroke improves the quality of care administered to acute stroke patients admitted to a community hospital and reduces the number of interhospital transfers (Zerna, Jeerakathil, & Hill, 2018; see Chapter 8 for more detail).

Here we present use cases to illustrate how subspecialty telehealth to the ED can impact care and outcome.

CASE STUDY 1: UPPER GI BLEED

A 35-year-old man presents to the ED with complaints of epigastric pain and melena for two days. He denies vomiting, hematemesis, dizziness, fatigue, chest discomfort, or shortness of breath. His past medical history is significant for chronic lower back pain, for which he takes ibuprofen daily. On examination, he appears alert and oriented with normal vital signs. Abdominal examination reveals mild tenderness in the epigastrium. The values in the comprehensive metabolic panel and lipase level are within normal limits. The complete blood count (CBC) reveals mild microcytic, hypochromic anemia (H/H: 11.2/36). Fecal occult blood tests positive, while a nasal gastric aspirate tests negative for blood.

The most likely diagnosis in this case is peptic ulcer disease secondary to chronic non-steroidal anti-inflammatory drug (NSAID) use. The ED clinician generally decides whether the patient requires in-patient admission versus outpatient follow-up to perform an endoscopy. The novel use of video capsule endoscopy (VCE) by ED physicians can improve the ability to detect active bleeding lesions and risk stratify patients. The diagnostic accuracy of VCE is comparable to

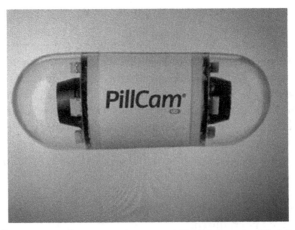

Figure 12.1 PillCam ™ capsule, 11mmx 26 mm. ©2020 Medtronic. All rights reserved. Used with the permission of Medtronic.

that of an esophagogastroduodenoscopy (EGD). Additionally, VCE offers several advantages, including a shorter learning curve, being a noninvasive procedure, and excellent tolerance in cases of active bleeding. This technology extends health care services to remote communities that have limited access to gastroenterologists by transmitting the video generated electronically to a secure cloud for remote interpretation by the gastroenterologist. Tele-interpretation of VCE represents cutting-edge work being undertaken at George Washington University (Meltzer et al., 2013). After the patient swallows the capsule, an on-call gastroenterologist reads the video in real time, evaluating for any active bleeding lesions in the stomach or small bowel that may require admission. This remote diagnostic modality could allow the patient to be safely discharged home with plans for out-patient follow-up endoscopy after a period of appropriate observation with medication changes (Figure 12.1).

CASE STUDY 2: FEVER AND SKIN LESIONS IN A RETURNED TRAVELER

A 47-year-old man who returned one week ago from South Africa presents to an ED in southern Virginia with a fever and rash over his left lower leg. These symptoms started three days after returning home and today are accompanied by headache and arthralgia. While traveling he went on safari and wildlife walks, on which he wore long trousers and hiking boots. He did not have direct contact with any of the animals and does not remember any specific insect bites. He took malaria prophylaxis throughout the trip. In the ED, he is febrile to 38.7°C with otherwise normal vital signs, appearing fatigued, mildly ill but nontoxic. Physical exam is remarkable only for two discrete raised skin lesions with some associated induration (Figures 12.2A and 12.2B). Blood work shows mild leukopenia, mild transaminitis, and mild thrombocytopenia. A malaria smear was performed and was negative. An infectious disease (ID) specialist teleconsultation is requested.

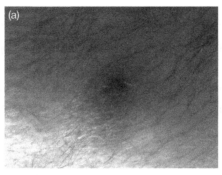

Figure 12.2A Skin lesion #1 in a febrile patient returning from South Africa

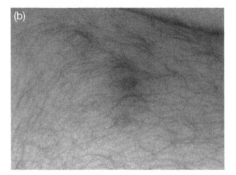

Figure 12.2B Skin lesion #2 in a febrile patient returning from South Africa

A real-time video or asynchronous image transfer allows the travel medicine or ID consultant to view the skin lesions. The patient's travel history, clinical presentation, and the characteristic eschar suggest a tick bite. In this particular case, asking for, finding, and seeing the eschars played a key role in making a diagnosis and recommending appropriate treatment. The specialist presumptively diagnoses the patient with African Tick Bite Fever due to *Rickettsia africae* and recommends starting the patient on oral doxycycline. The patient is instructed to follow up in three days, saving an observation admission.

CASE STUDY 3: PERITONEAL DIALYSIS CATHETER MALFUNCTION

A 56-year-old woman presents to the ED with complaints of leakage from her peritoneal dialysis catheter. She has end-stage renal disease from long-standing poorly controlled hypertension and started peritoneal dialysis about one year ago. She performs daily overnight peritoneal dialysis with a cycler. While sleeping, she was awakened by wet pajamas and bed sheets. Her peritoneal dialysis (PD) catheter was wet to touch. Concerned, she disconnected herself from the dialysis machine and went to the nearest ED.

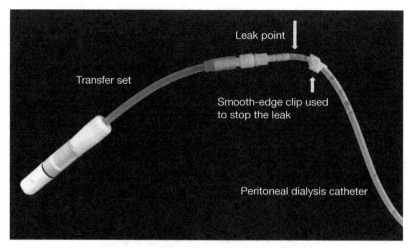

Figure 12.3 The leak point and proximally placed smooth-edge clip on a peritoneal dialysis catheter to stop the leakage

In the ED, she has stable vital signs, and physical examination is unremarkable. The PD catheter has a bead of fluid forming on the outside of the catheter and dripping off. The ED clinician diagnoses a leak in the PD catheter and plans admission for replacement. The patient, however, insists that before anything occurs, her nephrologist needs to be notified.

A telehealth consultation with video allows the nephrologist to observe the PD catheter leakage. The leakage is noted near the connection between the catheter and the transfer set. The nephrologist requests the ED clinician to place a no-teeth clamp proximal to the leak to stop the leakage. Alternatively, it is suggested to bend the catheter back on itself, proximal to the leak and secure it with tape or a rubber band. After brief observation, the nephrologist suggests discharging the patient to the peritoneal dialysis unit (PDU) later that morning. In the PDU, the PD nurse cuts the catheter with a sterile scissors proximal to the leak to obtain a new blunt edge and attaches a new transfer set after sterilizing the catheter tip with bleach per protocol.

Pin holes in the catheter occur in areas of high stress or frequent bending. This patient routinely bent the catheter back on itself to secure the tip under her bra to hold it in place. The telehealth encounter offered treatment options for PD catheter leakage without surgery or PD days lost awaiting a new catheter implantation. The telehealth encounter can facilitate outpatient dialysis care without interruption (Figure 12.3).

CASE STUDY 4: EVALUATION OF WEAKNESS

A 58-year-old female presents with sudden-onset mild right arm and leg weakness 20 minutes prior to arrival in a small rural hospital ED. She had difficulty speaking when she called 911. On arrival in the ED, her speech is slightly slurred, and she indicates her weakness is getting better but not normal. A telestroke consult is requested for possible administration of thrombolytics. Her BP is 170/100, and the CT scan and blood glucose are normal. The strokologist notes that the slurred speech and weakness are resolving during the encounter. By the end of the examination, the patient only has some very mild sensory deficit in the right upper and lower extremity; all other symptoms have cleared. The patient affirms that her remaining symptoms are not disabling and are merely a bit annoying. Thrombolytics are not recommended. With precise instructions from the strokologist, the patient is admitted by the hospitalist at the rural site for TIA/mild stroke workup and for initiation of secondary stroke prevention, including blood pressure management. MRI showed a small infarct in the left basal ganglia, while telemetry showed intermittent periods of atrial fibrillation. She is discharged three days later with blood pressure and anticoagulation medications. The rural hospital was able to provide and bill for diagnostic and treatment services. The patient was able to remain in her community, close to home, instead of being transported to the comprehensive stroke center 200 miles away.

CONCLUSION

These four cases illustrate how subspecialty telehealth can support treatment and disposition decisions made by emergency clinicians. Typically, this support is provided as an in-person consultation or via telephone; however, these case examples highlight the value of utilizing images and video to augment the consultation. The telestroke model has clearly demonstrated that specialty consultations to the ED can improve access to specialty care for patients, reduce time to consultation, be conducted safely, and improve compliance with treatment guidelines. However, much work remains to be done to further understand the clinical, financial, and satisfaction impacts of supporting teleconsultation to the ED beyond telestroke.

KEY TAKEAWAYS

➢ The use of asynchronous or real-time video consultation by medical specialists in the ED should be considered to augment phone-based communications.
➢ Providing telehealth options for consultants to the ED can reduce travel, reduce time to consult, and improve access to specialists.
➢ A telehealth consult can be used to provide care to new as well as established patients.
➢ Telehealth subspecialty consultation from the ED has unexplored potential, and its utilization may evolve with changing care models, payment structure, and transition or coordination of care.

REFERENCES

Demaerschalk, B. M., Miley, M. L., Kiernan, T. E., et al. (2009). Stroke telemedicine. *Mayo Clinic Proceedings*, 84: 53–64.

Meltzer, A. C., Ali, M. A., Kresiberg, R. B., et al. (2013). Video capsule endoscopy in the emergency department: A prospective study of acute upper gastrointestinal hemorrhage. *Annals of Emergency Medicine*, 61(4): 438–443.

Rheuban, K. S. (2006). The role of telemedicine in fostering health-care innovations to address problems of access, specialty shortages and changing patient care needs. *Journal of Telemedicine and Telecare*, 12(Suppl. 2): S45–50.

Zerna, C., Jeerakathil, T., & Hill, M. D. (2018). Telehealth for remote stroke management. *Canadian Journal of Cardiology*, 34: 889–896.

13

Telemedicine in the Surgical Disciplines

ARIEL SANTOS, DAVIN T. COMBS, YASSER AJABNOOR, AND CAMERON ONKS ∎

INTRODUCTION

Surgical telemedicine provides specialized care in medically underserved areas and facilitates intervention for time-sensitive surgical conditions such as leg ischemia, ischemic bowel, acute compartment syndrome and traumatic injuries. Recently, both synchronous and asynchronous telemedicine has captured the attention of surgeons as an alternative to the traditional clinic visit for low-complexity surgical care. Virtual visits offer patients several advantages. The University of Michigan finds that video visits of established patients are 72% shorter compared to standard established patient office visits (82 minutes vs 23 minutes, $p <0.001$) (Ellimootil & Boxer, 2018). The development and expansion of platforms for the delivery of virtual services and the resultant increase in capacity and readiness to sustain telemedicine might be a positive unintended consequence of population-wide social distancing due to COVID-19 (Hakim et al., 2020)). An online crowd source survey showed a high level of enthusiasm and acceptability, especially for noncomplex surgical consultations (Sorensen et al., 2020). If expanded telemedicine services are to persist beyond the pandemic, their impact and potential integration in the current surgical practice need to be evaluated as we gain more experience in technology-enabled surgical care.

Telemedicine technologies are used in preoperative, intraoperative and postoperative evaluations. During the COVID crises, telemedicine played an important role in providing surgical education, mentoring, preceptorship, and continuing medical education. Numerous surgical disciplines such as general surgery, trauma, and acute care surgery, burn management, plastic surgery, thoracic and cardiovascular surgery, pediatric surgery, colorectal surgery, endocrine surgery, orthopedic surgery, neurosurgery, urology, surgical oncology, and global surgery have all used and found utility in telehealth. There are also numerous studies on the implementation of artificial intelligence technology in surgery and surgical decision making. Teleconferencing, which falls under the umbrella of telehealth has been a great tool in specialty surgical consultation as well as in multidisciplinary conferences and tumor boards.

Telemedicine Applications in Surgical Practice

Telemedicine is an increasingly effective tool for providing pre- and postoperative care to surgical patients. It is a vital service to many who may find in-person clinical services prohibitive due to residence in distant or rural locations, difficulty in finding child care, inability to take off from work, health care provider shortages, transport logistics challenges, poor health state precluding long trips, and the cost of travel.

The use of telemedicine in pre- and postoperative care is associated with increased patient satisfaction, reduced hospital transfers, and decreased use of specialty services, while also providing access to specialty care and increasing opportunities for a multidisciplinary team approach. (Gunter et al., 2018; Miller et al., 2018) Preoperatively, telemedicine is an effective tool for making accurate diagnoses and treatment plans (Robie et al., 1998) Telemedicine can also reduce unnecessary hospital transfers for surgical subspecialties available at tertiary centers (e.g., neurosurgery and hand surgery), in fact, in 2014 it led to a 30% decrease in the rate of hand trauma transfers to the University of Arkansas for Medical Sciences (Wongworawat et al., 2017). Postoperatively, telemedicine can increase the catchment area for surgical services by improving patient satisfaction through access to safe and effective postdischarge or follow-up care for patients living in remote locations (Costa et al., 2015; Urquhart et al., 2011). It can also be an important tool for patient monitoring and early intervention for surgical complications. Furthermore, telemedicine can generally improve access to surgical health care, especially among underserved populations (Asiri et al., 2018).

PREOPERATIVE APPLICATIONS

For certain surgical subspecialties (e.g., plastic surgery, trauma/burn surgery, orthopedics, and neurosurgery), preoperative consultations are largely dependent on visual impressions and images; these include physical patient presentation, radiographs, and other readily transmissible data points such as laboratory values and vital signs. For patient cases that are primarily informed by these sources, telemedicine offers timely and accurate consultation in emergency department (ED) settings (Paik et al., 2017). Most of the preoperative questions and evaluations can be completed by the virtual surgeon consulting in the ED. This prevents unnecessary visits to tertiary care centers, can save time, and reduces the number of missed workdays (Asiri et al., 2018). Moreover, specialist job satisfaction may be higher when the option of utilizing telehealth is available (Postuma & Loewen, 2005). Preoperative activities such as reasons for referral, review of past medical history, initiation and review of workup, discussion of treatment options, risks and benefits of surgical treatment, explanation of the technical components of surgery, and follow-up can be adequately done virtually. Furthermore, initial tests and imaging can conveniently be done at the local hospital while helping small facilities that may be facing financial difficulties. Limitations include the establishment of trust and comfort with the surgeon and less comprehensive physical examination. Telemedicine is widely used in preoperative planning for general surgery, maxillofacial surgery (Wood et al., 2016), plastic and reconstructive surgery (Scerri, 1999), vascular surgery (Hands et al., 2004), bariatric surgery (Sudan et al., 2011), triaging trauma, burns, neurologic and orthopedic injuries (Wallace et al., 2008), endocrine surgery like pheochromocytoma (Heslin et al., 2019), neonatal and pediatric surgical consultation and operative planning, and global or overseas surgery (Robie et al., 1998).

INTRAOPERATIVE APPLICATIONS

Rapid growth has taken place in the use of robotic or robot-assisted surgery, given the ergonomic benefits for the surgeon and the advantages of a quicker recovery and smaller incisions for patients from minimally invasive procedures (Wee et al., 2020). Telesurgery or remote surgery is the use of wireless technology and remote-controlled robotic technology in operations to allow surgeons to operate on patients who are at a different physical location than the surgeon, which offers numerous benefits and might be the future of surgery (see Box 13.1; Choi et al., 2018). While intraoperative applications are seemingly not immediately applicable to the ED, given the expanding use of telesurgery, it may be expected that patients experiencing perceived or real complications of their procedure may not be able to resolve these issues via telefollow-up. They will by necessity often be directed to the closest ED where the clinician on duty will have to work up the patient and then consult with the remote surgeon. A basic familiarity of telesurgery by ED staff will greatly facilitate patient care. The telesurgeon may also guide the bedside clinician through procedures to better stabilize a patient who is experiencing unavoidable delays in transport to the higher-level facility.

While telesurgery was conceptualized in the 1970s by NASA and a transatlantic cholecystectomy operation was conducted in 2001 by Dr. Jacques Marescaux who was in New York City while operating on a patient in Strasbourg, France (Marescaux et al., 2002), currently, work in this surgical field has come to a halt. The industry awaits optimization of visual displays, latency time and haptic feedback technologies, design and publication of further randomized controlled trials, and minimization of the factors that limit its clinical translation. (Choiet al. 2018). Notwithstanding this

---

Box 13.1

FUTURE BENEFITS OF TELESURGERY

Reach medically underserved locations such as rural areas, battlefields, submarines and spacecraft.
Eliminates long-distance travel and associated financial burdens and/or dangers.
Allow for multi-surgeon collaborations utilizing 3-dimensional display systems.
Allows for collaboration amongst surgeons at different medical centers in real-time.
Operator's physiologic tremor can be counteracted in real-time with accelerometer technology improving surgical accuracy and reducing damage to adjacent healthy tissues which leads to faster patient recovery.

---

delay, the current technology can find applications for intraoperative consultations as well as for education of surgical residents and medical students without crowding the operating theater. These technologies can also be potential tools for operating on patients with contagious diseases while conserving personal protective equipment.

POSTOPERATIVE APPLICATIONS

Telemedicine in postoperative care has demonstrated excellent clinical outcomes, enhanced patient satisfaction, increased accessibility while reducing wait times, and imparted cost savings to patients and health care systems. Numerous reports show the benefits of telemedicine in postoperative follow-up after surgical procedures such as in parathyroidectomy (Urquhartet al. 2011), cleft lip and palate repair (Costa et al., 2015), colostomy or ileostomy care (Bednarskiet al.2018), and general wound care (Gunter et al., 2018).

In general surgery and other subspecialties with low complication rates, telemedicine is a safe and effective follow-up platform. Clinical results are similar between telemedicine and in-person follow-up visits. Patient satisfaction is high in studies examining postoperative use of telemedicine; however, the patient's ability to successfully navigate technology platforms is a challenge to visit completion (Forbes et al., 2020). Unique to telemedicine postoperative services is the opportunity for the surgeon to provide, train, and test technology with the patient prior to surgery to ensure they can use the technology after surgery. This is of particular importance for patients with limited technological literacy.

Unique to telemedicine postoperative services is the opportunity for the surgeon to provide, train, and test technology with the patient prior to surgery to ensure they can use the technology after surgery.

The use of telemedicine in postoperative settings can be generally divided into three categories: (1) follow-up (Hwa & Wren, 2013), (2) monitoring McGillicuddy et al., 2013), and (3) management of complications (Sidana et al., 2014).

1. Routine Scheduled Follow-up Visits via Telemedicine
   Previous studies have established that telemedicine is a suitable alternative to in-person routine postoperative visits. These studies have explored the efficacy of telephone, video internet conferencing, and instant messaging. Videoconferencing, the technology of choice if available, offers the provider the clearest view of the patient's general condition and surgical site. However, it is important to consider factors that could limit patient access to high-quality video such as restricted access to broadband internet. This is mostly a challenge for rural patients—a population that stands to gain the most through the use of telemedicine. The adoption of smart phones can help reduce the impact of this barrier (Williams et al., 2018).

2. Routine Postoperative Monitoring of the Surgical Patient
   Regular reporting of postoperative symptoms is another effective use of telemedicine in the postoperative setting. Many practices currently use automated telephone surveys or voice only telephone calls to assess complications in patients. Beyond this routine application, telemedicine-based routine monitoring has been effective at assessing key data points in surgery patients (Box 13.2).

The University of Kansas Medical Center's Department of Urology has piloted a telemonitoring program using wearable activity-tracking devices for postcystectomy patients to optimize recovery. In this program, the patients were sent home with software and devices capable of tracking weight, urine output, medication administration, and vital signs (Miller et al., 2018). Telemedicine can also serve as a tool to monitor ileostomy or ostomy output, thus possibly preventing dehydration, acute kidney injury, and possible readmission. Many of these functions are routinely performed by a home-health nurse, but telemedicine is especially effective in routine monitoring when patients lack access to home-health nursing, do not need it for other purposes, or live in geographically remote locations.

The use of telemedicine in these scenarios has repeatedly been shown to enable engagement between patient and provider and empower the patient through increased medical knowledge and information relevant to their self-care. Telemedicine was also demonstrated to be feasible for a variety of patients and for use in a variety of devices—factors that are key to its continued expansion into the treatment of at-risk populations who are disproportionately readmitted to the hospital for preventable causes (Williams, 2018).

3. Management of Postoperative Complications and Triage
   At many institutions in the United States, ED visits within 30 days of an elective procedure are a quality measure assessed by the Centers for Medicare and Medicaid Services (CMS). Postoperative complications are one cause of readmission. Telemedicine offers a platform to proactively manage patients after discharge and prevent costly readmissions for both the patient and the health care system. Risk factors for complications may not be addressable prior to patient discharge, but telemedicine is an effective tool to monitor for potential complications and holds promise for reducing ED utilization (Gillespie et al., 2016). A telemedicine service for the management of postoperative complications should be accessible by patients and be responsive to patient concerns. Considerations to account for in-program design include staffing, reimbursement and physician or advanced practice provider coverage. With good design, a telemedicine program aimed at addressing emerging postoperative complications can drive cost savings for both the patient and the organization.

Box 13.2

COMMON KEY DATA POINTS IN SURGICAL PATIENTS

Colostomy, ileostomy, or ostomy output
Digital imaging to assess patient's wound or surgical site
Medication adherence
Surgical drain output
Vital signs like blood pressure, heart rate, and temperature
Compliance with treatment
Gastrostomy or jejunostomy feeding tube functions

Telemedicine in Trauma

Increasingly, regional trauma centers and EMS providers are employing telemedicine technology, combined with evidence-based practices, in order to reduce response times, decrease costs, and improve outcomes of trauma victims. Implementation of telemedicine technology has been driven by a number of factors, including, but not limited to, public demand for better access and outcomes, improvements in telecommunication technologies, increased awareness of telemedicine as a solution, and the creation of innovative pilot programs such as the Next Generation 9-1-1 Telemedicine Medical Services Pilot Project (NextGen 9-1-1) at the Texas Tech University Health Sciences Center's F. Marie Hall Institute for Rural and Community Health.

In response to the implementation of telemedicine technologies, health care providers have had to rethink how to perform the primary and secondary evaluation of the patient. While the primary evaluation remains largely unchanged, the secondary evaluation can now be performed jointly by the originating site provider (often EMS personnel) and the distant site provider using telemedicine technology. Whereas the traditional primary and secondary evaluations are usually performed by a single individual, when making telemedicine-enabled evaluations, interprofessional team-based care is not only possible, it is highly encouraged. The originating site provider and the distant site provider are able to jointly review the findings of the primary and secondary evaluation and arrive at a consensus regarding the patient's condition. Based on the results of these evaluations, the distant site provider gives instructions for care and directs the originating site provider and the patient to the most appropriate source of care.

The NextGen 9-1-1 Telemedicine Medical Services Pilot Project (see Figure 13.1) provides a real-world demonstration of the application of telemedicine technology to the primary and secondary evaluations of the patient as well as the associated benefits. This project seeks:

1. To demonstrate whether telemedicine technology can establish and maintain connectivity between trauma centers in the region and EMS personnel in the field, both while on scene and in transit.
2. To improve patient outcomes by reducing the time between traumatic events and treatment.
3. To enable physicians to observe patients remotely to provide more effective pre-hospital care.
4. To improve communication between regional trauma centers and EMS personnel.
5. To achieve better outcomes and cost savings by directing patients to the most appropriate treatment facilities without prior screening in hospital EDs.

EMS providers who participate in the Next Gen 9-1-1 Project are located in rural counties in West Texas—defined as a county with a population of 50,000 people or fewer. Ambulances are equipped with a SwyMed DOT Telemedicine Backpack (http://swymed.com/dot-telemedicine-backpack/), ruggedized Windows 10 tablet,

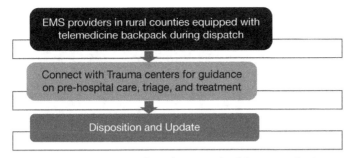

Figure 13.1 Next Generation 9-1-1 Telemedicine Medical Services Pilot Project (NextGen 9-1-1) at the Texas Tech University Health Sciences Center's F. Marie Hall Institute for Rural and Community Health Work flow

Yamaha speaker, PTZ camera, electronic stethoscope, dermatology camera, ultra-sound probe, USB hub, and camera switch. Likewise, participating trauma centers are required to have a trauma designation and are equipped with a tablet, SwyMed software, external speaker, and noise-canceling headphones. EMS providers use the telemedicine backpack to connect to workstations at area trauma centers both while on scene and in transit in order to receive instruction on prehospital care, guidance on treatment, and logistical support from regional trauma center staff.

At St. Michael's Hospital in Toronto, telemedicine was used to triage correct patients to the level 1 trauma center while helping the rural providers with limited trauma experience in resuscitation and performance of potential lifesaving procedures such as intraosseous line access, tube thoracostomy, basic airway management (i.e., endotracheal intubation), and fracture reduction for initial stabilization and eventual transfer (see Figure 13.2). Furthermore, specialists can remotely review laboratory results and radiographic imaging and facilitate transfer for specialized care if needed. Bullard et al. reported that mobile-phone images of CT scans appeared to be sufficient for neurosurgeons to make decisions about their patients and reduced the need to transfer patients from referring hospitals by 30–50% Bullard et al., 2013; Plant et al., 2016).

TELEMEDICINE FOR BURN CARE

There are about 128 trauma burn centers in the United States, yet there are still burn patients with limited access to specialized care due to geographic distribution. Telemedicine technology allows virtual consultation in order to diagnose, assess, stabilize, triage, and treat burn patients. Telemedicine facilitates accurate measurement of burn surface areas, helps guide optimal fluid management, and avoids treatment omissions (Giretzlehner et al., 2014). Teleburn services may lead to significantly different courses of burn care, including appropriately deferring intubation, facilitating correct fluid resuscitation rates, optimizing the route and timing of referral, and correctly triaging and avoiding unnecessary transfer of patients over long distances (Holt et al., 2012). Follow up can also be set up virtually for burn patients living

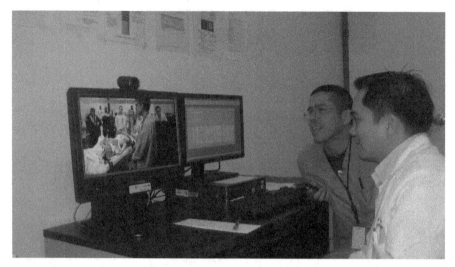

Figure 13.2 Use of telemedicine in real-time resuscitation and triaging of trauma patient at University of Toronto-St. Michael's Hospital

remotely to monitor wound healing, assess mental health, screen for posttraumatic stress disorders, and monitor for contractures and other complications of burn injuries. Physical and occupational therapists may use telemedicine to assess, treat, and rehabilitate the sequelae of burn injuries.

Telehealth Training Applications in Surgical Disciplines

Although telemedicine has great application in surgical fields, completing a physical exam is a big limitation in some telemedicine consultations. Telepresenters can be especially useful in those clinical situations that include assessment of burn wound, postop wound, and surgical drains. They may also be helpful in the assessment of skin and soft tissue infections like cellulitis and abscesses where they evaluate for signs of infections, including skin warmth, swelling, tenderness, and fluctuation. During real-time videoconferencing, telepresenters are needed to perform wound-care, including dressing, redressing, and wound cleaning (Theurer et al., 2016). They may also perform wound debridement, packing removal and repacking, and surgical drain removal under the supervision of the consulting provider (Theurer et al. 2016). Should the real-time video fail for technical reasons, they should be able to capture images of wounds, take measurements, and convey them to the consulting provider (Theurer et al.2016). Staff allocated for the telepresenting role should undergo specific relevant training in order to provide these assessments and assistance. Development of peripherals such as the stethoscope, ultrasound, and cameras can improve the physical examination, but it is limited by lack of olfactory and tactile findings. Eliciting peritoneal signs virtually is especially challenging but can be overcome by effective teamwork between the provider and site presenter.

CONCLUSION

Adoption of telemedicine in the surgical field is still evolving. Telemedicine services can be implemented in various surgical disciplines, including preoperative, intraoperative, and postoperative care. Telesurgery can be utilized in the ED in early diagnosis, triaging of trauma and burn patients, decreasing unnecessary transfers, as well as guiding providers with limited trauma experience in providing life-saving procedures. Telemedicine can provide solutions to physician shortages, and its wide adoption can improve surgical outcomes, increase physician productivity and satisfaction, and improve the patient's experience. Adoption of interstate licensure compacts may further increase the utility of surgical telemedicine and maximize its potential to provide health care access and promote health care equity. Appropriately used, telemedicine can potentially help prevent burnout by helping to create health care efficiency.

KEY TAKEAWAYS

➢ Surgical telemedicine can be incorporated into patient care via video visits, emergency and nonemergent teleconsultation, telerounding, intraoperative consultation, and even in surgical education and surgical mentoring.

➢ Telesurgery can play an important role in the triaging and management of postoperative complications and in preventing unnecessary ED visits.

➢ Telesurgery can be utilized in early assessment, triaging, and stabilization of trauma and burn patients, particularly the management of fluids, including crystalloids, blood products, thrombotic agents like tranexamic acid, and antibiotics.

➢ Telesurgeons can assist less experienced clinicians with infrequently performed resuscitative procedures, such as intraosseous line access, tube thoracostomy, basic and advanced airway management, and fracture reduction.

➢ Telesurgery is associated with increased patient satisfaction, reduced hospital transfers, and decreased use of specialty services. It is excellent for patients living far away from ready surgical access.

REFERENCES

Asiri, A., AlBishi, S., AlMadani, W., ElMetwally, A., & Househ, M. (2018). The use of telemedicine in surgical care: A systematic review. *Acta Inform Med.*, 26(3): 201–206.

Bednarski, B. K., Slack, R. S., Katz, M., You, Y. N., Papadopolous, J., Rodriguez-Bigas, M. A., et al. (2018). Assessment of ileostomy output using telemedicine: A feasibility trial. *Diseases of the Colon & Rectum.*, 61(1): 77–83.

Bullard, T. B, Rosenberg, M. S., Ladde, J., Razack, N., Villalobos, H. J., & Papa, L. (2013). Digital images taken with a mobile phone can assist in the triage of neurosurgical patients to a level 1 trauma centre. *Journal of Telemedicine and Telecare*, 19(2): 80–83.

Choi, P. J., Oskouian, R. J., & Tubbs, R. S. (2018). Telesurgery: Past, present, and future. *Cureus*, 10(5): e2716.

Costa, M. A., Yao, C. A., Gillenwater, T. J., Taghva, G. H., Abrishami, S., Green, T. A., et al. (2015). Telemedicine in cleft care: Reliability and predictability in regional and international practice settings. *Journal of Craniofacial Surgery*, 26(4): 1116–1120.

Ellimoottil, C., & Boxer, R. J. (2018). Bringing surgical care to the home through video visits. *JAMA Surgery*, 153(2): 177–178.

Forbes, R. C., Solorzano, C. C., & Concepcion, B. P. (2020). Surgical telemedicine here to stay: More support from a randomized controlled trial on postoperative surgery visits. *American Journal of Surgery*, 219(6): 880–881.

Gillespie, S. M., Shah, M. N., Wasserman, E. B., Wood, N. E., Wang, H., Noyes, K., et al. (2016). Reducing emergency department utilization through engagement in telemedicine by senior living communities. *Telemed J E Health*, 22(6): 489–496.

Giretzlehner, M., Dirnberger, J., Owen R., Haller H. L., Lumenta D. B., & Kamolz, L. P. (2014). The determination of total burn surface area: how big is the difference? *Burns,* 40(1): 170–171.

Gunter, R. L., Fernandes-Taylor, S., Rahman, S, Awoyinka, L., Bennett, K. M., Weber S. M., et al. (2018). Feasibility of an image-based mobile health protocol for postoperative wound monitoring. *Journal of American College of Surgeons*, 226(3): 277–286.

Hakim, A. A., Kellish, A. S., Atabek, U., Spitz, F. R., & Hong, Y. K. (2020). Implications for the use of telehealth in surgical patients during the COVID-19 pandemic. *American Journal of Surgery*, 220(1): 48–49.

Hands, L. J., Jones, R. W., Clarke, M., Mahaffey, W., & Bangs, I. (2004). The use of telemedicine in the management of vascular surgical referrals. *Journal of Telemedicine and Telecare*, 10 (Suppl 1): 38–40.

Heslin, M. J., Liles, J. S., & Moctezuma-Velazquez, P. (2019). The use of telemedicine in the preoperative management of pheochromocytoma saves resources. *Mhealth*, 5: 27.

Holt, B., Faraklas, I., Theurer, L., Cochran, A., & Saffle, J. R. (2012). Telemedicine use among burn centers in the United States: A survey. *Journal of Burn Care Research* 33(1): 157–162.

Hwa, K., &Wren S. M. (2013). Telehealth follow-up in lieu of postoperative clinic visit for ambulatory surgery: results of a pilot program. *JAMA Surgery*, 148(9): 823–827.

Marescaux, J., Leroy, J., Rubino, F., Smith, M., Vix, M., Simone, M., et al. Transcontinental robot-assisted remote telesurgery: Feasibility and potential applications. *Annals of Surgery*, 235(4): 487–492.

McGillicuddy, J. W., Gregoski, M. J., Weiland, A. K., Rock, R. A., Brunner-Jackson, B. M., Patel, S. K., et al. (2013). Mobile health medication adherence and blood pressure control in renal transplant recipients: A proof-of-concept randomized controlled trial. *JMIR Research Protocols* 2(2): e32.

Miller, A., Rhee, E., Gettman, M., & Spitz, A. (2018). The current state of telemedicine in urology. *Medical Clinics of North Ame*rica, 102(2): 387–398

Paik, A. M., Granick, M. S., & Scott, S. (2017). Plastic surgery telehealth consultation expedites emergency department treatment. *Journal of Telemedicine and Telecare*, 23(2): 321–327.

Plant, M. A., Novak, C. B., McCabe, S. J., & von Schroeder, H. P. (2016). Use of digital images to aid in the decision-making for acute upper extremity trauma referral. *Journal of Hand Surgery (European volume)*, 41(7): 763–768.

Postuma, R., & Loewen, L. (2005). Telepediatric surgery: Capturing clinical outcomes. *Journal of Pediatric Surgery*, 40(5): 813–818.

Robie, D. K., Naulty, C. M., Parry, R. L., Motta, C, Darling, B., Micheals, M., et al. (1998). Early experience using telemedicine for neonatal surgical consultations. *Journal of Pediatric Surgery*, 33(7): 1172–1176; discussion 7.

Scerri, G. V., & Vassallo, D. J. (1999). Initial plastic surgery experience with the first telemedicine links for the British forces. *British Journal of Plastic Surgery*, 52(4): 294–298.

Sidana, A., Noori, S., & Patil, N. (2014). Utility of smartphone camera in patient management in urology. *Canadian Journal of Urology*, 21(5): 7449–7453.

Sorensen, M. J., Bessen, S., Danford J., Fleischer C., & Wong S. L. (2020). Telemedicine for surgical consultations—Pandemic response or here to stay?: A report of public perceptions. *Annals of Surgery*, 272(3): e174–e180.

Sudan, R., Salter, M., Lynch, T., & Jacobs, D. O. (2011). Bariatric surgery using a network and teleconferencing to serve remote patients in the Veterans Administration Health Care System: feasibility and results. *American Journal of Surgery*, 202(1): 71–76.

Theurer L, Bashshur R, Bernard J, Brewer T, Busch J, Caruso D, Coccaro-Word B, Kemalyan N, Leenknecht C, McMillan LR, Pham T, Saffle JR, Krupinski EA.(2017). American Telemedicine Association Guidelines for Teleburn. *Telemedicine and e-Health*, 23(5): 365–375.

Urquhart, A. C., Antoniotti, N. M., & Berg, R. L. (2011). Telemedicine—An efficient and cost-effective approach in parathyroid surgery. *Laryngoscope*, 121(7): 1422–1425.

Wallace, D. L., Jones, S. M., Milroy, C., & Pickford, M. A. (2008). Telemedicine for acute plastic surgical trauma and burns. *Journal of Plastic, Reconstructive & Aesthetic Surgery*, 61(1): 31–36.

Wee, I. J. Y., Kuo, L. J., & Ngu, J. C. (2010). A systematic review of the true benefit of robotic surgery: Ergonomics. *The International Journal of Medical Robotics and Computer Assisted Surgery*, 16(4):e2113.

Williams, A. M., Bhatti, U. F., Alam, H. B., & Nikolian, V. C. (2018). The role of telemedicine in postoperative care. *Mhealth*, 4: 11.

Wongworawat, M. D., Capistrant, G., & Stephenson, J. M. (2017). The opportunity awaits to lead orthopaedic telehealth innovation: AOA critical issues. *Journal of Bone and Joint Surgery. American Volume*, 99(17): e93.

Wood, E. W., Strauss, R. A., Janus, C., & Carrico, C. K. (2016). The use of telemedicine in oral and maxillofacial surgery. *Journal of Oral and Maxillofacial Surgery*, 74(4): 719–728.

14

Pediatric Emergency Telehealth

KYLIE TAYLOR AND AMEER MODY ■

INTRODUCTION

Various iterations of telemedicine have been used for decades. Widespread use in the pediatric population has only recently been adopted, despite its potential for positive impact on pediatric care. The American Academy of Pediatrics (AAP) has stated that telemedicine could mitigate access barriers to and improve availability of pediatric-trained providers to underserved and remote regions. During the COVID-19 pandemic, pediatric telemedicine rapidly expanded and proved its value for patients, providers, and health care systems. This chapter discusses the significance of Pediatric Emergency Telehealth (PET), addresses barriers, and identifies clinical components unique to the pediatric population and the operationalization of a PET program.

Benefits of PET

PET can increase access to pediatricians who provide pediatric-specific emergency care as an adjunct to in-person care or as direct service to patients and families. The majority of pediatric injuries and illnesses are low acuity, and while stressful for families, many of these complaints are appropriate for telehealth visits that may allow for directly managing care or triage to the appropriate resource. Minor injuries tend to occur outside of primary care office hours, often making an emergency department (ED) visit the most convenient option for families. A focused remote visit can provide reassurance and appropriate anticipatory guidance. PET has the capacity to provide support and quality care to settings that lack clinicians with specialty training, such as community and rural hospital EDs that serve both adult and pediatric populations (Ray & Miller, 2020). One study investigated the effectiveness of a PET program operated by a large teaching hospital and reviewed 200 PET consultations. They found that 71% of patients were able to remain at the location where they initially presented for care, while only 29% of patients experienced a transfer to the PET site and change in treatment plan (Foster, 2020).

PET Models

There are a variety of uses and types for standard PET with special considerations during a pandemic. The most commonly used type is a visit initiated by a parent/caregiver or an adolescent as an adjunct service provided by a pediatric emergency department (PED) or urgent care center. This direct-to-patient service modality of telehealth extends the typical reach of a PED caring for low-acuity patients who cannot access their primary care physician, triaging patients who may require an ED visit, or facilitating access for adolescents and young adults in a confidential manner.

A remote health care facility or provider may also request PET services for consultation, subspecialty recommendations, or triage services. PET consultations are typically provided by an academic children's hospital setting. Triage services may be provided by a hospital interdisciplinary access center, PET physician, or pediatric nurse practitioner in the ED. This may be particularly useful in rural regions where access is limited due to geography and lack of physicians (Ray et al., 2015). In addition, pediatric patients who present to community hospital EDs with extraordinarily rare diagnoses like genetic syndromes or organ transplant and require tertiary care may benefit from access to PET. Pediatric tertiary care centers that provide telehealth to bordering states need to be cognizant of cross-state practice issues, like licensure and malpractice coverage.

PET may be used for PED follow-up visits when a primary care clinic is not available. Although this is not the traditional role for a PED, it may serve to improve access and prevent exacerbation of chronic illness or poor outcomes due to lack of access to care. During the COVID-19 pandemic, the AAP encouraged pediatric telehealth for a number of reasons, including family fear of presenting to pediatrician's office or ED due to risk of exposure (AAP Committee on Pediatric Workforce, 2015). Recent data from a study in Italy during the early months of the COVID-19 pandemic demonstrated a 73–88% decrease in pediatric ED visits due to fear. This study cited several cases of children with poor outcomes related to delays in seeking medical care—for example, children in severe diabetic ketoacidosis with the new onset of type 1 diabetes. Although their parents had recognized the classic symptoms of polyuria and polydipsia for several days, fear of exposure delayed seeking medical attention. Other children, with 5–7 days of fever, whose families avoided medical care, were noted to have severe bacterial pneumonias and pyelonephritis, requiring more aggressive treatment due to initial avoidance of the ED (Lazzerini et al., 2020). Barriers to PET include primary care offices lacking capacity to implement telehealth services on such short notice and low-income families lacking access to the technology required to participate in telehealth visits (AAP Committee on Pediatric Workforce, 2015).

Operationalizing PET

Launching PET requires important considerations for training, the care of adolescents, and billing. The process requires a multidisciplinary team that includes hospital administrators, community stakeholders, pediatric emergency staff, clerical staff, IT support, and billing resources. Quality improvement methods may be used to train staff and implement telehealth programs (Rosenthal, 2020). Training may include web-based courses, job aids available for online reference, in-person training, and real-time instruction by staff identified as superusers during the provider's shift. A key point of consideration for EDs and urgent care centers is whether to integrate telehealth services into the workflow of providers on shift seeing in-person visits or to create a separate work designation for telehealth providers. This decision will be largely affected by the ED census, the staffing model, and the demand for virtual services. At the initiation of PET services, it may be feasible to designate a provider on shift to field and perform the telehealth visits. As the program grows, demand for services may increase, and a dedicated telehealth shift clinician would be warranted. An alternative to the immediate access/integrated model would be an appointment-based workflow, similar to clinic visits. The benefits of this type of workflow include setting clear expectations for patients, having the convenience of scheduling for families, and optimizing staffing. Challenges for an appointment-based system include reduced access, depending on hours and potential delays in identifying emergent medical complaints (e.g., a head injury that requires emergent neuroimaging).

Reimbursement for Pediatric Telehealth

Billing and reimbursement often have been a barrier to widespread telehealth use in pediatrics and should be considered in the training and operationalization of a PET program. Federal programs that reimburse equally for pediatric telehealth visits do not exist, whereas adult populations see more standardized reimbursement through programs such as the Veterans Administration and Medicare (Sisk & Alexander, 2020). However, due to the COVID-19 pandemic and increasing support for telehealth from the AAP, reimbursement for pediatric telehealth visits by state programs and private insurers is experiencing an upward trend. Evidence suggests that implementing virtual care modalities may also decrease overall health costs for state or federally funded programs (Rea, Samuels, & Shah, 2020).

PET for Adolescent Patients

PET may provide a unique opportunity to improve care for adolescent patients. Providers must be aware of legislation regarding confidentiality. In many states, adolescents may initiate and attend a health visit without parental consent, if the visit pertains to sexual or mental health. Often, disclaimers accompany these laws, and it is imperative that the telemedicine clinician ensure privacy, with the exceptions of patients' intent to harm others or themselves. Research suggests that adolescents are more inclined to attend a health care visit if they feel their privacy will be maintained (Middleman & Olson, 2020). It has also been suggested that they will be more comfortable using a telehealth platform than an in-person visit, given their high rates of smart phone use, though more studies need to be completed. The Center for Adolescent Health and the Law (www.cahl.org) provides a detailed, state-by-state manual of practice laws that would be useful to organizations interested in starting a PET program (English, Bass, Boyle, & Eshragh, 2010).

PET-supported management of orthopedic injuries

Using PET consultation, a community hospital may manage pediatric orthopedic injuries such as angulated forearm fractures or Type I supracondylar humerus fractures (Woon, Souder, & Skaggs, 2020). These fractures do not require emergent evaluation by a pediatric orthopedist or transfer. They may be immobilized, and follow-up may be conducted in an out-patient orthopedics clinic. Conversely, fractures like Salter-Harris 3 or higher injuries may be misinterpreted as fractures that can be splinted, but in fact they require emergent orthopedic care. Telehealth consultation can provide a valuable backstop for these types of injuries. Similarly, PET can be valuable in collaborative discussions in the evaluation for possible nonaccidental trauma (NAT), for example, finding a spiral fracture on X-ray, which may or may not be NAT. These types of conversations, consultation, and care coordination can improve quality of care and patient safety, and can also provide cost savings. In the event that a patient does need to be transferred, the PET consult can provide guidance regarding stabilizing the patient prior to transfer such as c-spine precautions, fluid or antibiotic recommendations, burn management, and respiratory support.

CASE STUDIES

The following four cases of common medical concerns illustrate safe applications of PET: head injury, vomiting, rash, and ear pain. Note that each case is heavily reliant on taking a careful history looking for key elements. Similar to an in-person encounter, the history is typically more important than the examination. Next is the limited examination with (1) a general observation of the child's behavior and interaction with surroundings and (2) a family member/parent-guided physical examination while watching the response. More telehealth nuances are added to some of the cases. Without getting too far into the medical decision making, which is vital but beyond the scope of this text, we present examples of careful parental education, treatment plans, return precautions, and follow-up instructions, which can be provided virtually.

Head Injury: Although closed head injuries are alarming to parents, many are appropriate for telehealth visits and do not require imaging or intervention. In collaboration with a PET program, a mixed-population community hospital ED or urgent care center can likely reduce radiation exposure, decrease ED wait times, and cost. In this case, we see a three-year-old male who fell while running at the park and sustained a frontal contusion one hour prior to a telehealth call. The patient's mother denies loss of consciousness or vomiting. As the clinician, you are able to see that the child is interactive, his extraocular movements are intact, and mom affirms baseline mental status and denies the presence of nonfrontal scalp hematoma. Given this history and findings that were easily obtained via telehealth, the clinician may use the PECARN (Pediatric Emergency Care Applied Research Network) algorithm to help guide their decision making in identifying clinically significant head injuries (Kuppermann, Holmes, & Dayan, 2009). In this case, the clinician would provide reassurance and anticipatory guidance. Using this same tool in a four-month-old who rolled off the changing table onto hard flooring and sustained occipital scalp swelling, the telehealth clinician would direct the family to bring the patient into the ED for an in-person evaluation and likely radiologic studies.

Vomiting: Vomiting is a common PED complaint with a broad differential diagnosis. Certain red flag symptoms can quickly narrow the differential diagnosis, making it suitable for a PET triage or a completely virtual visit. In most cases, after history taking, clinicians will be able to guide families to assist in completing a physical examination and, if reassuring, provide anticipatory guidance and return precautions. However, vomiting in certain age groups should cause a higher suspicion of abdominal or other emergencies and warrant an ED evaluation.

Consider the case of a seven-week-old, previously healthy male, with a history of "spitting up" reported by patient's father with more frequent forceful vomiting over the past 36 hours, though his appetite remains good. The PET provider can ascertain key findings, including bilious vomiting, weight gain, and frequency of wet diapers to help guide management decisions. The most likely diagnosis is gastroesophageal reflux disease (GERD), and smaller, more frequent feeds may be indicated. However, given the patient's age and sex, pyloric stenosis may be the cause of progressive vomiting and must be ruled out via ultrasound, making an ED visit necessary.

In a 19-month-old with vomiting, a PET clinician will inquire about colicky pain, drawing legs up to the abdomen, or instruct the parent to palpate the abdomen to assess for pain. If present, intussusception may be the cause of the patient's symptoms, and the family should proceed to the ED.

Compared with infants and toddlers, vomiting in adolescents is slightly less concerning, especially given their ability to articulate pain. Certain red flags would warrant an in-person ED visit. These include vomiting that is accompanied by severe headache or early morning headaches that wake the patient from sleep, bilious emesis, and vomiting with unilateral lower quadrant pain.

Rash: Rashes in the pediatric patient are worrisome to parents, but they are rarely serious and can be amenable to telehealth. Consider a six-year-old male who came home from a field trip with what mom describes as "redness and swelling to his right arm and left ankle that is warm to touch." She denies new exposures such as sunscreen, soaps, or other topical products. She also denies trauma, fever, other contacts with the same rash, recent antibiotic use, or recent illness. The PET clinician is able to assess that the child has full range of motion of elbow and wrist and is ambulating well; also, the clinician sees two large areas of erythema without vesicles, scaling, or drainage. Obtaining images, still or video, is tricky, and many images initially provided are often out of focus. Directing bright lighting while minimizing reflection and glare is vital. Figure 14.1 shows multiple insect bites but includes glare on the skin, making it hard to observe the dimension, if any. Figure 14.2 has less light, making it easier to appreciate the raised quality of the lesion, which is also an insect bite.

En-face and tangential angles may be helpful. Using a ruler to measure the size rather than guessing or estimating is helpful for follow-up. Mom reports that the redness is about 5 x 5 cm to the arm and 4 x 4 cm to the ankle. Although these may look cellulitic as they are warm to touch, erythematous, and mildly indurated, a parent can palpate to assist the PET provider in noting whether or not the skin is blanching. If blanching is appreciated and palpation causes no significant discomfort, this helps rule out cellulitis. The presence of blanching erythema and rapid onset confirms

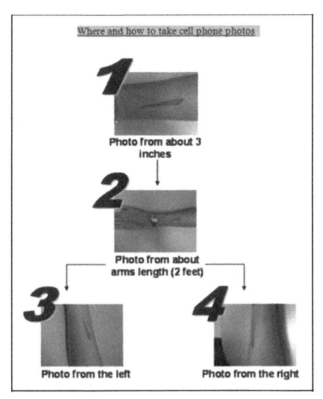

Figure 14.1 Telemed J E Health. 2012 Sep;18(7):554–7. doi: 10.1089/tmj.2011.0216. Epub 2012 Jul 23.PMID: 22823025.

a diagnosis of hypersensitivity reaction secondary to insect bite. Anticipatory guidance is imperative, as a cellulitis may still occur after the visit. Other return precautions specific to rashes include fever and rash for greater than or equal to five days, diffuse erythroderma, desquamation, and purpura (Hoffman & Wang, 2019). Additionally, novel Coronavirus-19 has posed new challenges to rash presentation in the pediatric patient as it may represent Multisystem Inflammatory Syndrome

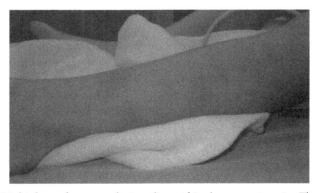

Figure 14.2 Multiple erythematous lesions (insect bites) on an extremity. The glare from excessive lighting creates a difficulty in assessing other qualities of the lesion such as raised, scaling, or vesicular characteristics.

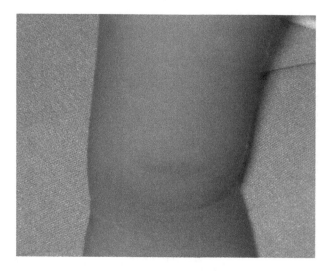

Figure 14.3 Less lighting on the photo of the insect bite allows observation of the raised dimension, central punctate lesion, and clear borders of the lesion. This may require guidance from the provider in assisting the parent or guardian capturing the photo or video for Pediatric Telehealth.

in Children (MIS-C) and should be evaluated with the help of an evidence-based algorithm, usually warranting an ED visit (Nakra, Blumberg, Herrera-Guerra, & Lakshminrusimha, 2020). Finally, rashes in genital or other private areas pose another challenge, including patient permission and archival or disposal of these image files. Processes for such circumstances should be thought out ahead of time. Best practices have not been uniformly disseminated, but it is recommended to use an encrypted, HIPAA compliant telehealth-specific platform.

Ear pain: A chief complaint of ear pain is also suitable for PET with certain clinical presentations. For example, the mother of a three-year-old female initiates a telehealth visit stating that her daughter has a one-day history of cough, congestion, right ear pain, and fever with a maximum temperature of 38.1°C. She denies recent ear infection, otorrhea, or pain, swelling, or redness behind the ear. Without the availability of visual inspection of the tympanic membrane (TM), a telehealth provider might suggest the family come in for a visit or, worse, prescribe an antibiotic without evaluating the TM in person. Although ear pain is a symptom of acute otitis media (AOM), it may be due to other causes such as viral upper respiratory infection, barotrauma from coughing or swimming, or cerumen impaction. Companies such as Tytocare and Cellscope sell devices that capture a picture or video of the ear canal and tympanic membrane that may be shared with the PET provider. These devices may be used by parents and general EDs alike, which may help prevent overuse of antibiotics or help streamline otolaryngology visits instead of the ED.

Ear pain and AOM have historically been overtreated with antibiotics, further contributing to antibiotic resistance (Lieberthal, 2013). The AAP recommends "Watchful Waiting" if the patient meets the following criteria: patient older than 24 months, unilateral ear pain without otorrhea, fever less than 39°C, symptoms present less than 48 to 72 hours, and access to close follow-up. In this case, the patient meets criteria, and pain should be treated with nonsteroidal anti-inflammatory analgesia in the interim. The telehealth provider must instruct the caregiver to follow up with their pediatrician if pain persists past the 48- to 72-hour mark, so the tympanic membrane can be evaluated and appropriate treatments initiated if needed. If that is not possible due to access issues, a safety net antibiotic prescription may be indicated. In the case of an older child who has been swimming and now complains of earache, guiding the parent to push on the tragus or tug gently on the helix and watch for a painful response, while having lack of tenderness over the mastoid, may diagnose a simple otitis externa.

CLINICAL PEARLS FOR PET PROVIDERS

Pediatric Assessment Triangle: Using this rapid evaluation tool, health care providers can reliably decide between acute and nonurgent patients (Horeczko, Enriquez, McGrath, & Gausche-Hill, 2013). In the PET setting, this tool may help clinicians distinguish patients who can remain at home and complete the telehealth visit from those who need emergent evaluation in the ED. The three components of this tool include general appearance, work of breathing, and color/circulation. In the infant/toddler population, it is important to instruct parents to remove extra layers of clothing or blankets in order to assess skin color and for the presence of retractions.

Assessment of Pain/Tenderness: Parents should palpate extremities or abdomen while the child is distracted (reading a book, watching a video, playing with a toy) while the physician assesses for guarding or wincing.

Rash Tips: Instruct parents to palpate to assess for blanching and pain. Instruct parents to expose palms and soles for the PET clinician to inspect.

CONCLUSION

The integration of an emergency telehealth visit into the typical workflow of the ED could be a significant factor in improving multiple issues in pediatric emergency medicine. With appropriate prompts and screening, a family can have their initial triage and registration done remotely, from a general pediatrician's office, a general ED, or home. Wearable technology can potentially allow for the recording of heart rate, temperature, and pulse oximetry. Depending on the remote triage assessment, the patient can be directed to:

1. Call EMS for emergent transport, or
2. Be preregistered, transported by family, and brought immediately to ED room, or
3. Be preregistered at home for direct admit from a community hospital ED. This option may require collaboration with the hospital medicine team, specialty teams, bed supervisor, and PET team. Stable patients suitable for this option could include those who require IV antibiotics or are waiting for surgery such as stable fractures or appendicitis, or

4. Be placed in a virtual waiting room queue by the registration team and have the telehealth visit completed remotely by a PET clinician. This option is available when PET teams offer on-demand services in real time similar to ED arrival, as opposed to scheduled appointments.

To accomplish this degree of integration would require a significant investment in infrastructure but would likely result in improvements in waiting room crowding, patient/family satisfaction, reduced "left without being seen" rates, and improved revenue capture.

KEY TAKEAWAYS

➤ PET is a safe tool to provide timely consultations to clinicians, parents, and adolescents, who may not otherwise have access to these expert resources readily available.

➤ The patient history is the most important element of a PET encounter, often more important than the physical examination.

➤ When assessing for pain and tenderness, parents should palpate extremities or abdomen while the child is distracted at the same time that the physician is watching for guarding or wincing.

➤ When assessing rashes, good lighting and in-focus images are vital. Instruct parents to palpate to assess for blanching and pain. Be sure palms and soles are exposed for inspection.

➤ Rapport is established with the parents through careful listening, good parental education, with simple treatment plans, return precautions, and follow-up instructions.

REFERENCES

AAP Committee on Pediatric Workforce. (2015). The use of telemedicine to address access and physician workforce shortages. *Pediatrics*, 136(1).

English, A., Bass, L., Boyle, A., & Eshragh. (2010, January). *State minor consent laws: A summary*. Retrieved September 10, 2020, from Center for Adolescent Health: https://www.freelists.org/archives/hilac/02-2014/pdftRo8tw89mb.pdf.

Foster, C. (2020). Emergency care connect: Extending pediatric emergency care expertise to general emergency departments through telemedicine. *Academic Pediatrics*, 20(5): 1–8.

Hoffman, R., & Wang, V. (2019). *Fleisher and Ludwigs 5 minute pediatric emergency medicine consult*. Philadephia: Lippincott Williams & Wilkins.

Horeczko, T., Enriquez, B., McGrath, N., & Gausche-Hill, M. L. (2013). The pediatric assessment triangle: Accuracy of its application by nurses in the triage of children. *Journal of Emergency Nursing*, 39(2): 182–189.

Kuppermann, N., Holmes, J., & Dayan, P. (2009). Identification of children at very low risk of clinically important brain injuries after a head trauma: A prospective cohort study. *Lancet*, 374(9696): 1160–1170.

Lazzerini, M., Barbi, E., Andrea, A., et al. (2020). Delayed access or provision of care in Italy resulting from fear of COVID-19. *The Lancet Child and Adolescent Health*, 4(5), e10–e11.

Lieberthal, A. S.(2013). The diagnosis and management of acute otitis media. *Pediatrics*, 131(3): 964–999.

Middleman, A., & Olson, K. (2020, April 7). *Confidentiality in adolescent health care.* Retrieved July 12, 2020, from Up To Date: https://www.uptodate.com/contents/confidentiality-in-adolescent-health-care.

Nakra, N., Blumberg, D., Herrera-Guerra, A., & Lakshminrusimha, S. (2020). Multi-system inflammatory syndrome in children following SARS-CoV2 infection: Review of clinical presentation, hyporthetical pathogenesis and proposed management. *Children*, 7(7): 69.

Ray, K., & Miller, E. (2015). Optimizing telehealth strategies for subspecialty care; recommendations from rural pediatricians. *Telemedicine and e-Heath*, 21(8): 622–629.

Rea, C., Samuels, R., & Shah, S. (2020). Electronic consultation: Latest evidence regarding the impact on referral patterns, patient experience, cost and quality. *Academic Pediatrics*, 20(7): 891–892.

Rosenthal, J. (2020). Testing pediatric telehealth implementation strategies using quality improvement methods. *Telemedicine and e-Health,* 27(4): 459–463.

Sisk, B., & Alexander, J. B. (2020). Pediatrician attitudes toward and experiences with teleheath use; Results from a national survey. *Academic Pediatrics*, 20(5): 628–635.

Woon, C., Souder, C., & Skaggs, D. (2020). *Supracondylar fracture—Pediatric.* Retrieved September 5, 2020, from Ortho Bullets: https://www.orthobullets.com/pediatrics/4007/supracondylar-fracture--pediatric

PART III

Distant Site Services

(Section Editor: Neal Sikka)

15

Teletriage

MATTHEW LAGHEZZA, PETER GREENWALD, ETHAN BOOKER,
DAVID MISHKIN, AND RAHUL SHARMA ■

INTRODUCTION

Triage is not only important to assign treatment priorities, but can be engineered to improve operational efficiency and the patient experience in the emergency department (ED). With telemedicine quickly becoming a mainstream method of health care delivery, many institutions are considering a combination of a provider-in-triage (PIT) model with telemedicine to improve patient throughput. To understand the potential role of telemedicine in this context, it is helpful to first review the history of triage, regulatory parameters, and the provider-in-triage model.

TRIAGE

The notion of triage derives from the French word "trier," meaning "to sort." It was originally applied to a process of medical sorting in the late eighteenth century by Baron Dominique Jean Larrey, Surgeon in Chief to Napoleon's Imperial Guard (Iserson & Moskop, 2007).

The core function of triage at ED arrival is the clinical assessment of the individual's presenting signs and symptoms at the time to prioritize when and by whom the individual will be seen (State Operations Manual, 2019). In the early 1900s, a triage system evolved in emergency departments in the United States, United Kingdom, and Europe, to include a brief clinical assessment that determined the time and sequence in which the patient should receive a complete evaluation due to limited resources. Analogous processes are applied in the prehospital environment to determine the speed of transport and the choice of hospital destination for initial treatment.

In 1999, the Emergency Severity Index (ESI) was developed and is maintained by the Agency for Healthcare Research and Quality (AHRQ). ESI has been widely adopted in the United States as a five-level ED triage algorithm that provides clinically relevant stratification of patients into five groups from 1 (most urgent) to 5 (least urgent) on the bases of acuity and resource needs (Emergency Severity Index, 2018).

ENSURING ACCESS TO EMERGENCY CARE: EMTALA AND ED REGULATION

In 1986, Congress enacted the Emergency Medical Treatment and Labor Act (EMTALA) to prevent the dangerous practice of patient transfers from hospitals based on patients' financial status, a practice that included pregnant women in labor being turned away from EDs and some patients being redirected to charity and public hospitals (Emergency Medical Treatment and Labor Act, 2019). Today, Medicare and Medicaid participating hospitals that offer emergency services are obligated to evaluate patients who present to the ED with a medical screening examination (MSE). MSE is the process required to decide, with "reasonable clinical confidence," whether an emergent medical condition (EMC) exists. Hospitals are also required to provide stabilizing care for the EMC identified regardless of an individual's ability to pay (Emergency Medical Treatment and Labor Act, 2019).

A hospital must formally determine the qualified medical personnel to perform the initial medical screening examinations. While a hospital is permitted to designate a nonphysician practitioner as the qualified medical person, the designated nonphysician practitioners must be identified in a document that is approved by the governing body of the hospital (Emergency Medical Treatment and Labor Act, 2019).

PUBLICLY REPORTABLE QUALITY MEASURES

The Centers for Medicare and Medicaid Services (CMS), a federal agency within the United States Department of Health and Human Services, and the Joint Commission on Accreditation of Healthcare Organizations (JCAHO), an independent not-for-profit organization that certifies health care organizations, are two organizations that rate and evaluate hospitals (The Center for Consumer Information & Insurance Oversight, 2019; The Joint Commission Mission Statement, 2009). Since 2003, CMS and JCAHO have worked to align their evaluations, resulting in a unified set of criteria periodically updated and published as the *Specifications Manual for National Hospital Inpatient Quality Measures* (The Joint Commission Website, 2018). Good (or poor) performance on quality measures has implications for hospital accreditation, public insurance payments, and hospital reputation. Several CMS core quality measures focus on the efficiency and effectiveness of ED care delivery. One example is measure OP-20: "Door to diagnostic evaluation by a qualified medical professional," widely known as "door to provider time." Medicare- and Medicaid-certified hospitals began publicly reporting data on these measures in October 2013 (Hesse et al., May 2017). With these metrics being publicly reported, hospital administrators had to prioritize operational efficiency and develop better systems to reduce this "door to provider time."

EMERGENCY DEPARTMENT VOLUME AND CROWDING

There were 145.6 million ED visits in 2016, which is an increase of 5.6% since 2014 (Sun, Karaca, & Wong, 2018). Increased access to health insurance, decreased avail-ability of primary care providers, and changing societal preferences for immediate care all contribute to this trend (Abdulwahid, Booth, Kubzawski, et al., 2015). While overall ED visits are increasing, the number of EDs has been decreasing. Between 1990 and 2009, there was a 27% decrease in the number of nonrural EDs in the United States, and from 2013 to 2017, rural hospitals closed at a rate nearly double that of the previous five years (Hsia, Kellerman, & Shen, 2011; *Rural Hospital Closures,* 2018). More visits and fewer EDs result in ED overcrowding, which in turn can lead to delays in care, errors, and other negative patient-oriented outcomes (Morley, Unwin, Peterson, Stankovich, & Kinsman, 2018).

The COVID-19 pandemic developed and intensified throughout 2020, resulting in a substantial decrease in ED visits across the country (Hartnett, 2020). With patients not seeking as much emergency care, there has been an increase in the use of telemedicine.

PROVIDER IN TRIAGE AND MEDICAL SCREENING EXAMS

Interventions designed to improve ED efficiency often require additional resources and labor, but they can also include improvements in the sophistication of queuing. One common intervention is the placement of a provider in triage, (the provider in triage, or PIT model) in which a physician or advanced practice provider (APP) is positioned within the intake process to rapidly evaluate patients. The goals of the PIT model can be broken down into four domains:

1. MSE and immediate treatment: Immediate disposition with all evaluation, testing, and disposition (usually discharge) managed by the initial PIT; ensures that all patients arriving to the ED get an MSE (limits opportunity to walk out of ED before MSE performed).
2. Initiation of simple testing and interventions with triage to a low acuity, "fast-track" area.
3. Initiation of diagnostic testing and interventions for patients who are not critically ill but will require comprehensive evaluation and possibly consultation, advanced imaging, and hospitalization.
4. Recognition of the critically ill or emergent patients not identified by the nurse intake process for immediate bypass to comprehensive evaluation.

The PIT model moves the medical screening exam earlier to earlier in the ED pro-cess, resulting in a decreased "door to provider time" and a reduction in the number of patients who leave without being seen.

CASE STUDIES: PROVIDER IN TRIAGE

Presbyterian Hospital Matthews, North Carolina PIT (Love, Murphy, Lietz, & Jordan, 2012)

In 2011, Presbyterian Hospital Matthews placed an APP in triage during high-volume hours, 12 hours per day, 7 days per week. In this model, the triage area was staffed with one APP, one registered nurse, one patient care technician, one phlebotomist/electrocardiogram technician, and one financial registrar. Upon arrival, the APP would initiate MSE and order appropriate radiologic exams and laboratory studies, while the RN would complete the triage. The average door-to-provider time decreased from 75 to 25 min, and the percentage of patients who left without being seen decreased from 3.6% to 0.9%.

Northwestern Delnor Emergency Department PIT (Duarte, 2019)

In 2018, the Delnor Emergency Department placed a nurse practitioner (NP) as an additional provider in the triage process, six hours per day, four days per week, during peak times. In this model, after patients were triaged by an RN, the NP would perform a medical screening exam, order appropriate testing, and patients would either return to the waiting room, be discharged, or wait for an ED bed to become available. Through implementation of the PIT process, the Delnor ED was able to decrease Left Without Being Seen (LWBS) rates by 0.45% and decrease the average door-to-provider time by 30%.

TELEMEDICINE IN TRIAGE: A VARIATION ON THE PIT MODEL

A provider who joins the triage process by telemedicine can provide many of the same services as a face-to-face PIT provider, and potentially do so with some efficiency advantages. By using telemedicine, this provider has the ability to cover more than one ED, making it possible for institutions with lower volume to justify the expense of a PIT provider and for institutions with higher volume to be able to expand PIT hours to off-hour periods, where presentations occur less frequently. In addition, as more institutions adopt telemedicine as part of their health care delivery, there will be opportunities to deploy providers engaged in other telemedicine activities to do PIT between cases in their other telemedicine workflows; such dual usage may help the institution justify having a dedicated telemedicine provider.

IMPLEMENTATION OF TELEMEDICINE IN TRIAGE/MSE BY TELEMEDICINE

Many of the workflow and clinical processes of a teletriage system are the same as in-person PIT processes, but some unique aspects need to be addressed. In what follows, we lay out the fundamental components of a telehealth-enabled provider in the triage process.

Required Technology

An integral part of teletriage is the ability to communicate with both the clinical staff and the patient. This includes being in a private area with a high-quality camera for visualization and a microphone that provides clear audio communication. Audio connections to triage areas can be challenging because these areas often have high ambient noise. Optimizing microphone placement and limiting sound from other areas are essential. Successful systems use triage areas in a room with a closing door on either side.

Communication Devices

In order to provide medical treatment as well as one would in-person, the remote provider has to have a means to communicate with the treatment team that is in-person. This communication should be through HIPAA-secure devices, which allow the provider, who is present by telemedicine, to have close contact with the treatment teams for delivery of time-sensitive information. This is most easily accomplished with mobile devices using either a secure text message or a phone call.

Documentation

The remote provider needs to be able to document in the same medical record that will be visible to the treatment team and also needs to be able to place orders for radiologic exams, laboratory studies, and medications. Standardization of the documentation template, history taking, and exam components of an MSE will ensure more consistent care.

Quality Assurance

All new care pathways require assessment and evaluation. This should follow a rigorous standardized process for review of the telemedicine MSE, including checking the charting for compliance with documentation standards and evaluating the medical care initiated to ensure it is in keeping with local standards. (See Box 15.1.)

CASE STUDIES: TELEMEDICINE TRIAGE

The following institutions all transformed their in-person PIT model into a telemedicine triage as an innovative solution to the rise in volume, so that they could continue to provide compassionate, efficient, and high-quality medical care to ED patients.

Box 15.1

TeleMSE Quality Assurance Grading

Was the approved template used?
Was a chief complaint documented?
Were there two elements of a history of present illness?
Were there two elements of a physical exam?
Were vital signs reviewed/addressed?
Was there an assessment and plan?

TeleMSE Overall Quality Scale

A—appropriate care; no adverse outcome
B—area to improve care; no adverse outcome
C—significant deviation from care standard; possible adverse outcome
D—significant deviation from care standard; adverse outcome
E—care inconsistent with standards; any outcome

Triage/Intake Nurse Advocacy Telepresentation at MedStar Health, DC Metro Area

In September 2016, MedStar Health implemented a teletriage process covering peak volume hours, 11 a.m.–8 p.m. on weekdays. The telemedicine platform allowed for assessments by the telemedicine physician in a designated office within the hospital with audio/video capabilities, as well as ready access to medical records.

A standardized reporting methodology was developed for the triage/intake nurse to communicate via telemedicine video portal with a remote provider. Nurses sent the consult request to the telemedicine physician while still in the process of completing the intake. The nurse provided a summary with the patient name and age, brief description of the HPI, and vital signs. The physician then interviewed the patient for any necessary additional details and ordered appropriate laboratory or radiologic exams. Phone numbers for ED areas and tech support were available for rapid communication or to facilitate the movement of critically ill patients.

A patient advocacy-centered approach for nurse telepresentation incorporates the lessons of bedside reporting, namely, that patient satisfaction can be improved, information can be conveyed succinctly, and provider time can be minimized while employing a technology that brings additional resources to the patient rather than moving them.

MedStar found that in a high-volume, high-acuity, tertiary care ED, a telemedicine model for the physician intake process can positively impact door-to-provider time when compared with traditional physician intake with similar time to disposition decision metrics (Izzo et al., 2018; see Table 15.1).

Table 15.1 Comparing In-Person versus Telemedicine Provider in Triage Models

	Institution	Provider in Triage Process	Schedule	Door-to-Provider Time	Left Without Being Seen
In-Person	Presbyterian Hospital Matthews North Carolina	Upon arrival, the APP would initiate the MSE and order appropriate radiologic exams and laboratory studies, while the RN would complete the triage.	12 hours per day 7 days per week	Average door-to-provider time decreased from 75 min to 25 min	LWBS decreased from 3.6% to 0.9%
	Northwestern Delnor Emergency Department	After patients were triaged, the NP would perform a medical screening exam, order appropriate testing, and patients would either return to the waiting room, be discharged, or wait for an ED bed to become available.	6 hours per day 4 days per week	Decreased average door-to-provider by 30%	Decreased LWBS by 0.45%
Telemedicine	MedStar Health	A standardized reporting methodology was developed for the triage/intake nurse to communicate via telemedicine video portal with a remote provider. Nurses sent the consult request to the telemedicine physician while still in the process of completing the intake.	11 a.m.–8 p.m. Monday–Friday	Decreased from 44min with traditional PIT to 32min with Telemedicine	
	Baptist Hospital of Miami Emergency Department	Nurse would greet the patient and introduce the technology. The physician would receive a summary of the reason for the visit and would then be able to interview the patient for additional details and order appropriate laboratory or radiologic exams.	Covering surge times in 4-hour shifts	Improved door-to-provider times	
	TeleMSE for Ambulance Arrivals Weill Cornell Medicine	The triage nurse, the patient, and emergency medical services staff have a video interaction with the APP through a HIPAA-secure videoconferencing unit physically located at a remote centralized location in the ambulance bay.	10 a.m. – 10 p.m. Monday–Friday	Decreased from 38 min to 4 min for ambulance arrivals	

Teletriage at Baptist Hospital of Miami Emergency Department, Florida

In 2016, Baptist Hospital of Miami started a teletriage process covering surge times in 4-hour shifts. The telemedicine platform allowed for assessments from a designated office within the hospital with audio/video capabilities, as well as ready access to medical records.

The physician worked with the triage nurse, who acted as the catalyst for the program. The nurse would greet the patient, introduce the technology, and make sure that the patient was comfortable using it. The physician would receive a summary of the reason for the visit and would then be able to interview the patient for additional details, if needed, and order appropriate laboratory or radiologic exams.

Teletriage was used for all patients outside of ESI Level I's and was found to be most helpful for patients with chest pain and epigastric pain. Teletriage improved door-to-provider times and received excellent feedback from both patients and providers who participated in the pilot.

New York Presbyterian Weill Cornell Medicine TeleMSE for Ambulance Patients, New York

In 2018, NewYork Presbyterian Weill Cornell started a teletriage process with an APP covering two different EDs during peak arrival hours, 10 a.m.–10 p.m. on weekdays. The telemedicine platform allowed for assessments from a designated office in a remote location outside of the hospital with audio/video capabilities, as well as ready access to medical records.

An APP began performing Telemedicine Medical Screening Exams (TeleMSE) for patients arriving by ambulance using a videoconferencing platform available at two different EDs. In this program, the triage nurse, the patient, and emergency medical services (EMS) staff have a video interaction with the APP through a HIPAA-secure videoconferencing unit physically located at a remote centralized location in the ambulance bay. The APP receives pertinent documents with on-scene information from EMS, as well as any prehospital intervention. A virtual physical exam by visual inspection, sometimes assisted by the triage nurse or EMS provider, is performed via a high-definition camera remotely controlled by the APP. The APP documents this interaction in the electronic medical record and may enter orders such as labs, point-of-care testing, and ECGs, before the patient is transported to the treatment area. For higher-acuity patients, the APP can rapidly place orders for stroke, STEMI, sepsis, or trauma patients and activate the alert that triggers treatment pathways and communicates with care teams through the department's HIPAA-secure process for each of these time-sensitive pathways.

One APP is able to observe two ambulance arrival areas simultaneously and rapidly switch back and forth to interact with patients while RNs and EMS personnel are at both locations. The APP is seeing approximately five patients per hour with a median "door to provider time" of 4 minutes.

FUTURE OF THE TELETRIAGE MODEL

The future of teletriage is closely related to our growing understanding of the strengths and weaknesses of provider-in-triage models. The COVID-19 pandemic presented an opportunity to explore innovative strategies with telemedicine and highlighted the strength of remote patient care. Using a teletriage model during the COVID-19 pandemic allowed providers the opportunity to work remotely, which decreased staff exposures and limited use of PPE while still providing high-quality medical care to patients.

The PIT model can be considered beneficial in three distinct ways: a financial perspective, a quality of care perspective, and a publicly reportable metrics perspective.

FINANCIAL PERSPECTIVE

PIT models allow a medical screening exam to be initiated within the first few minutes of a patient's arrival into the ED. The conversion of LWBS patients to ED visits allows the institution to bill for that part of the ED evaluation, therefore increasing revenue. Health Care Cost Institute (HCCI) analyzed 70 million insurance bills for ED visits for the 2009–2015 period, focusing on the prices that health plans paid hospitals for facility fees. The average ED facility charge was found to be $1,322. The rising ED facility fees coupled with the growing usage of the most expensive codes means it is significantly more expensive to go to an ED now than it was six years ago. (ER facility prices grew in tandem with faster-growing charges from 2009–2016, 2018.) Whether or not the introduction of a PIT system is a net positive for the institution's bottom line depends in part on the institution's LWBS rate.

Considered in this financial context, converting the provider in triage model to one where the provider in triage is present by telemedicine has the advantage of allowing one provider to staff more than one institution, bringing added financial efficiency and making it possible for lower-volume institutions (and higher-volume institutions during off hours) to have a financially justifiable PIT process.

QUALITY PERSPECTIVE

PIT models have been shown in randomized controlled trials to correlate with reduced Length of Stay (LOS), reduced waiting time, and reductions in LWBS rates, although results even in these measures are less clear when all study types are considered, and performance may vary depending on the severity of the patient's illness and the details of the PIT model that was evaluated (Abdulwahid, Booth, Kuczawski, et al., 2016). It is less clear whether the PIT model has any benefit with respect to patient satisfaction or efficiency of resource use.

In a systematic review of PIT model care, 33 studies that included over 800,000 patients in total were reviewed regarding triage-related interventions to improve patient flow in the ED. Results showed that team triage that includes a physician most likely leads to shorter waiting times, shorter lengths of stay, and fewer patients leaving without being seen (Oredsson, Jonsson, Rognes, et al., 2011).

The future of telemedicine triage will require consensus that placing a provider into the triage process provides a similar benefit to in-person PIT. If studies are done demonstrating comparable efficacy and quality between in-person PIT and telemedicine provider in triage, it will be more likely that the telemedicine PIT models will be widely adopted.

PUBLICLY REPORTABLE METRICS PERSPECTIVE

According to the CDC, the national average time to be seen in an ED is between 15 and 59 minutes (National Hospital Ambulatory Medical Care Survey, 2019). In a high-volume, high-acuity, tertiary care ED, a telemedicine model of a physician intake process can positively impact door-to-provider time when compared with traditional physician intake, using similar time to disposition decision metrics (Watson et al., 2017).

Publicly reportable metrics related to ED care include length of stay for both admitted and discharged patients, Left Without Being Seen rate, median time to pain medication for long bone fractures, median time to troponin result for chest pain patients, and median time to provider evaluation (Section 3. Measuring Emergency Department Performance, 2018). How a hospital preforms on these statistics is visible to the public on a variety of news and rating sites. Having a provider in triage is one way that an institution can ensure that time to provider is short, and some of the enthusiasm for teletriage providers relates to a desire to perform well on these metrics. If the CMS emphasis on these reporting statistics should change, some of that current enthusiasm regarding both PIT models and their telemedicine provider in triage equivalent would diminish.

CONCLUSION

Future studies of teletriage should focus on the promotion of patient-centered care. Patient satisfaction, time to diagnosis, time to discharge or admission, and efficiency and appropriateness of laboratory and radiology test ordering would all fall into this category. In addition, further research is required for techniques on improving the process of teletriage itself. Although there may be advantages inherent in the initial provider triage being remote, it would be intuitive to think that technology that brings the experience of teletriage closer to that of an in-person evaluation from both the provider and patient experience would be valuable.

The future adoption of teletriage based on patient-centered care will depend on developments in the understanding of both the effect of PIT on patient evaluation and how well teletriage replicates the PIT model, as well as direct assessment of the value of teletriage concerning patient outcomes. One recent study during the pandemic showed that implementing a telehealth-enabled workflow in ED triage areas could enable remote providers to collaborate with nursing to evaluate and discharge well-appearing, low-risk COVID-19 ED patients while identifying more serious illness for expedited in-person care (Carlberg, 2020). As of the time of this writing, there is still little literature regarding teletriage concerning patient outcomes, although it appears that teletriage providers can see roughly the same number of patients per hour as in-person providers and that teletriage may have high accuracy and ordering patterns that are similar to in-person triage (Rademacher, Cole, Psoter, et al., 2019; Polinski et al., 2016).

KEY TAKEAWAYS

> - Medical Screening Exams are a vital component of the emergency department evaluation
> - Medical Screening Exams performed via telehealth help reduce door-to-diagnostic evaluation times and decrease Left Without Being Seen rates
> - Patients should receive the same level of care regardless of whether the service is in-person treatment or a virtual telehealth service.
> - A variation on the provider in a triage model using telemedicine allows a provider to be present in more than one location.
> - All new care pathways require assessment and evaluation.

REFERENCES

Abdulwahid, M., Booth, A., Kuczawski, M., Mason, S. (2016). The impact of senior doctor assessment at triage on emergency department performance measures: Systematic review and meta-analysis of comparative studies. *Emergency Medicine Journal*, 33(7): 504–513.

Carlberg, D. J. (2020). Preliminary assessment of a telehealth approach to evaluating, treating, and discharging low-acuity patients with suspected COVID-19. *Journal of Emergency Medicine*, 59(6): 1–7.

Center for Consumer Information & Insurance Oversight. (2019, September 20). Retrieved from Centers for Medicare and Medicaid Services at https://www.cms.gov/CCIIO/Resources/About-Us/index.html.

Duarte, C. (2019). *Emergency medicine benchmarking alliance 2019 innovations in emergency medicine poster session runner-up*. Retrieved from Emergency Medicine Benchmarking at https://www.edbenchmarking.org/assets/docs/EDBA%20Poster%3D%20Carlos.pdf.

Emergency Medical Treatment and Labor Act (EMTALA). (2019, January 10). Retrieved from Centers for Medicare and Medicaid Services at https://www.cms.gov/Medicare/Provider-Enrollment-and-Certification/CertificationandComplianc/Downloads/EMTALA.pdf.

Emergency Medical Treatment and Labor Act (EMTALA). (2019, September 20). Retrieved from Centers for Medicare and Medicaid Services at https://www.cms.gov/Regulations-and-Guidance/Legislation/EMTALA/index.html.

Emergency Severity Index (ESI): A triage tool for emergency departments. (2018, May). Retrieved from Agency for Healthcare Research and Quality at https://www.ahrq.gove/professionals/systems/hospital/esi/index.html.

ER *facility prices grew in tandem with faster-growing charges from 2009–2016.* (2018, September 11). Retrieved from Health Care Cost Institute at https://www.healthcostinstitute.org/blog/entry/er-facility-prices-charges-2009-2016.

Hartnett, K. P.,(2020). Impact of the COVID-19 pandemic on emergency department visits—United States, January 1, 2019–May 30, 2020. *MMWR Morbidity and Mortality Weekly Report*, (69), 699–704.

Hesse, C., Assid, P., Jackson, P., Schmitz, J., Stigdon, T., Solheim, J., & lson, C. (2017, May). Emergency department throughout emergency. Nurses Association: Brief Topic (https://www.ena.org/docs/default-source/resource-library/practice-resources/topic-briefs/ed-throughput.pdf). Retrieved from https://www.ena.org/docs/default-source/resource-library/practice-resources/topic-briefs/ed-throughput.pdf.

Hsia, R., Kellerman, A., & Shen, Y. (2011). Factors associated with closures of emergency departments in the United States. *Journal of American Medical Association*, 305(19): 1978–1985.

Iserson, K., & Moskop, J. (2007). Triage in medicine, part I: Concept, history, and types. *Annals of Emergency Medicine*, 49: 275–281.

Izzo, J., Watson, J., Bhat, R., Wilson, M., Blumenthal, J., Houser, C., et al. (2018). Diagnostic accuracy of a rapid telemedicine encounter in the emergency department. *American Journal of Emergency Medicine*, 36(11): 2061–2063.

The Joint Commission Mission Statement. (2009, August 15). Retrieved from the Joint Commission at https://www.jointcommission.org/about-us/

The Joint Commission Website. (2018, December 18). Retrieved from Specifications Manual for National Hospital Inpatient Quality Measures at https://www.jointcommission.org/specifications_manual_for_national_hospital_inpatient_quality_measures.aspx.

Love, R., Murphy, J., Lietz, T., & Jordan, K. (2012). The effectiveness of a provider in triage in the emergency department: A quality improvement initiative to improve patient flow. *Advanced Emergency Nursing Journal*, 34(1): 65–74.

Morley, C., Unwin, M., Peterson, G., Stankovich, J., & Kinsman, L. (2018). Emergency department crowding: A systematic review of causes, consequences and solutions. *PLoS one*, 13(8): e0203316.

National Hospital Ambulatory Medical Care Survey. (2019, September 20). Retrieved from Centers for Disease Control and Prevention website at https://www.cdc.gov/nchs/data/nhamcs/web_tables/2016_ed_web_tables.pdf

Oredsson, S., Jonsson, H., Rognes, J., et al. (2011, July 19). A systematic review of triage-related interventions to improve patient flow in emergency departments. *Scandinavian Journal of Trauma, Resuscitation and Emergency Medicine*, 19: 43. (https://sjtrem.biomedcentral.com/articles/10.1186/1757-7241-19-43).

Polinski, J., Barker, T., Gagliano, N., Sussman, A., Brennan, T., & Shrank, W. (2016). Patients' satisfaction with and preference for telehealth visits. *Journal of General Internal Medicine*, 31(3): 269–275.

Rademacher, N., Cole, G., Psoter, K., et al. (2019, May 8). Use of telemedicine to screen patients in the emergency department: Matched cohort study evaluating efficiency and patient safety of telemedicine. *JMIR Medical Informatics*, 7(2): e11233.

Rural Hospital Closures: Number and characteristics of affected hospitals and contributing factors. (2018, August). Retrieved from United States Government Accountability Office at https://www.gao.gov/assets/700/694125.pdf.

Section 3. Measuring emergency department performance. (2018, July). Retrieved from Agency for Healthcare Research and Quality at https://www.ahrq.gov/research/findings/final-reports/ptflow/section3.html.

State Operations Manual. (2019). Retrieved from Centers for Medicare and Medicaid Services at https://www.cms.gov/regulations-and-guidance/guidance/manuals/downloads/som107ap_v_emerg.pdf.

Sun, R., Karaca, Z., & Wong, H. (2018, March). *Trends in hospital emergency department visits by age and payer, 2006–2015 Statistical Brief#238.* Retrieved from Healthcare Cost and Utilization Project at https://www.hcup-us.ahrq.gov/reports/statbriefs/sb238-Emergency-Department-Age-Payer-2006-2015.jsp.

The Center for Consumer Information & Insurance Oversight. (2019, September 20). Retrieved from Centers for Medicare and Medicaid Services at https://www.cms.gov/CCIIO/Resources/About-Us/index.html.

Izzo, J., Watson, J., Bhat, R., Descallar, E., Hoffman, D., Booker, E., (2017, October). 325 Telemedicine model of physician intake decreases door-to-provider time. *Annals of Emergency Medicine,* 70(4): S128–S129.

16

Telehealth for Medication for Opioid Use Disorder Treatment

BILL WAYNE CHAN, JAVAD JOHN FATOLLAHI,
NATALIE LYNN KIRILICHIN, AND ZEINA SALIBA ■

INTRODUCTION

With an 80% retention rate in opioid use disorder (OUD) treatment after 30 days, emergency department (ED)-initiated buprenorphine has shown to be efficacious as an entryway into formal addiction treatment (D'Onofrio et al., 2015). Medication for Opioid Use Disorders (mOUD), particularly buprenorphine, has proven to be the gold standard in managing opioid addiction. As telehealth expands its reach to a growing number of EDs across the country, its utility in treating OUD grows in a similar fashion (Wicklund, 2018). While current models of care integrating telehealth and mOUD are predominantly in outpatient office-based settings, modifications to existing models offer potential ways to implement telehealth and mOUD in point-of-care settings, including the ED. This chapter outlines existing models of care for bridging telehealth and mOUD, barriers addressed with these models, potential cost reductions, and legal constructs regarding its implementation.

MEDICATION FOR OPIOID USE DISORDER

Compared to counseling and behavioral therapies alone, mOUD prevails as the gold standard for managing opioid addiction (U.S. Department of Health and Human Services [HHS], 2018). Studies suggest that over 80% of patients will return to opioid use with behavioral interventions alone (Bart, 2012). Buprenorphine, even at low doses (2–6 mg), retains more patients in treatment compared to placebo, and at high doses (> 16 mg), suppresses illicit opioid use (Mattick, Breen, Kimber, & Davoli, 2014). Compared to flexibly adjusted low-dose buprenorphine, fixed low-dose methadone (< 40 mg) has shown to be superior at retaining patients in treatment (Mattick, Breen, Kimber, & Davoli, 2014). At fixed higher doses, buprenorphine and methadone are equally effective in retention in treatment (Mattick, Breen, Kimber, & Davoli, 2014). Furthermore, mOUD has been shown to reduce overdose death due to opioid use (Larochelle et al., 2018). Medications to treat OUD include methadone, buprenorphine, and naltrexone and are described in Table 16.1.

BUPRENORPHINE: THE BEST OPTION FOR TELEHEALTH

While all three medications have demonstrated effectiveness in treating OUD, buprenorphine is the only realistic option for emergency telehealth. By law, methadone, for the treatment of OUD (as opposed to pain), must be dispensed by a Substance Abuse and Mental Health Services (SAMHSA)-certified opioid treatment program (OTP), currently rendering it incompatible with the concept of remote prescribing. Naltrexone's biological requirement of opioid-abstinence for 7–14 days prior to initiation of treatment limits its utility in point-of-care settings, such as the ED or urgent care centers. Methadone and naltrexone are better suited for in-person longitudinal care settings.

Buprenorphine has proven utility in point-of-care settings for both treatment of opioid withdrawal and maintenance treatment of OUD. In 2015, research at Yale New Haven Hospital showed that ED-initiated buprenorphine significantly increased patients' engagement in formal addiction treatment, reduced illicit opioid use, and decreased the use of in-patient addiction treatment services. Compared to brief negotiated interview (BNI) and facilitated referral only, ED-initiated buprenorphine with BNI resulted in 80%, or twice as many patients, in OUD treatment at 30 days post-ED visit (D'Onofrio et al., 2015). Over 100 sites across the country have adopted this practice and have found similar rates of success following ED-initiated

Table 16.1 MEDICATIONS FOR OPIOID ADDICTION TREATMENT

	Methadone	Buprenorphine	Naltrexone
Mechanism of Action	μ-Opioid Receptor Full Agonist	μ-Opioid Receptor Partial Agonist and kappa-opioid receptor antagonist	μ-Opioid Receptor Full Antagonist
Effect	Reduces opioid cravings and withdrawal	Reduces opioid cravings and withdrawal	Reduces reinforcing effects of opioids
Route of Administration	Oral	Oral, buccal, sublingual	Oral, intramuscular injection
Dosing*	Taken once per day	Variable from once every other day to 3–4 times daily, with BID dosing common	Taken once per day (Oral) or once every 4 weeks (Intramuscular)

*Dosing differs when used for pain; for example, buprenorphine is dosed more frequently in that case.

buprenorphine with referral to specific community-based opioid treatment clinics/ providers. As of September 2019, the National Institute on Drug Abuse (NIDA) has supported ED-initiated buprenorphine and has supported four clinical trials to further prove its efficacy (National Institute on Drug Abuse, 2019).

According to SAMHSA, a total of 102,570 practitioners were eligible to prescribe buprenorphine as of August 2020 (Substance Abuse and Mental Health Services, 2020), though many do not citing lack of exposure to addiction medicine and perception of patients with addiction as "difficult" as primary reasons (Andraka-Christou & Capone, 2018). One study estimates that 55% of eligible practitioners do not prescribe buprenorphine to capacity primarily due to "not having time for more patients" (Huhn & Dunn, 2017). With nearly 2 million people in the United States suffering from OUD (Substance Abuse and Mental Health Services, 2019), the number of eligible practitioners and those willing to prescribe simply do not meet the need. In addition, many practitioners who do prescribe buprenorphine do not take insurance, creating a financial barrier for patients. Furthermore, the geographic distribution of providers concentrated in urban settings further exacerbates access to mOUD. More than half of all rural counties (56.3%) lack an eligible mOUD provider. Almost one-third of rural Americans compared to less than 3% of urban Americans live in a county without a buprenorphine prescriber (Andrilla, Moore, Patterson, & Larson, 2019). Limited availability of treatment options contributed to a nationwide opioid-related ED utilization of 225 visits per 100,000 in 2017, with some states exceeding 500 visits per 100,000 (Agency for Healthcare Research and Quality, 2020). The following section outlines two models of care integrating telehealth and MAT and describes how each can be tailored to point-of-care settings.

TELEHEALTH AND MAT: SELECT MODELS OF CARE

Rural Maryland

Developed by the University of Maryland in collaboration with an addiction treatment center in rural Maryland, this model consists of program coordinators at an originating (rural) site and a distant (university) site facilitating ongoing communication and scheduling (Figure 16.1). Originating site coordinators arrange,

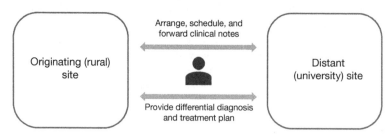

Figure 16.1 Model of care for rural Maryland.

schedule, and forward substance use counselors' clinical notes and patients' urine toxicology results to the distant site coordinator. Patients are initially screened by the originating site's substance use counselor. Through videoconferencing, physicians at the distant site conduct a full diagnostic evaluation, including psychiatric, medical, and substance use history. The physician then provides a diagnosis and treatment plan, including a medication dose. Through the distant site coordinator, notes are sent to the originating site coordinator following each encounter and are placed in charts at both sites with subsequent follow-up appointments scheduled. Other staff members include social workers and part-time nurses, particularly at the originating site (Weintraub, Greenblatt, Chang, Himelhoch, & Welsh, 2018).

Since its inception in 2015, a retrospective review showed patients had a 98% retention in treatment at 1 week, 91% at 1 month, 73% at 2 months, and 57% at 3 months. As of January 2019, the success of this program had led to expansion into other counties of rural Maryland. Specifically, in rural settings, the use of video telehealth has shown to be a valuable tool to expand mOUD in underserved rural populations. A reported key advantage of this program is its use of program coordinators at the originating and distant sites to coordinate ongoing care (Weintraub et al., 2018).

In point-of-care settings, this model could be leveraged to utilize ED physicians as the distant site and advanced practitioners from rural health clinics as the originating site. In this scenario, advanced practitioners from rural health clinics could collaborate with ED physicians capable of prescribing buprenorphine. Via videoconferencing, an ED physician can see the patient in clinic, collaborate with the advanced practitioner, and prescribe buprenorphine if appropriate. The ED physician would also facilitate subsequent referral to community-based opioid treatment clinics or providers for long-term management.

Community Hospital of the Monterey Peninsula and Bright Heart Health

Another model of integrating telehealth, specifically emergency telehealth, and mOUD is displayed by Bright Heart Health and CHOMP (Figure 16.2).

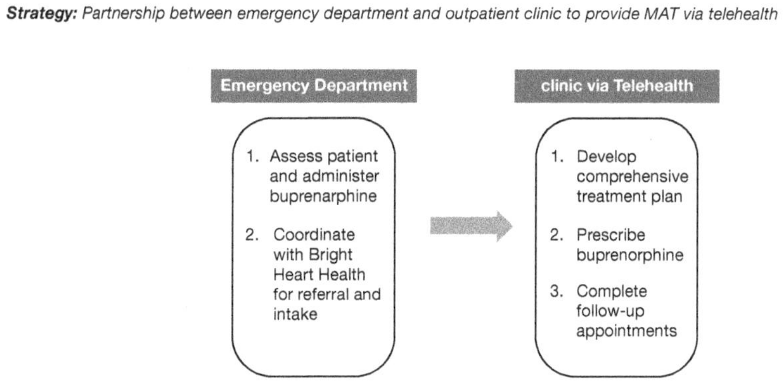

Strategy: *Partnership between emergency department and outpatient clinic to provide MAT via telehealth*

Emergency Department

1. Assess patient and administer buprenarphine

2. Coordinate with Bright Heart Health for referral and intake

clinic via Telehealth

1. Develop comprehensive treatment plan

2. Prescribe buprenorphine

3. Complete follow-up appointments

Figure 16.2 Community Hospital of the Monterey Peninsula and Bright Heart Health.

Bright Heart Health is marketed as the first nationwide opioid use treatment program via telehealth. In this model, a patient suffering from OUD or opioid withdrawal presents to the ED at CHOMP. The patient is then immediately assessed by an ED physician and if in withdrawal, the patient is started on buprenorphine with reassessment in one hour (SHOUT Support for Hospital Opioid Use Treatment, 2020). During this time, ED physicians refer patients to Bright Heart Health and explain their telehealth model of addiction treatment. With the help of ED staff, patients call Bright Heart Health and complete intake paperwork. Appointments with Bright Heart Health are typically set up within the next 48 hours. Upon discharge, an ED-case manager facilitates discharge paperwork, documents the date of the patient's next appointment with Bright Heart Health in the ED health portal, and ensures the patient knows how to virtually attend their appointment (Bright Heart Health, 2018).

Via videoconferencing, patients meet with Bright Heart Health medical staff and substance use counselors to develop a comprehensive treatment plan. Bright Heart Health physicians prescribe buprenorphine following evaluation and initial drug screening at an outside laboratory service provider. Patients meet with their physicians once a week or every two weeks to discuss treatment progress and to renew their prescription. Patients are also required to have random monthly drug screenings. Urine test kits are mailed to patients' addresses. After receipt of the urine test kit, patients attend a virtual clinic appointment via videoconferencing, privately provide a urine sample, and review the results together with Bright Heart Health staff, who then share the results with the physicians. In addition, patients are required to meet with a primary therapist individually twice a month and attend weekly group sessions via videoconferencing (Bright Heart Health, 2020). Within the first months, the collaboration between CHOMP and Bright Heart Health displayed 95% retention in addiction treatment at 30 days, even higher than seen in the 2015 Yale study (Bright Heart Health, 2018).

A key advantage in partnering ED-initiated buprenorphine with telehealth-based opioid treatment clinics/providers is the immediate access that ED physicians and patients have to OUD specialists for scheduling follow-up maintenance appointments. The strength of this partnership is contingent upon the 24/7 access ED physicians have to the telehealth-based treatment program and the comfort and reassurance physicians have that the needs of their patients in times of crisis will be addressed as soon as possible. Another reported advantage of this model is the ability for patients to receive addiction treatment from the privacy of their home, at their own schedule. Lastly and perhaps most importantly, consistent messaging from the ED physicians to patients, in which patients are reassured that they will get into treatment when they are ready, has also been reported as an advantage of this model (Bright Heart Health, 2018). Overall, the role of the ED physician is twofold: treat patients who present to the ED with OUD and withdrawal symptoms and directly refer them from the ED to telehealth-based outpatient opioid treatment clinics/providers.

BARRIERS TO TREATMENT

Barriers to mOUD are numerous and can broadly be classified as those faced by patients in receiving treatment (e.g. lack of available providers, transportation, stigma, etc.) and those faced by physicians in prescribing medications (e.g. lack of comfort with addiction medicine, time and staff limitations, funding, stigma etc.) (Bunting, Oser, Staton, Eddens, & Knudsen, 2018; Andraka-Christou & Capone, 2018). While telehealth does not solve all barriers, it addresses several of them, such as access to care and stigma.

Telehealth has been shown to address geographical and temporal barriers to care, such as clinic hours of operation, travel time to appointments, and long wait times for appointments. Patients suffering from OUD, especially those who have lost driving privileges, report the distance from treatment centers/providers and the need to rely on family and friends for transportation as contributing factors for missed appointments or not scheduling appointments at all (Pullen & Oser, 2014). Particularly in rural settings, where public transportation is limited, lack of transportation is a significant limiting factor to accessing care. Patients in mouD programs should not have to rely on others for transportation as a long-term solution (Pullen & Oser, 2014). Research indicates that shorter travel distances have been associated with longer duration of treatment and greater completion rates in substance use treatment (Beardsley, Wish, Fitzelle, O'Grady, & Arria, 2003). Long clinic wait times at treatment facilities have also been reported to deter patients from treatment (Pullen & Oser, 2014). Telehealth enhances the availability of addiction specialists by removing many of the external barriers that deter patients from treatment.

Stigma is another well-documented deterrent to substance use treatment that manifests in multiple forms. The stigma of having OUD alienates patients, 74% of whom avoid others for fear of being looked down upon (Ahern, Stuber, & Galea, 2007). The stigma of receiving opioid agonist therapy, such as methadone or buprenorphine, which some believe is simply a way of substituting one drug for another, deters patients from seeking treatment. One qualitative study found that among people who injected drugs, methadone maintenance therapy was more stigmatized than injection drug use and ultimately discouraged participation in treatment (Paquette, Syvertsen, & Pollini, 2018). Lastly, the language used by the health care system surrounding addiction further perpetuates stigma. Urine test results are routinely referred to as "clean" or "dirty," judgmental terms not used in the management of other medical condition (Olsen & Sharfstein, 2014). One study found that 54% of ED physicians agreed that they "prefer not to work with patients with substance use with pain" and 54% agreed that "patients like this irritate me"(Mendiola, Galetto, & Fingerhood, 2018). These stigmatizing attitudes toward patients suffering from OUD are documented to evoke judgment in providers and produce suboptimal care for patients (Kelly & Westerhoff, 2010; van Boekel, Brouwers, van Weeghel, & Garretsen, 2013).

While telehealth does not promote appropriate and affirming language by providers, telehealth and its remote delivery of services have been shown to remove the barrier of lack of confidentiality and to increase privacy (King et al., 2009). In addition, telehealth has been associated with an increase in patient perception of comfort, security, and satisfaction (Matusitz & Breen, 2007). One systematic review found that patient satisfaction was associated with the modality of telehealth and that patient expectations were adequately met with videoconferencing (Kruse et al., 2017). Through telehealth, the ability of patients to receive addiction treatment in the comfort and privacy of their own home has been noted as a reason for high retention in treatment.

COST REDUCTION

As of 2013, the total economic burden of the opioid epidemic was estimated to be nearly $80 billion, with one-third of the burden due to health care and substance use treatment costs (Florence, Luo, Xu, & Zhou, 2016). While comprehensive economic evaluations of medications for opioid use treatment are lacking, preliminary studies have described methadone and buprenorphine as cost-effective options (Chalk et al., 2013). According to one health plan, members receiving methadone treatment had a nearly 50% lower cost when compared to those with two or more outpatient addiction treatment programs but no methadone (McCarty et al., n.d.). One study, examining how buprenorphine impacts costs from the health system perspective, found that patients receiving buprenorphine with counseling had statistically significant lower health care costs compared to patients receiving little or no addiction treatment (Lynch et al., 2014). Considering only health care system costs, by converting health care use to dollar values and creating cost-effectiveness acceptability curves, one study found that ED-initiated buprenorphine treatment in the 2015 Yale study was more cost-effective at 30 days than both brief intervention (BNI) with referral and referral to community-based treatment (Busch et al., 2017). Telehealth programs for mOUD are still relatively new, and further studies are indicated to facilitate cost-benefit analyses.

Funding for mOUD in the telehealth setting can potentially be achieved via grants and insurance reimbursement. Grants, specifically through SAMHSA, offer start-up funding to expand mOUD into the telehealth realm (Substance Abuse and Mental Health Services, 2020). Cost and insurance coverage for telehealth services for mOUD vary from state to state. Depending on the model of care implemented, telehealth costs will vary for patients. All state Medicaid programs currently cover at least one mOUD medication as well as naloxone, an opioid antagonist that reverses opioid overdose. However, only 42 state Medicaid programs cover methadone for treatment of OUD (in contrast to reimbursing for the use of methadone to treat pain and other conditions), and fewer than 70% of states cover implanted or extended-release injectable buprenorphine. Federally qualified health centers could also use a Medicaid prospective payment system, which allows greater flexibility in funding telehealth services. A prospective payment system is a method of reimbursement in which payment is made based on a predetermined, fixed amount. The payment amount for a particular service is derived based on the classification system of that service (Centers for Medicare and Medicaid Services, 2020). A viable Medicaid reimbursement plan is thought to be crucial for the success of mOUD treatment in the telehealth setting.

LEGAL CONSIDERATIONS REGARDING MOUD

Since its inception, multiple legal constructs have been in place to regulate the dissemination of mOUD services. Some of the medications are controlled substances governed by the Controlled Substances Act. This act regulates the manufacture, importation, possession, use, and distribution of controlled substances. The Drug Addiction Treatment Act of 2000 (DATA, 2000) allows physicians who meet certain qualifications to treat opioid addiction with FDA-indicated schedule III, IV, and V controlled medications in office-based settings, instead of OTPs. They are permitted to do so by applying for a waiver from the registration requirements required by the Narcotic Addict Treatment Act of 1974.

Regulations for OTPs include the Certification of Opioid Treatment Programs—42 Code of Federal Regulations (CFR) 8, which provides for an accreditation and certification-based system for OTPs, overseen by SAMHSA, and includes regulations for using narcotic drugs to treat opioid addiction (Code of Federal Regulations, 2018). The regulations acknowledge that OUD is a medical disorder and that patients could need vastly different treatment services. DATA 2000 requires that the practitioner prescribing buprenorphine have the capacity to refer patients to "appropriate counseling," and many insurers require therapy or counseling when patients are getting medication for addiction (Congressional Research Service, 2020). The regulations also preserve states' authority to regulate OTPs. The Certification of Opioid Treatment Programs—42 Code of Federal Regulations Part 2—protects patient confidentiality through restrictions concerning the disclosure and use of patient records pertaining to substance use treatment (Code of Federal Regulations, 2018).

The Substance Use Disorder Prevention that Promotes Opioid Recovery and Treatment (SUPPORT) for Patients and Communities Act of 2018 increased the maximum number of patients that practitioners could initially treat under the buprenorphine waiver from 30 up to 100 if they met at least one of two conditions: (1) physician certification in addiction medicine or addiction psychiatry, and (2) usage of medication (buprenorphine) in a qualified practice setting (e.g., emergency departments; Congressional Research Service, 2018). This Act also added buprenorphine-prescribing eligibility for clinical nurse specialists, certified registered nurse anesthetists (CRNAs), and certified nurse midwives (CNMs). After one year at the 100-patient limit, physicians and other qualifying practitioners who meet the above criteria can apply to increase their patient limit to 275.

There is an exception to the registration requirements listed above which allows the prescribing of buprenorphine without a waiver in emergency settings. The "three-day rule" (Title 21, Code of Federal Regulations, Part 1306.07(b)) is an exception to the registration requirement, which allows practitioners who are not registered in a narcotic treatment program and not DATA-waivered, to administer (but not prescribe) buprenorphine or methadone (one day at a time for up to 72 hours, or three days) to a patient for the treatment of acute withdrawal symptoms, while arranging for the patient's referral to treatment (DEA Diversion Control Division, 2020).

The Ryan Haight Act

The Ryan Haight Online Pharmacy Consumer Protection Act of 2008, created to regulate online and internet prescriptions, requires practitioners prescribing controlled substances to have conducted at least one in-person evaluation of the patient before or prior to prescribing. There are several telemedicine exceptions to this requirement, but they are narrow, limited to a subset of practitioners, settings, and situations, as defined by one of the following conditions (per 21 U.S.C. § 802(54)): The patient is located in a DEA-registered hospital or clinic; the patient is in the presence of a DEA-certified practitioner; the remote practitioner is an Internet Eligible Controlled Substances Provider for the Indian Health Service or a tribal organization; the telemedicine consult is conducted during an HHS-declared public health emergency; the practitioner has a special DEA telemedicine registration; and the telemedicine consult is conducted by a VA practitioner during a VHA-declared medical emergency (DEA Diversion Control Division, 2016). In other words, outside of emergencies, a patient located at home, for example, for a telemedicine consultation would still require an in-person evaluation prior to the practitioner prescribing them a controlled substance. Practitioners must also be registered with the DEA in the state where they are physically located and in the state where their patient is physically located. Practitioners must still comply with state controlled substance and telehealth laws, which can be more restrictive.

The in-person examination requirement became an especially significant barrier to treatment of OUDs during the COVID-19 pandemic, with quarantining and shelter-at-home orders. On March 16, 2020, the public health emergency exception to the Ryan Haight Act was designated as active by the DEA, in response to the 2019 novel Coronavirus emergency declared by the Secretary of Health and Human Services on January 31, 2020; it allows qualified practitioners to prescribe controlled substances via telemedicine without first conducting an in-person examination for the duration of this public health emergency. On March 31, 2020, the DEA issued a letter announcing the increase in flexibility, allowing the prescribing of buprenorphine (without in-person examination) by audio-only telemedicine, or telephone evaluation, instead of requiring a video component (DEA Diversion Control Division, 2020). About a week earlier, on March 23, the DEA granted DEA-registered practitioners permission to prescribe controlled substances by telemedicine to patients in states where the practitioners are not registered (DEA Diversion Control Division, 2020). There have been efforts, such as the introduction of Senate bill S.4103, the Telehealth Response for E-prescribing Addiction Therapy Services (TREATS) Act on June 30, to ensure that some of these temporary changes become permanent (Congressional Research Service, 2020).

CASE STUDY

The case study presented in this section proposes how DEA-registered ED physicians can be leveraged via telehealth in treatment of patients suffering from OUD. For example, a patient suffering from OUD presents to a rural health clinic staffed by an advanced practitioner who does not have the DATA 2000 waiver to prescribe buprenorphine (Figure 16.3). The rural health clinic has a working collaboration with a distant ED, staffed by DEA-registered ED physicians. Via telehealth, a DEA-registered ED physician can assess the patient, who is in the clinic, discuss treatment options with

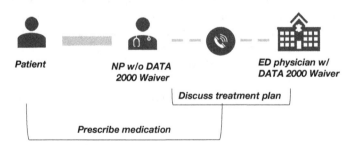

Strategy: *Collaboration between clinic and DATA waivered ED physicians to provide MAT via telehealth*

Figure 16.3 Case Study: DATA 2000 Waiver Workflow Strategy.

the advanced practitioner, and prescribe buprenorphine if appropriate. Subsequent referral to opioid treatment clinics/providers can be made by the ED physician and or advanced practitioner to ensure maintenance therapy is achieved.

CONCLUSION

Medication for Opioid Use Disorder, specifically buprenorphine, is the gold standard for treatment of opioid use disorder. The ability to provide early initiation of treatment via telehealth services in point-of-care settings, like an ED, has been shown to correlate with higher retention rates in treatment. Additionally, telehealth addresses common barriers to mOUD such as transportation and stigma. Funding for these services can be procured through a variety of government programs. There are existing models of care in place to bridge telehealth and mOUD services, along with legal constructs that guide their implementation. The COVID-19 pandemic allowed the public health emergency exemption to go into effect, authorizing practitioners to prescribe controlled substances without a prerequisite in-person evaluation. This exemption has given patients greater access to care through the removal of common barriers to treatment initiation, and legislation has been introduced to permanently lift the in-person evaluation requirement.

KEY TAKEAWAYS

➤ ED-initiated buprenorphine has been shown to be an effective entryway into formalized addiction treatment.

➤ There are multiple models of care that integrate mOUD and telehealth in point-of-care settings. Models can be adjusted to best fit one's clinical practice.

➤ Funding for mOUD treatment in the telehealth setting can be achieved through government grants and insurance reimbursements.

➤ Multiple legal constructs are in place to regulate the dissemination of mOUD services. The Ryan Haight Act of 2008 regulates online prescribing of controlled substances and requires that the prescribing practitioner conduct at least one in-person evaluation of the patient prior to prescribing a controlled substance.

➤ The DEA activated the public health emergency exemption to the Ryan Haight Act on March 16, 2020, in response to the COVID-19 pandemic and allowed practitioners to prescribe controlled substances via telehealth without the requirement of an initial in-person examination.

REFERENCES

Agency for Healthcare Research and Quality. (2020, April 29). *HCUP fast stats—Opioid-related hospital use*. Retrieved from Healthcare Cost and Utilization Project at https://www.hcup-us.ahrq.gov/faststats/OpioidUseServlet?radio-3=on&location1=

US&characteristic1=01&setting1=ED&location2=&characteristic2=01&setting2=I
P&expansionInfoState=hide&dataTablesState=hide&definitionsState=hide&export
State=hide.

Ahern, J., Stuber, J., & Galea, S. (2007). Stigma, discrimination and the health of illicit drug users. *Drug and Alcohol Dependence*, 88(2-3): 188–196. doi:10.1016/
j.drugalcdep.2006.10.014. Epub 2006 Nov 21. PMID: 17118578.

Andraka-Christou, B., & Capone, M. J. (2018). A qualitative study comparing physician-
reported barriers to treating addiction using buprenorphine and extended-release
naltrexone in U.S. office-based practices. *International Journal of Drug Policy*, 54: 9–
17. doi:10.1016/j.drugpo.2017.11.021. Epub 2018 Jan 8. PMID: 29324253.

Andrilla, C. H., Moore, T. E., Patterson, D. G., & Larson, E. H. (2019, January).
Geographic distribution of providers with a DEA waiver to prescribe buprenorphine
for the treatment of opioid use disorder: A 5-year update. *Journal of Rural Health*,
35(1): 108–112.

Bart, G. (2012). Maintenance medication for opiate addiction: The foundation of recovery. *Journal of Addictive Diseases*, 31(3): 207–225.

Beardsley, K., Wish, E. D., Fitzelle, D. B., O'Grady, K., & Arria, A. M. (2003, December).
Distance traveled to outpatient drug treatment and client retention. *Journal of
Substance Abuse Treatment*, 25(4): 279–285.

Bright Heart Health. (2018). *Telemedicine case study for emergency departments*.
Retrieved from Bright Heart Health at https://www.brighthearthealth.com/
telemedicine-case-study-for-emergency-departments.

Bright Heart Health. (2020). *Rapid access opioid use disorder treatment*. Retrieved from https://
www.brighthearthealth.com/services/rapid-access-opioid-use-disorder-treatment.

Bunting, A. M., Oser, C. B., Staton, M., Eddens, K. S., & Knudsen, H. (2018). Clinician
identified barriers to treatment for individuals in Appalachia with opioid use disorder following release from prison: a social ecological approach. *Addiction Science
and Clinical Practice*, 13(1): 23. doi:10.1186/s13722-018-0124-2.

Busch, S. H., Fiellin, D. A., Chawarski, M. C., Owens, P. H., Pantalon, M. V., Hawk, K.,
et al. (2017, November). Cost-effectiveness of emergency department-initiated treatment for opioid dependence. *Addiction*, 112(11): 2002–2010.

Centers for Medicare and Medicaid Services. (2020, November 13). *Prospective Payment
Systems—General Information*. Retrieved from https://www.cms.gov/Medicare/
Medicare-Fee-for-Service-Payment/ProspMedicareFeeSvcPmtGen#:~:text=A%20
Prospective%20Payment%20System%20(PPS,groups%20for%20inpatient%20
hospital%20services).

Chalk, M., Alanis-Hirsch, K., Woodworth, A., Mericle, A., Curtis, B., & McLoyd, K.
(2013). *Advancing access to addiction medications*. American Society of Addiction
Medicine.

Code of Federal Regulations. (2018, October 1). *Part 8—Medication assisted treatment
for opioid use disorders*. Retrieved from https://www.govinfo.gov/content/pkg/CFR-
2018-title42-vol1/xml/CFR-2018-title42-vol1-part8.xml.

Congressional Research Service. (2018, October 24). *H.R.6—SUPPORT for Patients and
Communities Act*. Retrieved from https://www.congress.gov/bill/115th-congress/
house-bill/6?q=%7B%22search%22%3A%5B%22hr6%22%5D%7D&s=3&r=2.

Congressional Research Service. (2020, July 19). *H.R.2634—Drug Addiction Treatment
Act of 2000*. Retrieved from https://www.congress.gov/bill/106th-congress/house-
bill/2634.

Congressional Research Service. (2020, June 30). *S.4103—TREATS Act*. Retrieved from https://www.congress.gov/bill/116th-congress/senate-bill/4103.

DEA Diversion Control Division. (2016). *Title 21 United States Code (USC) Controlled Substances Act*. Retrieved from https://www.deadiversion.usdoj.gov/21cfr/21usc/802.htm.

DEA Diversion Control Division. (2020, March 25). Retrieved from https://www.deadiversion.usdoj.gov/GDP/(DEA-DC-018)(DEA067)%20DEA%20state%20reciprocity%20(final)(Signed).pdf.

DEA Diversion Control Division. (2020, November 2). *Title 21 Code of Federal Regulations*. Retrieved from https://www.deadiversion.usdoj.gov/21cfr/cfr/1306/1306_07.htm.

DEA Diversion Control Division. (2020, March 31). *Use of telephone evaluations to initiate buprenorphine prescribing*. Retrieved from https://www.deadiversion.usdoj.gov/GDP.

D'Onofrio, G., O'Connor, P. G., Pantalon, M. V., Chawarski, M. C., Busch, S. H., Owens, P. H., et al. (2015, April 28). Emergency department-initiated buprenorphine/naloxone treatment for opioid dependence: a randomized clinical trial. *JAMA*, 313(16): 1636–1644.

Florence, C., Luo, F., Xu, L., & Zhou, C. (2016). The economic burden of prescription opioid overdose, abuse and dependence in the United States, 2013. *Medical Care*, 54(10): 901–906.

Huhn, A. S., & Dunn, K. E. (2017). Why aren't physicians prescribing more buprenorphine? *Journal of Substance Abuse Treatment*, 78: 1–7. doi:10.1016/j.jsat.2017.04.005. Epub 2017 Apr 12. PMID: 28554597; PMCID: PMC5524453.

Kelly, J. F., & Westerhoff, C. M. (2010, May). Does it matter how we refer to individuals with substance-related conditions? A randomized study of two commonly used terms. *International Journal of Drug Policy*, 21(3), 202–207.

King, V. L., Stoller, K. B., Kidorf, M., Kindbom, K., Hursh, S., Brady, T., & Brooner, R. K. (2009). Assessing the effectiveness of an Internet-based videoconferencing platform for delivering intensified substance abuse counseling. *Journal of Substance Abuse Treatment*, 36(3): 331–338. doi:10.1016/j.jsat.2008.06.011. Epub 2008 Sep 4. PMID: 18775625.

Kruse, C. S., Krowski, N., Rodriguez, B., Tran, L., Vela, J., & Brooks, M. (2017). Telehealth and patient satisfaction: a systematic review and narrative analysis. *BMJ Open*, 7: e016242. doi:10.1136/bmjopen-2017-016242.

Larochelle, M., Bernson, D., Land, T., Stopka, T., Wang, N., Xuan, Z., et al. (2018). Medication for opioid use disorder after nonfatal opioid overdose and association with mortality. *Annals of Internal Medicine*, 169(3): 137–145. doi:10.7326/M17-3107. Epub 2018 Jun 19. PMID: 29913516; PMCID: PMC6387681.

Lynch, F. L., McCarty, D., Mertens, J., Perrin, N. A., Green, C. A., Parthasarathy, S., et al. (2014). Costs of care for persons with opioid dependence in commercial integrated health systems. *Addiction Science and Clinical Practice*, 9(1): 16.

Mattick, R. P., Breen, C., Kimber, J., & Davoli, M. (2014, February 6). Buprenorphine maintenance versus placebo or methadone maintenance for opioid dependence. *Cochrane Database of Systematic Reviews*, (2): CD002207. doi:10.1002/14651858.CD002207.pub4. PMID: 24500948.

Matusitz, J., & Breen, G.-M. (2007). Telemedicine: Its effects on health communication. *Health Communication*, 21(1): 73–83.

McCarty, D., Perrin, N. A., Green, C. A., Polen, M. R., Leo, M. C., & Lynch, F. (2010). Methadone maintenance and the cost and utilization of health care among individuals dependent on opioids in a commercial health plan. *Drug and Alcohol Dependence*, 111(3): 235–240. doi:10.1016/j.drugalcdep.2010.04.018. PMID: 20627427; PMCID: PMC2950212.

Mendiola, C. K., Galetto, G., & Fingerhood, M. (2018). An exploration of emergency physicians' attitudes toward patients with substance use disorder. *Journal of Addiction Medicine*, 12(2): 132–135. doi:10.1097/ADM.0000000000000377. PMID: 29351141.

National Institute on Drug Abuse. (2019, September 26). *Initiating buprenorphine treatment in the emergency department.* Retrieved from National Institute on Drug Abuse Advancing Addiction Science at https://www.drugabuse.gov/nidamed-medical-health-professionals/discipline-specific-resources/emergency-physicians-first-responders/initiating-buprenorphine-treatment-in-emergency-department.

Olsen, Y., & Sharfstein, J. M. (2014). Confronting the stigma of opioid use disorder— and its treatment. *Journal of the American Medical Association*, 311(14): 1393–1394. doi:10.1001/jama.2014.2147. PMID: 24577059.

Paquette, C. E., Syvertsen, J. L., & Pollini, R. A. (2018). Stigma at every turn: Health services experiences among people who inject drugs. *International Journal of Drug Policy*, 57: 104–110. doi:10.1016/j.drugpo.2018.04.004. Epub 2018 Apr 30. PMID: 29715589; PMCID: PMC5994194.

Pullen, E., & Oser, C. (2014, June). Barriers to substance abuse treatment in rural and urban communities: A counselor perspective. *Substance Use Misuse*, 49(7): 891–901.

SHOUT Support for Hospital Opioid Use Treatment. (2020). *Quick guide: Buprenorphine starts in the hospital.* Retrieved from SHOUT Support for Hospital Opioid Use Treatment at https://static1.squarespace.com/static/5acbce828f51302409d8bdcb/t/5ad817f403ce646d1a1f4646/1524111350276/QUICK+GUIDE-+Buprenorphine+-+04-18-18.pdf.

Substance Abuse and Mental Health Services. (2019). *Key substance use and mental health indicators in the United States: Results from the 2018 National Survey on Drug Use and Health.* Retrieved from https://www.samhsa.gov/data/sites/default/files/cbhsq-reports/NSDUHNationalFindingsReport2018/NSDUHNationalFindingsReport2018.pdf.

Substance Abuse and Mental Health Services. (2020). *Opioid treatment program directory.* Retrieved from https://dpt2.samhsa.gov/treatment/directory.aspx.

Substance Abuse and Mental Health Services. (2020, April 29). *Targeted capacity expansion: medication assisted treatment—prescription drug and opioid addiction.* Retrieved from https://www.samhsa.gov/grants/grant-announcements/ti-18-009.

U.S. Department of Health and Human Services (HHS). (2018*). Facing addiction in America: The surgeon general's spotlight on opioids.* Washington, DC: U.S. Department of Health and Human Services.

van Boekel, L., Brouwers, E. P., van Weeghel, J., & Garretsen, H. F. (2013). Stigma among health professionals towards patients with substance use disorders and its consequences for healthcare delivery: Systematic review. *Drug and Alcohol Dependence*, 131(1-2): 23–35. doi:10.1016/j.drugalcdep.2013.02.018. Epub 2013 Mar 13. PMID: 23490450.

Weintraub, E., Greenblatt, A. D., Chang, J., Himelhoch, S., & Welsh, C. (2018, December 27). Expanding access to buprenorphine treatment in rural areas with the use of tel-emedicine. *American Journal on Addictions*, 8: 612–617.

Wicklund, E. (2018, September 18). *HHS makes a pitch for telemedicine in substance abuse treatment*. Retrieved from mHealthIntelligence: https://mhealthintelligence.com/news/hhs-makes-a-pitch-for-telemedicine-in-substance-abuse-treatment.

17

Supporting Advance Practice Providers in the Emergency Department Using Telehealth

L. KENDALL MCKENZIE, TEARSANEE CARLISLE, LISA HAYNIE, JASON MCKAY, GREG HALL, AND ROBERT GALLI ■

INTRODUCTION

Projections for health care needs in the United States are concerning due to a significant shortage of primary care and specialty physicians, including residency-trained emergency physicians. These shortages are contributing to a mismatch between supply and demand for emergency department (ED) services (Klauer, 2013). A 2018 analysis of Medicare claims from the 2014 data set identified the ED workforce as comprising 61% emergency physicians, 14.3% nonemergency physicians, and 24.5% advanced practice providers (APPs; Hall, 2018). The analysis further suggests that rural areas staff EDs with larger proportions of nonemergency physicians and APPs (Hall, 2018; Pines, 2020). The distribution of medical providers to rural and urban areas is multifactorial; however, the availability and lower cost of staffing with APPs are drivers in rural hospitals (Pines, 2020).

According to the National Hospital Ambulatory Medical Care Survey in 2016, APPs see between 12 and 16% of ED patients (Rui, 2016). While there is large variability in EDs with collaborative staffing models and onsite emergency physician (EP) supervision of APPs, APPs tend to see fewer patients per hour with lower acuity (Pines, 2020). The American College of Emergency Physicians permits both collaborative practice, where the EP also evaluates each patient the APPs sees, as well as indirect supervision models in which the APP seeks supervision from the EP as needed (*Advanced Practice Providers*, 2016). Supervision of APPs is influenced by licensing requirements, state regulation, and local hospital policy (Ward, 2018). In 2013, the Centers for Medicare and Medicaid Services (CMS) clarified Emergency Medical Treatment and Labor Act (EMTALA) rules that allow telemedicine physicians at a hub to meet the requirements of physician availability for APP supervision at critical access hospitals (CAHs) with telemedicine equipment (Ward, 2018). The staffing needs of rural hospital EDs are often met by APPs. Emergency telehealth is an emerging model designed to provide cost-effective supervision, but despite reduced regulatory barriers, the model has not yet been widely adopted (Ward, 2018).

The following case study describes an emergency telehealth program that focuses on the remote supervision of APPs that staff rural EDs across an entire state. Later sections of the chapter refer to this model to demonstrate the effectiveness and operational considerations of this type of telemedicine program.

CASE STUDY

Telemedicine was first considered at the University of Mississippi Medical Center (UMMC) in 1999 but was tabled because of the uncertainty of the model and inadequate technology. By 2001, Mississippi Critical Access Hospital (CAH) administrators were struggling to find 24-hour ED coverage to fulfill the Medicare requirement for certification due to very limited staffing options. Contract ED staffing companies were too expensive to staff low-volume, rural EDs. Physician assistants (PAs) were not yet licensed in Mississippi. The solution was nurse practitioners (NPs), many of whom returned to their home communities after training (Graves, 2016). Early on it was recognized that NPs were staffing several EDs across the state, and they would be transferring critically ill patients to UMMC with little evaluation or resuscitation.

In some states, NPs have privileges to practice as independently licensed health care providers; in Mississippi, however, they must work in cooperation with and under the direct supervision of physicians. At the time, NPs could work with a collaborating physician available within 15 miles due to the Board of Medical Licensure's position that physician "presence" within 15 miles meant the physician would be able to leave the office, hospital, or clinic to assist the NP as needed. Despite this requirement, often the collaborating physician was not able to attend at the bedside to assist with care in a timely fashion. UMMC argued to the Board that telehealth supervision would allow the NP and the patient 24/7 access to a board-certified emergency physician over video to examine the patient in real time.

After 11 months of consideration, UMMC was given a one-year probation period to test the telehealth model. After successfully reporting the UMMC experience and passing site visits, UMMC telemedicine physicians enjoy full privileges, including telemedicine-based APP supervision. Between 2003 and 2006, the UMMC TelEmergency program evaluated 40,000 patients located in rural EDs via telemedicine (Galli, 2008).

The first major component of the program was NP training in emergency medicine. In addition to completing a master's level NP program, UMMC TelEmergency provided 40 hours of continuing medical education on the evaluation and treatment of the ED patient and tested for competency (Galli, 2008). Additionally, NPs were provided with procedural training for common and critical ED procedures, and they spent over 135 hours and saw at least 100 patients in the UMMC ED. This training is similar to a clinical fellowship in emergency medicine (Sterling, 2017). All UMMC ED attending physicians and senior residents completed an orientation to the program and learned about rural hospital capabilities. The initial program provided

Table 17.1 Top Reasons for Patient Receiving
a TelEmergency Consult

Diagnosis	Frequency
Chest Pain	11%
Blunt Trauma	7%
Abdominal Pain	6%

dedicated physician coverage from 10 a.m. to 2 a.m., with as needed coverage from 2 a.m. to 10 a.m.

The second major component of the program was telemedicine and information technology infrastructure. The goal was to design a simple, user friendly system that allowed the physician to adequately evaluate the patient. At that time, the technology infrastructure was a complicated web of cameras, monitors, conference bridges, and a controller system. The program's paramount issues were image quality, reliability, and HIPAA (Health Insurance Portability and Accountability Act) matters. The ready solution at the time was hardwired T1 broadband lines. It was critical that the consulting physician could identify the appropriate patient in the appropriate room. Pan-tilt-zoom cameras allowed for more complete evaluation of the patient.

The third component of the program was a viable business model. The premise of the model was based on the delta cost between staffing an NP and staffing a physician in the ED. By utilizing a subscription model that reimbursed UMMC by hour of coverage, the cost of the coverage was divided among multiple sites. This created a sustainable model for both rural sites and the hub.

Over time, the clinical care model evolved to a tiered system of patients treated by the NP alone, those treated collaboratively with the telemedicine physician, and those requiring immediate consultation. Engagement is now high, with 54% of NPs reporting use of the video telemedicine system on every shift and 91% collaborating with an EP by phone multiple times per shift (Sterling, 2017). Detailed analysis and quality improvement regarding ED care were enabled by implementation of the TelEmergency program. The program has led to an increased volume of patients presenting to the ED with higher-risk complaints. For example, 23% of patients require admission and 34% require transfer (Sterling, 2017). One study on the impact of TeleEmergency demonstrated statistically similar hospital cardiac arrest survival in rural hospitals to survival in urban hospitals (Henderson, 2014). Other important metrics include high patient satisfaction and high hospital administrator satisfaction. The TelEmegency program has made UMMC a leader in emergency telehealth and is recognized as one of only two federally designated Centers of Excellence in Telehealth by HRSA (Telehealth Center of Excellence, n.d.).

RURAL ED WORKFORCE AND EMERGENCY CARE QUALIFIED APPS

All states, especially rural ones, face issues of health care coverage based on geography. The principal concern in rural areas is the patient's distance from a tertiary center, which is often located in an urban area. It is difficult to recruit primary care and specialty physicians to rural areas. Many physicians with young families seek career opportunities in locations with high-performing school systems, career options for spouses, and entertainment to foster wellness when not at work (Ludwig, 2018). While similar hurdles are found in urban environments as well, it remains that there are special challenges in recruiting physicians to rural hospitals (Sukel, 2019).

All EDs serve as safety nets for acute unscheduled care. Given the staffing challenges rural EDs face in hiring board-certified EPs, they must seek alternatively trained nonemergency physicians to meet this need. Nonemergency trained physicians with ambulatory experience are one option (Hall, 2018). In EDs with volumes of over 20,000 annual visits, there has been a growing trend of staffing APPs with physicians (*Advanced Practice Providers*, 2016). Similarly, rural EDs can staff with APPs, PAs, or NPs supervised via telemedicine.

NPs are registered nurses who have completed master's or similar high-level degrees. Once certified, an NP may pursue specialization. NPs interested in becoming emergency nurse practitioners (ENPs) first train as a family nurse practitioner (FNP), who provides adult and pediatric care training critical to emergency medicine. Alternatively, NPs could pursue the critical care (CCNP) pathway, learning to care for sicker patients and adopting certain emergency procedures specific to the ED, with adult patients only. Since FNP training is geared to outpatient clinic care, they were historically encouraged to cover the ED where many patients had clinic or urgent care complaints (*Advanced Practice Providers*, 2016).

PAs typically have prior medical exposure, such as serving as medical scribes, nurses, technicians, or prehospital care providers. The training programs require a bachelor's degree and a master's degree. Graduates must pass a national certifying exam and may pursue a Certificate of Added Qualification (CAQ) in emergency medicine. In addition to 150 emergency medicine continuing medical education credits, the PA must complete 3,000 hours in the ED. The requirements for both PA- and NP-supervised clinical practice in the ED to receive certification have led to the development of structured emergency medicine training programs or residencies (*Advanced Practice Providers*, 2016).

ADDITIONAL EDUCATIONAL REQUIREMENTS AND EXPERIENCE FOR APP PRACTICE UNDER TELEMEDICINE SUPERVISION

The National Organization of Nurse Practitioner Faculties (NONPF) supports new strategies that will effectively address the national health care provider shortage, complexity of disease, aging of the population, as well as the limited access to care. In accordance with the Institute of Medicine's (IOM's) latest nursing goals, innovative solutions for providing patient care such as telehealth offer a unique answer to these current challenges. In order to meet these challenges head on, it is imperative that APPs possess the education and clinical background necessary to utilize such technologies in practice (Rutledge, 2018).

In addition, APP students should possess the knowledge to competently utilize telehealth modalities by the time they graduate. NONPF recommends incorporating creative and innovative ways to include telehealth into the APP education curriculum in both didactic and clinical settings. There are telehealth technologies that allow faculty to conduct site visits and provide support to preceptors/clinical sites.

APP education should also include effective use of videoconferencing devices to connect patients, providers, and faculty for evaluation, management, and education. Also, interprofessional clinical experiences utilizing telehealth technologies between providers as well as face-to-face encounters are imperative. These experiences better prepare APPs with the skills to care for patients in rural and underserved areas where specialty health care services might not be available. Lastly, competency should be assessed throughout the APP education program to ensure that the student has the knowledge and skill to effectively deliver health care, utilizing telehealth modalities.

APP PRACTICE REGULATIONS

State nursing and medical boards regulate NP and PA practice in all venues. A delegation or supervisory agreement codifies how the APP will be supervised by the physician. Further, these documents should be regarded as essential when developing a telehealth program for APP supervision. Through such documents, clear expectations can be defined. Key topics to include are basic practice standards, responsibility for liability malpractice coverage, availability for and methods of collaboration, quality assurance and performance improvement processes, and basic functions of the APP. The section on basic functions should describe in detail which patients require collaborative interaction with the physician. This is most useful if patients are subcategorized based on presenting complaints, diagnoses, and/or acuity level. However written, the overarching goal of providing a safe practice environment that is patient-centric must be clearly understood through these documents. In the case of emergency telehealth, the supervision should be defined as virtual supervision by real-time audio-video connection. Just as in an in-person collaborative practice, it is imperative that the APP feel no barriers to consulting with the physician.

The rural hospital has full responsibility for the APP, including liability insurance, and must ensure that the APP complies with the ongoing educational requirements set forth by the medical center. Each member of the collaborative team must adhere to the rules and regulations presented by their respective licensing boards. The use of telemedicine does not supersede any state's rules for practice. Any requirements specific to oversight, collaboration, and quality assurance must be maintained; however, there may be additional requirements to ensure patient safety and quality care (Committee, 2008).

TECHNOLOGY

More than any other area, technology has been the greatest challenge and has evolved the fastest during the 17 years of TelEmergency. Early programs relied on T1 lines that provided a fixed wire from ED to ED with 99% reliability. This ensured HIPAA compliance, as it isolated audio and video to and from the station. Still, 24-hour IT availability was required to troubleshoot transmission interruptions and evoke the backup plan if necessary.

Newer wireless technologies enable reliable, portable, and cost-effective solutions that maintain all the security requirements for telehealth. During UMMC's third

Box 17.1

TECHNOLOGY CONSIDERATIONS FOR EMERGENCY TELEHEALTH
FOR APP SUPERVISION

Teleconferencing in each ED room with a pan-tilt-zoom camera (originating site)
Command center or dedicated telemedicine area in the ED for distant site
Mechanisms to manage sound in from ambient noise in a busy ED
Systems for easy activation of the TM service and to manage notifications
The expected response time from the TM physician
Management of simultaneous consultations (both originating and distant site)
Technology and training need to assist with procedures (including tele-ultrasound)

iteration, the IT team stepped back and simplified the components. As an example, TelEmergency's latest technology update utilized the Polycom Group Series in order to provide the video and audio streams for each of the sites. Each room at the rural sites that needed to be equipped simply had a Polycom Group Series installed with a monitor and a microphone.

At UMMC, all hardware codecs were replaced in the TelEmergency room with the Polycom RealPresence Application. This application allowed a webcam and microphone to be used with a standard PC enabling the rural hospital to see and hear the physician. This simple setup allows for rapid deployment of technology to multiple areas of the spoke hospital and allows physicians to conduct telemedicine consults. It is important that all physicians have training in virtual presence and that the utilization of remote control for the pan-tilt-zoom camera to optimize the physician–patient interaction. Depending on the need for supervision of procedures, specific technologies may be required for real-time supervision, for example, for endotracheal intubation (Sakles, 2011; Van Oeveren, 2017). See Box 17.1 for technologies to consider for APP supervision.

CONTRACTS AND BUSINESS MODELS

Another essential document to generate when developing any telehealth-based service is a contract between the involved parties, in this case the hub hospital/company where the EM-boarded physician practices, and the spoke hospital where the patient is physically located. Depending on the underlying relationship of the two entities (subsidiary vs. independent facilities), this document may take the form of a simple memorandum of agreement or a more formalized contract. Several key topics must be contractually addressed. Equipment ownership, as well as maintenance and replacement responsibilities, must be defined. Access to distant site records for quality assurance review should be contractually ensured. Likewise, timely submission of clinical documentation from the hub facility to the spoke site should be guaranteed through the contract. Receipt of this documentation is essential for third-party reimbursement of spoke site charges. Employment arrangements of the APPs and ongoing training requirements of these non-physician providers should also be addressed contractually. Administrative processes such as transmission of patient demographic information from the originating site to the hub facility for registration/documentation purposes should be addressed. Another reasonable approach to such topics would be a separately generated standard operating procedure manual.

There continue to be limited mechanisms to bill CMS or private payers for an emergency provider consultation to another emergency provider. However, state regulations regarding the billing for telehealth as well as the billing of medical services provided by APPs, both under direct supervision and telemedicine, are evolving.

The simplest business model remains a subscription or hourly rate for coverage. The assignment of all billing is returned to the rural facility and can offset some or all of the cost of the telemedicine services. The return on investment (ROI) for rural hospitals is seen in the increases in the scope of services, the volume of patients in the ED, the volume of patients retained for inpatient admission, and reduced risk. The community benefits from improved access to high-quality care.

IMPACT OF COVID-19

The response to the COVID-19 global pandemic was a series of emergency waivers for telehealth utilization for emergency care. While this chapter describes the remote supervision of APPs in rural EDs, the pandemic ushered in the opportunity for the use of real-time video to supervise another provider inside a patient care room from the outside of the patient care room. The pandemic also enabled the provision of emergency care by telehealth directly to the patient while in the ED and for EPs to provide emergency care to patients at a variety of other originating sites, including the home. All these functions were necessary in the setting of a highly infectious disease; as of this writing, it remains unclear whether they will be made permanent.

COMMUNITY PARAMEDICINE

Broader application of telehealth with remote physician supervision may expand the use of telehealth in community paramedicine. The availability and capability of community paramedicine as an integrated healthcare system resource have gained momentum in the United States since its debut in 2001. After completing additional training, prehospital paramedics (under the medical direction of their EMS agency or Mobile Integrated Healthcare system protocol) utilize an expanded scope of practice to increase access to primary care and reduce ED encounters. Remote patient monitoring, laboratory collection with point-of-care testing, procedural wound care, and preventative medicine are just some of the tools available to the community paramedic. Existing models have demonstrated significant reductions in ambulance transports to the ED (Langabeer, 2016) in both rural and urban areas of implementation. Subsequent benefits to CAH and metropolitan hospitals can be observed through measured improvements in the health of community participants, specifically, the management of chronic disease (Bennett, 2018). Reductions in cost associated with ED encounters and readmissions present additional economic relief and resource conservation for these regions. Data from homogeneous, international programs with longer operational histories (specifically the United Kingdom, Canada, and Australia) demonstrate similar, durable benefits of community paramedicine when incorporated into integrated health care systems. The efficacy of online medical direction between EPs and community paramedics via telemedicine, specifically the use of real-time video, is promising but requires further investigation.

CONCLUSION

TelEmergency at UMMC provides reliable adjunctive health care to 18 hospitals across the state of Mississippi. This long-standing program demonstrates the broad opportunities available for sustained business models providing emergency telehealth services. The combination of technology and advanced training opportunities support the utilization of APPs and board-certified emergency physicians in a collaborative model for rural and less resourced hospitals. In addition, staffing that includes APPs provides financial advantages. Many visits to the ED are low acuity. It is feasible to staff the ED with clinicians who are trained to appropriately treat the majority of the complaints while providing additional support to them using technology for more complex conditions. In order to implement a collaborative model that ensures patient safety and health care quality, effort must be placed on creating a structure for education and real-time support for the APP working with an EP through telehealth.

KEY TAKEAWAYS

- ➢ For a critical access hospital, emergency telemedicine could mean survival. By federal rules, they must provide 24/7 emergency care. A telehealth link with an experienced ED physician provides specialty backup for an APP known to the community in a cost-effective manner that the hospital administrator desires.
- ➢ An emergency telehealth program for APP supervision relies on the development of strong relationships between EPs and APPs. Critical to success are onsite training and orientation periods, open lines of communication, and a culture that promotes consultation.
- ➢ Scaling emergency telehealth coverage for a small number of hospital partners can be challenging. Program design, business model, and staffing should be flexible to accommodate growth.
- ➢ The complicated regulatory environment for telehealth requires that telehealth programs have dedicated business managers who can stay current on evolving rules and payment restrictions and serve as advocates.
- ➢ It is critical to ensure an optimal patient experience, including virtual presence training for distant site EPs, as well as proper design and setup of technology.

REFERENCES

Advanced Practice Providers (physician assistant and nurse practitioner) medical-legal issues. (2016). Information paper reviewed by the ACEP Board of Directors. Retrieved October 2, 2020, from https://www.acep.org/globalassets/uploads/uploaded-files/acep/clinical-and-practice-management/resources/medical-legal/mlc_adv-prac-prov-ip_final_nov-2016.pdf.

Bennett, K. J. (2018, February). Community paramedicine applied in a rural community. *Journal of Rural Health* (Suppl. 1): s39–s47.

Committee, A. C. (2008, July 7). *Consensus model for APRN regulation: Licensure, accreditation, certification and education.* Retrieved October 2, 2020, from https://ncsbn.org/Consensus_Model_for_APRN_Regulation_July_2008.pdf.

Galli, R. K. (2008, March). TelEmergency: A novel system for delivering emergency care to rural hospitals. *Annals of Emergency Medicine*, 51(3): 275–284.

Graves, J. (2016, January). Role of geography and nurse practitioner scope-of-practice in efforts to expand primary care system capacity: Health reform and the primary care workforce. *Medical Care*, 54(1): 81–89.

Hall, M. K. (2018). State of the national emergency department workforce: Who provides care where? *Annals of Emergency Medicine*, 72(3): 302–307.

Henderson, K. (2014). Relative survivability of cardiopulmonary arrest in rural emergency department utilizing telemedicine. *Journal of Rural Emergency Medicine*, 1(1): 9–12.

Klauer, K. (2013). Innovative staffing in emergency departments: The role of midlevel providers. *Canadian Journal of Emergency Medicine*, 15(3): 1340140.

Langabeer, J. (2016, November). Telehealth-enabled emergency medical services program reduces ambulance transport to urban emergency departments. *Western Journal of Emergency Medicine*, 17(6): 713–720.

Ludwig, K. (2018, November 15). Barriers to practicing general practice in rural areas—Results of a qualitative pre-post-survey about medical students during their final clinical year. *GMS Journal of Medical Education*, 35(4).

Pines, J. M. (2020). The impact of advanced practice provider staffing on emergency department care: Productivity, flow, safety, and experience. *Academic Emergency Medicine*, 1–10.

Rui, P. (2016). *National Hospital Ambulatory Medical Care Survey: 2016 emergency department summary tables.* Retrieved from https://www.cdc.gov/nchs/data/nhamcs/web_tables/2016_ed_web_tables.pdf.

Rutledge, C. (2018, February 27). *Papers/Statements.* Retrieved October 27, 2020, from National Organization of Nurse Practitioner Faculties at https://cdn.ymaws.com/www.nonpf.org/resource/resmgr/2018_Slate/Telehealth_Paper_2018.pdf.

Sakles, J. C. (2011, April). Telemedicine and telepresence for prehospital and remote hospital tracheal intubation using a GlideScope™ Videolaryngoscope: A model for tele-intubation. *Telemedicine and e-Health*, 17(3): 185–188.

Sterling, S. (2017). Case study 10 coordinating emergency care through telemedicine. In J. L. Wiler (Ed.), *Value and quality innovations in acute and emergency care* (pp. 139–147). Cambridge: Cambridge University Press.

Sterling, S. A. (2017). The impact of the TelEmergency program on rural emergency care: An implementation study. *Journal of Telemedicine and Telecare*, 23(6): 588–594.

Sukel, K. (2019, September 10). Dealing with the shortage of rural physicians. *Medical Economics*, 96(17): 18–21. Retrieved from Medical Economics: https://www.medicaleconomics.com/view/dealing-shortage-rural-physicians.

Telehealth Center of Excellence. (n.d.). Retrieved September 23, 2020, from the University of Mississippi Medical Center, UMMC Center for Telehealth: https://www.umc.edu/Research/Centers-and-Institutes/Centers/Telehealth_Center_of_Excellence/Home.html.

Van Oeveren, L. (2017, April). Telemedicine-assisted intubation in rural emergency departments: A National Emergency Airway Registry Study. *Telemedicine and e-Health*, 23(4): 290–297.

Ward, M. M. (2018). Use of telemedicine for ED physician coverage in critical access hospitals increased after CMS policy clarification. *Health Affairs*, 37(12): 2037–2044.

18

Emergency Telehealth Services in the Correctional Setting

NEWTON E. KENDIG, DAVID G. ELLIS, RENOJ VARUGHESE, AND OBINNA M. OME IRONDI ■

INTRODUCTION

The incarceration rate in the United States has declined since 2009 and is currently at its lowest since 1996. Yet over two million persons were housed in a U.S. jail or prison at year-end 2016 (Kaeble & Cowhig, 2018). U.S jails in 2,800 different jurisdictions house local county and urban inmate populations, the majority of whom are unconvicted with brief incarcerations of less than one year. In mid-year 2017, U.S. jails housed 745,200 inmates and reported 10.6 million annual admissions, with an average time in jail of 26 days (Zeng, 2019). In contrast to jails, prisons house mostly sentenced inmates who have received a court-ordered term of imprisonment of more than one year. At the end of 2017, nearly 1.5 million inmates resided in state or federal prisons (Bronson & Carson, 2019).

The over 2 million patients who receive their health care within a U.S. correctional setting are disproportionately male and members of ethnic and racial minorities (Bromson & Carson, 2019). (See Table 18.1.) Inmates often live lives of poverty

Table 18.1 Incarcerated and General Population Demographic Comparisons

	Incarcerated	General
Gender		
Male	93%	49.2%
Female	7%	50.8%
Race		
Black	32%	12.8%
Hispanic	22%	18.4%
White	29%	72%
Total Population	1,489,400	328,239,523

Table 18.2 HEALTH CONDITIONS OF PRISONERS AND JAIL INMATES COMPARED TO THE
GENERAL POPULATION*

	Prisoners	Jail Inmates	General Population*
Meet criteria for drug dependence or abuse	58%	63%	5%
Psychological distress	14%	26%	5%
History of chronic medical condition	44%	45%	27%–31%
Hypertension	30%	26%	14%–18%
Infectious disease	21%	14%	5%
Obese or overweight	74%	62%	72%

*Standardized to match the incarcerated populations by sex, age, race, and Hispanic origin.

with limited engagement with the health care system prior to incarceration. They frequently suffer from serous health conditions, particularly addiction disorders, mental illness, and chronic medical issues. Between 2007 and 2009, 58% of state prisoners and 63% of sentenced jail inmates met the DSM-IV criteria for drug dependence or abuse (Bronson, Stroop, Zimmer, & Berzofsky, 2017). A later survey, conducted in 2011–2012, reported that every one in seven state and federal prisoners (14%) and one in four jail inmates (26%) had experienced serious psychological distress (Bronson & Berzofsky, 2017) (see Table 18.2). In a special report from the Bureau of Justice Statistics, state and federal prisoners and jail inmates had rates of self-reported histories of chronic diseases, infectious diseases, or overweight that equaled or far exceeded general population percentages when standardized to match the incarcerated populations by sex, age, race, and Hispanic origin (Maruschak, Berzofsky, & Unangst, 2016). Lastly, the aging of the incarcerated patient population further complicates their health care needs. The number of state prisoners age 55 or older sentenced to more than one year increased 400% between 1993 and 2013, from 26,300 to 131,500 (Carson & Sabol, 2016).

HEALTH CARE IN THE CORRECTIONAL SETTING CONTEXT

State correctional systems currently employ a variety of health care delivery models to care for incarcerated patient populations. Recent surveys indicate that 17 states provide the majority of health care services through department of corrections staff; 20 states contract out the majority of health services to private providers; 8 states use a hybrid model of public and private health care services; and 4 states deliver health care through academic medicine affiliations (Prison Health Care Costs and Quality, 2017). The Pew Survey also reported contract requirements for 30 states' correctional systems with contracted or hybrid models. Four states included contract financial incentives; 20 included contract financial penalties; and 25 included contract quality metrics.

States diverge widely in their approaches to staffing correctional health care services. Across multiple state prison systems, the number of health care employees, measured as full-time equivalents (FTEs) for every 1,000 inmates, ranged from 18.6 to 86.8, with a median of 40 FTEs. The majority of correctional health care professionals were registered nurses or licensed practical nurses. Prescribing clinicians represented the smallest portion of health care staffing in every state (Prison Health Care Costs and Quality, 2017). Patient care in correctional medicine is provided mostly in outpatient health care units within the facilities. In-patient care may also be available in prison infirmaries, with skilled and long-term nursing care provided 24 hours a day, 7 days a week. Access to onsite subspecialty care and diagnostic services is highly variable across systems, as reported in a national survey of 45 state prisons (Chari, Simon, DeFrances, & Maruschak, 2016).

In contrast to prisons, health care delivery models within U.S. jails have not been as carefully assessed. In an analysis of one state's jail system, 84% of local jails had private contracts for at least some health care services (Jails: Inadvertent Health Care Providers, 2018). Other models employed by jails include health care delivery by jail employees or agreements with local county health departments to provide medical care. The focus of health care in the jail setting is also different from the prison setting. Incarcerated jail patients frequently enter the facility directly from the community, potentially with serious unmet medical and mental health care needs that require stabilization or urgent interventions. Withdrawal from substances, contagious disease detection, and suicidal ideation are of particular concern. The recurrent, short-term incarcerations that frequently affect jail patient populations may result in lapses in care and curtail the opportunity for chronic disease management.

Providing value-based health care to incarcerated patients can be challenging considering the high prevalence of chronic medical and behavioral health conditions. Health care delivery may also be compounded by severe health care staffing shortages, lack of community hospital and subspecialty care in rural areas where many jails and prisons are located, and burgeoning health care costs that exceed allocated budgets. A survey of state departments of corrections determined that $8.1 billion was spent on prison health care in fiscal year 2015. Per capita inmate costs ranged from $2,173 in Louisiana to $19,796 in California. The median per capita cost for inmate health care was $5,720 (Prison Health Care Costs and Quality, 2017).

EMERGENCY CARE IN THE CORRECTIONAL SETTING

The delivery of timely and adequate emergency care to incarcerated patients is a core component of medically necessary and constitutionally required health care in the correctional setting. The emergency health care needs of incarcerated patients are rarely reported on, however. One retrospective review characterized New York Department of Corrections' jail and prison patients who were treated in an academic Level I Trauma Center during 2013. Table 18.3 summarizes the most common presenting complains for 576 emergency department (ED) visits (Koester, Brenner, Goulette, Wojcik, & Grant, 2017).

The high frequency of trauma visits to the ED is not surprising considering the frequency of injuries documented during incarceration. An analysis of 2004 survey data of 14,449 inmates from 287 state prisons reported that 3,117 inmates (21.5%) had an accident-related injury during incarceration and that 2,129 inmates (14.7%)

Table 18.3 PRESENTING COMPLAINTS FOR NEW YORK DEPARTMENT OF CORRECTIONS
PRISONER ED VISITS

Complaint	%
Trauma	16.8%
Abdominal pain	13.5%
Chest pain	9.0%
Self-injury	8.7%
Neurologic symptoms	7.1%
Hematologic symptoms	4.0%

had a violence-related injury during incarceration (Sung, 2010). Self-injurious behaviors also frequently affect inmate populations, who have high rates of serious mental illness and personality disorders. In a national survey, state prison systems reported that inmate self-injuries occur weekly in at least 85% of systems, although the types and severity of injuries were largely uncharacterized (Appelbaum, Savageau, Trestman, Metzner, & Baillargeon, 2011). A separate targeted analysis in California, however, assessed 704 state inmates taken to the hospital for toxic ingestion. Compared to controls, inmates had a much higher rate of toxic drug exposures, with a high morbidity associated with body stuffing and packing (Butterfield et al., 2015).

Providing high-quality emergency care to inmates can be challenging in the correctional setting. Physician-level expertise is frequently unavailable 24 hours a day, 7 days a week. Onsite emergency equipment and response capabilities may also be quite limited. In the 2016 Centers for Disease Control (CDC) survey of prison health care, 18 state correctional systems reported that onsite emergency care was restricted to patient triage, stabilization, and basic suturing (Chari, Simon, DeFrances, & Maruschak, 2016). For rural jails and prisons, community-based emergency medical transport services (EMS) and hospital emergency services may be distantly located and have limited capabilities. Not infrequently, security requirements for outside transports may delay or complicate emergency transportation. Additionally, community-based emergency care may be costly depending on the degree of necessary medical care and the extent of required correctional officer security. Reducing outside medical trips for incarcerated patient populations may also have relevant public health implications. The disparate impact of the COVID-19 pandemic on congregate settings highlighted the importance of minimizing the movement of patients into and out of correctional facilities (Reinhart & Chen, 2020). Lastly, outside medical trips of incarcerated patients pose an inherent public safety risk for the community at large.

TELEHEALTH IN THE CORRECTIONAL SETTING

Correctional systems are increasingly using telemedicine to support primary care providers based in U.S. jails and prisons. A 2016 CDC survey indicated that 30 of 45 state correctional systems used telemedicine for at least one subspecialty, with the most common being psychiatry or cardiology (Chari, Simon, DeFrances, & Maruschak, 2016) (see Table 18.4).

Table 18.4 NUMBER OF STATES REPORTING SERVICES FOR A SPECIALTY VIA
TELEMEDICINE

Specialty	Number of states
Psychiatry	28
Cardiology	12
Orthopedics	7
Oncology	7
Obstetrics	3
Ophthalmology	3
Gynecology	2

Some state correctional telehealth programs are quite comprehensive, serving multiple facilities throughout the state's correctional system and providing a wide range of subspecialty services through university-based providers (Rappaport, Reynolds, Baucom, & Lehman, 2018). This access to academic medicine subspecialty care in areas such as infectious diseases and psychiatry has improved clinical outcomes for incarcerated patients (Zaylor, Nelson, & Cook, 2001; Young et al., 2014; Sterling et al., 2018). An additional benefit of university partnerships has been the upskilling of correctional providers in disease management that evolves with telementoring by subspecialists (Arora et al., 2011). Over time, correctional practitioners become more independent, reducing the need for less complicated consultations.

Despite the tangible benefits of telemedicine for correctional health care, potential barriers to effective implementation must be recognized and addressed. Concerns include lack of collaborative engagement and commitment from key stakeholders; underestimation of the administrative and training required by prison personnel; equipment compatibility and connectivity issues; patient privacy concerns; and hidden financial costs (Doarn, Justis, Chaudhri, & Merrell, 2005; Edge et al., 2019). Overall, correctional telemedicine programs can be cost-effective, but multiple factors must be considered in the analysis.

Correctional systems have not widely adopted telemedicine to support emergency care for incarcerated patients. Successful programs have been described in the New York state correctional system, in adolescent detention facilities in Tennessee, and in Italian penitentiaries (Ellis, Mayrose, & Phelan, 2006; Fox, Somes, & Waters, 2007; Brunetti, Dellegrottaglie, Si Giuseppe, De Gennaro, & Di Biase, 2013). The New York telehealth model has provided emergency consultations 24 hours a day to over 50,000 inmates in 51 correctional facilities over the last 20 years through real-time videoconferencing (Ellis, 2003). Emergency care is provided by physicians, physician assistants, or nurse practitioners with emergency medicine expertise who are located at an academic center. An evaluation of 1,522 teleconsultations over 52 weeks indicated that 38% of incarcerated patients avoided outside transportation to the ED (Ellis, 2003). In Tennessee, Fox described a more limited, 7% reduction in ED visits with implementation of behavioral telehealth services for patients in juvenile detention. In the Apulia region of Italy, cardiologists provide 24/7 ECG interpretations and case consultations for 12 penitentiaries. Over a three-year period, 2,015 ECGs were taken on incarcerated patients presenting with acute cardiac conditions. Only 4% of patients required urgent hospitalization.

OPERATIONAL CONSIDERATIONS

A number of considerations can assist the emergency provider to be most effective at providing care in a correctional setting using telemedicine technologies. It is important to recognize the role of identifying an emergency condition that would require the patient to be transported outside the facility to an ED or alternatively, determining which patients can be managed using the resources of the correctional facility. Construction of an appropriate and adequate differential diagnosis should be as important in the correctional telemedicine setting as it is in the ED (Sandhu, 2006).

Emergency telehealth providers can confidently state that they would treat the patient in a very similar fashion if they saw them in their ED utilizing the same evidence base for treatment decisions. An important risk management rule in the system has been that the correctional facility providers and nursing staff always have the last word in decisions to transport to an ED. Nursing staff, particularly those working off-hours when a local facility provider is not present, are encouraged to use their clinical judgment when deciding whether they should wait for emergency telemedicine direction or initiate an EMS response and transport to the ED by calling 911.

The practice of emergency telehealth in a correctional setting is unique due to its secure environment. Patients are housed in cells and may not easily be constantly observed. Nursing staff have multiple nonemergency care duties, such as passing medications, that limit their ability to support patients with ongoing medical needs. Patients should be placed in infirmaries with the confidence that the patient's condition is relatively stable, with a low likelihood of deterioration. The distance of the correctional facility from the nearest ED is an important factor when considering facility management of potentially rapidly exacerbating conditions such as asthma, chronic obstructive pulmonary disease (COPD), or altered mental status. Furthermore, triaging patients directly to tertiary medical centers with multispecialty on-call coverage while avoiding referral to small, rural hospital EDs for stable patients may be a win–win for the facilities and the patients who have a high likelihood of needing specialty care or admission.

The correctional care nurse at the facility routinely serves as the telepresenter. The emergency telehealth provider is required to oversee and manage the clinical examination using available peripheral devices and the participation of telepresenting nursing staff (Weinstein, 2018).

Operationally, understanding the pretest probability of an abnormal exam and the sensitivity and specificity of the physical examination will help determine if performing that physical exam component will make the diagnostic possibilities more or less likely. In the New York experience, the correctional facility nursing staff was especially helpful in facilitating the physical examination using their hands, ears, and eyes with their close-up visual resolution, and advocacy to assist in the patient examination. In this situation, it is critical that the examining telehealth provider utilize specific directions and questioning in conjunction with the telepresenter in order to facilitate the history, physical exam, and resulting patient care decisions. An example might be the examination for hyphema, hemotympanum, tympanic rupture, or septal hematoma by having the telepresenter look at the likely normal unaffected eye, ear, nose, or throat to assist in comparison (see Table 18.5). If the telehealth provider is not confident in the information being relayed by the telepresenter, they should always have the option of referring to the facility provider or transferring to the ED.

Table 18.5 KEY EXAM FINDINGS FACILITATED BY THE TELEPRESENTER

Area of Exam	Diagnoses/Key Findings	Telepresenter, Nurse Instruction/Facilitation
Vitals	Hypertensive emergency, hypotension, temperature	BP cuff size, position, repeat vitals, temperature method
Eye	Hyphema, abnormal pupil, scleral redness, corneal abrasion	Visual acuity, compare eyes, blood/fluid level in anterior chamber, fluorescein stain
ENT	Hemotympanum, ruptured TM, septal hematoma	Compare ears, describe Tympanic Membrane, hole in TM, compare nostrils, describe septum (grapelike)
Lungs	Bronchospasm, pneumothorax, consolidation	Air entry, equal bilateral, wheeze, rhonchi, rales
Heart	Pericardial tamponade, ruptured valve	Muffled heart sounds, machine-like murmur
Abdomen	Obstruction/perforation, AAA, ischemic bowel	Deep palpation, four-quadrant exam, rebound tenderness
Musculoskeletal	Dislocation, fracture, spinal injury	Patient/camera positioning, range of motion, strength against resistance
Skin	Laceration depth, "fight bite," rash, lesions	Manage camera/lighting, skin warmth, feel patient for clammy skin, describe lesion (vesicle/pustule)
Neuro	Delirium, CVA, psychosis, excited delirium	Mental status assess (voice/pain stimulus) gait, assist limited NIH Stroke Scale (NIHSS), motor strength assess

Diagnostic testing may be limited by onsite availability and turnaround time. Point-of-care testing can be relatively simple and include electrocardiogram, vital signs with pulse oximetry, fingerstick glucose, urine dipsticks, and spirometry. The electrocardiogram is a frequently used and useful tool in the practice of correctional care emergency telehealth. Other prison clinical environments may provide iSTAT™ or other Clinical Laboratory Improvement Amendments of 1988 "CLIA"-waived tests in addition to urine test strips. The reduced cost of portable ultrasound with limited training and remote supervision may help make it a more common diagnostic tool.

Methods by which inmates or their clinical samples are transported is also an important consideration for the emergency telehealth provider. Whereas many large correctional facilities will be in rural locations, a small, rural hospital and ED are usually relatively close by, which will serve as the destination for most emergent referrals or problems such as lacerations that might require attention followed by return of the inmate to the facility. The laboratories in these local facilities can also be used for STAT blood tests, such as troponin in certain clinical scenarios. The emergency telehealth program can prove valuable if it can save an extra transfer by identifying relatively stable but urgent medical concerns that can be transported by corrections vehicle a longer distance to a tertiary care facility rather than to the local hospital ED. Patients who likely require a specialist or admission to a secure locked ward in the tertiary hospital may benefit from this direct referral. Decisions over transport via correctional vehicle versus Basic Life Support (BLS) or Advanced Life Support (ALS) ambulance transfer should be based on an assessment of patient stability (e.g., chest pain, possible acute coronary syndrome (ACS) via ALS, trauma in cervical collar (C-collar) via BLS). The majority of cases can occur via correctional vehicle but should be predefined by policy to avoid confusion and delay. The use of telehealth in correctional care populations for common complaints may require a strategic approach to diagnosis and treatment (Table 18.6).

Patient privacy should be protected with health care policies that are informed by the Health Insurance Portability and Accountability Act (HIPAA). The HIPAA Privacy Rule has exceptions for correctional facilities that allow the disclosure of personal health information for significant public safety reasons. However, correctional

Table 18.6 EMERGENCY TELEHEALTH CORRECTION CARE DIAGNOSTIC STRATEGIES FOR COMMON COMPLAINTS

Complaint	Diagnostic Considerations	Management Strategy
(Atypical) Chest pain	Consider broad differential in potentially high-risk population (AMI, PE, aortic dissection); Utilize risk assessment tools (e.g., HEART Score, GRACE, mini Grace)	POC cardiac enzyme testing On-site chest X-ray, transport bloods locally for STAT testing
Abdominal pain	Leverage telepresenter abdominal examination; treat and reevaluation strategies for nonemergent diagnoses (GERD, renal colic, GE)	POC urine testing; follow-up effect of GI Cocktail, PPI, H2 blockers; delayed CT, or POC US for renal colic
Pneumonia	Evaluate appropriateness for outpatient treatment of pneumonia, Consider viral syndromes (including COVID-19); Consider sepsis possible	Clinical exam, vital signs, pulse ox, comorbidities
Cellulitis	Evaluate for sepsis, Fournier's gangrene Evaluate for appropriateness of outpatient treatment with clinical monitoring Consider risk for MRSA infections	Antibiotics; warm soaks/ compresses; elevation; wound care; incision, and drainage Pain control
Extremity injuries	Evaluate for unstable fractures, open fractures, dislocation, and neurovascular injuries	Clearly document lack of deformity, intact mobility, intact motor and sensory function; Immobilization and nonweight-bearing; delayed X-ray (next a.m.)

Table 18.6 CONTINUED

Complaint	Diagnostic Considerations	Management Strategy
Eye, ear, nose and throat	Consider that evaluation occurs prior to significant swelling and edema	Utilize visual acuity and visual inspection to rule out severe eye injuries
	Fundoscopy and intraocular pressure measuring devices are typically not available	Utilize fluorescein and Woods Lamp for corneal abrasions
	Be vigilant for symptoms concerning for glaucoma that need ED	
Foreign body ingestion	Consider ASGE standards for which ingestions require emergent removal (button batteries, sharp objects, objects larger than 5 cm)	Utilize serial X-rays to document passage of foreign body; Delayed transfer for removal depending on object and size
Medication / contraband drug ingestion	Stable patients without toxidrome, bezoar, and nonlethal ingestions may be observed; K2 or Spice ingestions common; Consider excited delirium with fever, tachycardia and AMS	Utilize vital signs, EKG and mental status; Evaluate for toxidrome; Assess for role of Narcan; Access poison control; Consider ED evaluation
Cardiac arrest	Comprehensive cardiac resuscitation is likely outside the scope of facility medical services; limited ACLS trained staff along with lack of support for in-facility IV meds or airway intervention	Response and telehealth guidance should focus on high-quality CPR, early defibrillation with AED, therapeutic hypothermia, transport to a STEMI-capable ED

systems must still strive to protect patient privacy in accordance with HIPAA (Barraza, Collmer, Meza, & Penunuri, 2015). Patient privacy can be respected and managed by actively limiting and identifying persons in the rooms at either end, keeping patient records secure, providing translation services in consultation, or obtaining patient permission for translation services in the jail and by provider/ nurse reports when transferring the patient for emergency care. Information technology systems in jails may vary greatly with respect to which entity, jail or contractor, provides support and upgrades the availability of electronic health records and wireless connectivity. Therefore, often medical records are still on paper or have limited accessibility.

CONCLUSION

The provision of emergency telehealth care services in the correctional setting is an underutilized capability that could enhance the quality of care provided to incarcerated patients in certain U.S. jails and prisons. The limited available reports suggest that emergency telehealth can substantively reduce outside medical trips and prove cost-effective in some correctional settings. Correctional facilities or systems that could potentially benefit most from emergency telehealth services include those with large patient populations; those with high-security inmates who require significant security escort costs; those located in remote locations without nearby EDs; and those that have an in-state telehealth provider with proven capabilities for providing emergency telehealth services. Implementing an emergency telehealth program in the correctional setting, however, requires a significant investment of time and resources. Key requirements include developing telehealth policies and procedures; obtaining necessary funding; formalizing a relationship with the telehealth provider through contracts or other means; securing the telehealth infrastructure and equipment to ensure connectivity; and providing training to health care personnel. These investments should be strongly considered for certain jails and prisons, as they will improve access to quality patient care in a value-based manner while promoting public safety.

KEY TAKEAWAYS

> Correctional care telehealth requires collaborative stakeholder engagement between the correctional facility leadership, the correctional care health contractor, and telehealth services provider.
> Telehealth model cost-effectiveness can be assessed by major cost drivers, such as the anticipated volume and types of outside emergency medical trips, the associated security escort requirements, contractual costs for emergency care services provided by the community hospital ED provider or the telehealth provider, equipment procurement and maintenance costs, and other administrative costs.
> Reliable telehealth compatibility and connectivity between the correctional facility and the telehealth provider should be ensured.
> Correctional health care staff serve as telepresenters that should be provided with the competencies to effectively assess medical emergencies and communicate with emergency telehealth personnel.
> Emergency telehealth diagnostic and management protocols for commonly occurring emergencies that are approved by both the local medical director and the telehealth provider should be developed.

REFERENCES

Appelbaum, K. L., Savageau, J. A., Trestman, R. L., Metzner, J. L., & Baillargeon, J. (2011, March 1). A national survey of self-injurious behavior in american prisons. *Psychiatric Services*, 62(3): 285–290.

Arora, S., Thorton, K., Murata, G., Deming, P., Kalishman, S., Dion, D., et al. (2011, June 9). Outcomes of treatment for hepatitis c virus infection by primary care providers. *New England Journal of Medicine*, 364: 2199–2207.

Barraza, L., Collmer, V., Meza, N., & Penunuri, K. (2015, July). The legal implications of HIPAA privacy and public health reporting for correctional facilities. *Journal of Correctional Health Care*, 21(3): 213–221.

Bronson, J., & Berzofsky, M. (2017). *Indicators of mental health problems reported by prisoners and jail inmates, 2011–12*. Bureau of Justice Statistics, U.S. Department of Justice.

Bronson, J., & Carson, E. A. (2019). *Prisoners in 2017*. Bureau of Justice Statistics, U.S. Department of Justice.

Bronson, J., Stroop, J., Zimmer, S., & Berzofsky, M. (2017). *Drug use, dependence, and abuse among state prisoners and jail inmates, 2007–2009*. Bureau of Justice Statistics, U.S. Department of Justice.

Brunetti, N. D., Dellegrottaglie, G., Di Giuseppe, G., De Gennaro, L., & Di Biase, M. (2013, October 3). Prison break: Remote tele-cardiology support for cardiology emergency in Italian penitentiaries. *International Journal of Cardiology*, 168(3): 3138–3140.

Butterfield, M., Al-Abri, S., Huntington, S., Carlson, T., Geller, R. J., & Olson, K. R. (2015, September). Symptomatic exposures among california inmates 2011–2013. *Journal of Medical Toxicology*, 11(3): 309–316.

Carson, E. A., & Sabol, W. J. (2016). *Aging of the state prison population, 1993–2013*. Bureau of Justice Statistics, U.S. Department of Justice.

Chari, K. A., Simon, A. E., DeFrances, C. J., & Maruschak, L. (2016). *National survey of prison health care: Selected Findings*. U.S. Department of Health and Human Services, Centers for Disease Control and Prevention, National Center for Health Statistics.

Doarn, C. R., Justis, D., Chaudhri, M. S., & Merrell, R. C. (2005, April 1). Integration of telemedicine practice into correctional medicine: An evolving standard. *Journal of Correctional Health Care*, 11(3): 253–270.

Edge, C., Black, G., King, E., George, J., Patel, S., & Hayward, A. (2019, October 22). Improving care quality with prison telemedicine: The effects of context and multiplicity on successful implementation and use. *Journal of Telemedicine and Telecare*, 1357633X19869131.

Ellis, D. G. (2003, Spring). The success of emergency telemedicine at the State University of New York at Buffalo. *Telemedicine Journal and E-Health*, 9(1): 73–79.

Ellis, D. G., Mayrose, J., & Phelan, M. (2006, September 1). Consultation times in emergency telemedicine using realtime videoconferencing. *Journal of Telemedicine and Telecare*, 12(6): 303–305.

Fox, K. C., Somes, G. W., & Waters, T. M. (2007, August 1). Timeliness and access to healthcare services via telemedicine for adolescents in state correctional facilities. *Journal of Adolescent Health*, 41(2): 161–167.

Jails: Inadvertent health care providers. (2018). The Pew Charitable Trusts. The Pew Charitable Trusts. https://www.pewtrusts.org/-/media/assets/2018/01/sfh_jails_in-advertent_health_care_providers.pdf

Kaeble, D., & Cowhig, M. (2018). *Correctional populations in the United States, 2016*. Bureau of Justice Statistics, U.S. Department of Justice.

Koester, L., Brenner, J. M., Goulette, A., Wojcik, S. M., & Grant, W. (2017, April). Inmate health care provided in an emergency department. *Journal of Correctional Health Care*, 23(2): 157–161.

Maruschak, L. M., Berzofsky, M., & Unangst, J. (2016). *Medical problems of state and federal prisoners and jail inmates, 2011–12*. Bureau of Justice Statistics, U.S. Department of Justice.

Prison health care costs and quality. (2017). The Pew Charitable Trusts. The Pew Charitable Trusts. https://www.pewtrusts.org/-/media/assets/2017/10/sfh_prison_health_care_costs_and_quality_final.pdf

Rappaport, E. S., Reynolds, H. N., Baucom, S., & Lehman, T. M. (2018, January). Telehealth support of managed care for a correctional system: The open architecture telehealth model. *Journal of Telemedicine and e-Health*, 24(1): 54–60.

Reinhart, E., & Chen, D. L. (2020, June 4). Incarceration and its disseminations: COVID-19 pandemic lessons from Chicago's Cook County jail. *Health Affairs*, 39(8): 1412–1418.

Sandhu H, C. C. (2006, December). Clinical decisionmaking: Opening the black box of cognitive reasoning. *Annals of Emergency Medicine*, 48(6): 713–719.

Sterling, R. K., Cherian, R., Lewis, S., Genther, K., Driscoll, C., Martin, K., et al. (2018, April). Treatment of HCV in the Department of Corrections in the era of oral medications. *Journal of Correctional Health Care*, 24(2): 127–136.

Stobo, J. D., & Raimer, B. G. (2004, July 28). Health care delivery in the Texas prison system: The role of academic medicine. *JAMA*, 292(4): 485–489.

Sung, H.-E. (2010, May 12). Prevalence and risk factors of violence-related and accident-related injuries among state prisoners. *Journal of Correctinoal Health Care*, 12(3): 178–187.

Weinstein, R. S. (2018, May). Clinical examination component of telemedicine, telehealth, mHealth and connected health medical practices. *Medical Clinics of North America*, 102(3): 533–544.

Young, J. D., Patel, M., Badowski, M., Mackesy-Amiti, M., Vaughn, P., & Shicker, L., et al. (2014, July 1). Improved virologic suppression with HIV subspecialty care in a large prison system using telemedicine: An observational study with historical controls. *Clinical Infectious Diseases*, 59(1): 123–126.

Zaylor, C., Nelson, E.-L., & Cook, D. J. (2001, January 1). Clinical Outcomes in a Prison Telepsychiatry Clinic. *Journal of Telemedicine and Telecare*, 7(S1): 47–49.

Zeng, Z. (2019). *Jail inmates in 2017*. Bureau of Justice Statistics, U.S. Department of Justice.

19

Extending Care Team Access to Out-of-Hospital Settings via Telehealth

DENISE WASSENAAR, PAUL KNIGHT, MARK A. HANSON, AND JEFFREY D. WESSLER ∎

INTRODUCTION

Within the spectrum of senior care and specifically long-term care (LTC), telehealth is beginning to demonstrate its value as social, financial, workforce, and regulatory factors are influencing adoption by health care providers. In the United States, people over 65 years of age make up the fastest-growing population segment. By 2030, this segment will increase by 20%, as every baby boomer will have reached the age of 65 (Bureau, n.d.).

As the older population continues its extraordinary growth, national health expenditures as a percent of gross domestic product (GDP) "is projected to grow at an average annual rate of 5.5 percent for 2018–27 and represent 19.4 percent of gross domestic product in 2027" (Keehan et al., 2020). Concomitantly, by 2030 the United States will face a significant shortage of physicians (Research shows shortage . . . , n.d.). Although these statistics present a challenge to the health care system and out-of-hospital (OOH) provider, they are also an opportunity for innovation around digital technology.

The signing of the Affordable Care Act (ACA) in March 2010 launched the transformation of health care by influencing the transition from fee for service to value-driven care (Scott & Eminger, 2016). Within value-based care, providers are reimbursed based on patient outcomes. Consequently, the LTC industry has experienced tremendous change in health care delivery, daily operations, and regulatory implementation, with an emphasis on quality. The prevention of hospital readmissions and emergency department (ED) visits is the primary focus of LTC providers. Therefore, telehealth has the potential to revolutionize the delivery of care in this health care space with on-demand access to physician services.

Throughout this chapter, the reader will gain a better understanding of the landscape of eldercare, as well as barriers and opportunities for telehealth, and learn how the focus on quality will benefit the role of the emergency physician (EP) within the framework.

OVERVIEW OF OUT-OF-HOSPITAL SETTINGS

The following acronyms are used in this chapter:

AL	Assisted living
CMS	Centers for Medicare and Medicaid Services
HHA	Home health agency
IL	Independent living
OOH	Out of hospital
PAC	Post-acute care
SNF	Skilled nursing facilities

The term *post-acute care (PAC),* as defined by CMS, represents the settings or services a patient receives following an acute care stay and includes long-term care hospitals, in-patient rehabilitation facilities, skilled nursing facilities (SNFs), and home health agencies (HHAs) (Morley et al., 2014). This CMS definition assumes a Medicare recipient has had a previous acute care stay. However, when considering opportunities to expand the use of telehealth, it is imperative to look beyond this narrow scope and include providers serving the elderly in residential care settings such as independent and assisted living. Additionally, one must consider patients in their homes receiving home care or palliative care services. Historically, an older adult would be admitted to an acute care setting, be transferred to a skilled nursing facility, and then sent home with home care. However, alternate payment models such as accountable care organizations, bundled payments, and the increased prevalence of managed care have been disruptive to the traditional concept of transitions of care. Changes to the health care delivery model have resulted in more care being provided in home or residential settings, which would benefit from telehealth services.

Using the term *out of hospital* provides a broader view of health care sites for older adults, which includes (1) CMS-defined PAC settings, (2) independent and assisted living, and (3) community living. All OOH settings face similar challenges in providing care, such as inadequate transition of care coordination, limited staff resources, access to physician services, and poor communication with physicians, resulting in the inability to manage changes in condition and geographic barriers adequately. Providers are working to find solutions to these challenges, and telehealth is receiving more attention as a strategy to extend health care delivery effectively. Another consideration for employing telehealth in OOH settings, especially for IL, AL, and home settings, is the need for patient engagement and assessment of their comfort with technology.

REGULATORY AND LEGISLATIVE LANDSCAPE OF
VALUE-BASED CARE PAC SETTINGS

Understanding PAC's regulatory landscape provides the context for the value telehealth will provide to this segment of our health care delivery system. Only federally funded PAC settings are subject to federal regulations, while other OOH such as IL and AL are governed by state and local regulations. Since the signing of the ACA, there has been unprecedented growth in the development of alternative payment models and innovation in care delivery that affects all health care, including PAC (*Home Health Value-Based Purchasing Model | CMS Innovation Center*, n.d.). However, two pieces of legislation, the Improving Medicare Post-Acute Care Transformation (IMPACT) Act and Value-Based Purchasing, have been the most influential on quality initiatives in PAC by emphasizing outcome management, workflow redesign, and process improvements (https://www.cms.gov/Medicare/ Quality-Initiatives-Patient-Assessment-Instruments/Post-Acute-Care-Quality- Initiatives/IMPACT-Act-of-2014/IMPACT-Act-of-2014-Data-Standardization-and- Cross-Setting-Measures). The Nursing Home Compare website provides publicly available data on the quality and staffing of U.S. nursing homes: https://www.med- icare.gov/NursingHomeCompare/About/howcannhchelp.html. Consequently, a negative quality rating can affect census, hospital relations, market perception, and revenue losses.

THE IMPROVING MEDICARE POST-ACUTE CARE
TRANSFORMATION ACT

The ACA intended to "expand access to insurance, increase consumer protections, emphasize prevention and wellness, improve quality and system performance, expand the health workforce, and curb rising health care costs," thereby assuring the transformation of health care in the United States (*The Affordable Care Act*, n.d.). In the years following implementation of the ACA, several fundamental PAC-specific federal laws were implemented which focused primarily on quality and system performance. In 2014, the Improving Medicare Post-Acute Care Transformation Act of 2014 was signed into law. The IMPACT Act requires the standardization of data across all PAC settings with the goal "to improve Medicare beneficiary outcomes through shared-decision making, care coordination, and enhanced discharge planning" (*IMPACT Act of 2014 Data Standardization & Cross Setting Measures | CMS*, n.d.-b). This law gives CMS the ability to monitor quality throughout PAC by collecting patient assessments and claims data and converting it to patient outcomes. The collected data and, ultimately, quality outcomes are publicly available and provide insight into crucial quality domains within these settings (*Data.Medicare.Gov | Data.Medicare.Gov*, n.d.). The use of telehealth by SNFs and HHAs by providers would impact the key quality measures of the IMPACT Act, which includes the all-condition risk-adjusted potentially preventable hospital readmissions rate.

Value-Based Purchasing Programs

Two other laws specific to PAC are the Skilled Nursing Facility Value-Based Purchasing (SNF VBP) Program (*The Skilled Nursing Facility Value-Based PurchasingProgram,* n.d.-a) and the Home Health Value-Based Purchasing (HHVBP) Model (*Home Health VBP,* n.d.). According to CMS, "The SNF VBP Program rewards skilled nursing facilities (SNFs) with incentive payments based on the quality of care they provide to Medicare beneficiaries, as measured by a hospital readmissions measure" (*The Skilled Nursing Facility Value-Based Purchasing (SNF VBP) Program | CMS,* n.d.-b). The SNF-VPB was designed to withhold 2% of Fee-for-Service (FFS) Medicare A claims for all SNFs and to use 60% of the withholding to incentivize SNFs who better-managed SNF 30 day All-Cause Readmission Measures (SNFRM). Beginning October 1, 2018, CMS utilized 60% of the withholding pool to incentivize SNFs that met the readmission performance measure calculated by the risk-standardized re-admission rate. The SNF-VBP financial penalty facilitated SNF operators to focus on the quality of care and avoidable readmissions to the hospital. In CMS fiscal year 2020, 77% of SNFs that had reported sufficient data did not receive any incentive, indicating providers failed to meet the national average readmission rate (*Proportion of Skilled Nursing VBP Losers Grows as 77% Receive Medicare Payment Cuts—Skilled Nursing News,* n.d.). Utilizing telehealth to manage change in condition and to min-imize care setting transfers from the SNF to the hospital is a valuable tool to help decrease financial penalties.

The HHVPB demonstration model was implemented on January 1, 2016, in Medicare-certified HHAs in Arizona, Florida, Iowa, Maryland, Massachusetts, Nebraska, North Carolina, Tennessee, and Washington. The intent of the model is similar to that of all other CMS value-based programs where payment is connected to quality performance and improved efficiency, as demonstrated through standardized quality outcome and process measures (Pozniak et al., 2018; *Home Health Quality Measures | CMS,* n.d.). Failure of HHAs to meet the national standards for quality results in having their Medicare payment adjusted by a specific percentage. Since the program is in demonstration status, the final penalty amount is not yet deter-mined (*Home Health Value-Based Purchasing Model | CMS Innovation Center,* n.d.). Although financial penalties directly impact traditional Medicare providers, all settings defined as PAC are responsible for the delivery of quality care.

Pay for performance can be viewed as an incentive for out-of-hospital providers to explore the use of technology, and specifically telehealth, to mitigate the financial impact of value-based penalties to improve the care treatment of chronic conditions prevalent in the older adult.

Medicare Advantage Plans

Although Medicare Advantage Plans are not a regulation, they need to be discussed within the context of telehealth and OOH. Over the last 20 years, Medicare Advantage plans have experienced steady, continuous growth. Among Medicare enrollees, 24 million of the 68 million, or 36% of the total Medicare-eligible pop-ulation, participate in these plans (*Medicare Advantage Growth Higher for 2020 |*

ForeSee Medical, n.d.). This statistic is important because Medicare Advantage plans can provide benefits not available to original Medicare enrollees. In 2019, CMS confirmed policies that allow Medicare Advantage plans to add telehealth services to their benefit packages without the rural location requirements of original Medicare (*CMS Finalizes Policies to Bring Innovative Telehealth Benefit to Medicare Advantage |* *CMS*, n.d.). The availability of telehealth to Medicare Advantage recipients provides an additional opportunity for EPs to work with residential communities and consult before a potential unnecessary trip to the ED.

VALUE PROPOSITION OF TELEHEALTH IN OUT-OF-HOSPITAL SETTINGS

The value proposition for telehealth within OOH care settings has evolved as a result of multiple factors: health care regulatory changes, emphasis on value-driven care, reduced healthcare costs, and improved patient engagement. Hospital readmissions and ED visits present the most significant risk to OOH providers in a value-driven health care system. Providers are incentivized to avoid transfer by managing the care onsite. Since these settings often do not have medical staff on premises 24/7, telehealth becomes a possible alternative. Through emergency physician engagement, providers have access to specialists in triaging care needs and guiding the appropriate interventions, which could result in avoiding a trip to the hospital.

Skilled Nursing Facilities

Skilled nursing facilities (SNFs) are using telehealth to connect third-party physician services, payers, acute care partners, and the existing care team members to deliver care for change in condition management. Examples of telehealth use in skilled nursing include monitoring and managing patients' change in vital signs, mental status, pain, and respiratory and cardiovascular status. Traditionally, when a patient develops an acute change in condition, the nurse's only option is to contact the primary care physician by phone. The phone-based approach often leaves the physician to rely on verbal information to triage symptoms, with limited access to the patient's health record. Telehealth platforms, coupled with EHR interoperability and connected diagnostic devices, add real-time clinical data with face-to-face capabilities for physicians to see and hear their patients to deliver comprehensive virtual care. Telehealth, which provides access to their patients' health records along with video and diagnostic capabilities, is an immediate improvement in health care delivery.

CASE STUDY

Year over year, the number of patients admitted to SNFs following hospitalizations has been growing. Despite this development, over 22% of patients in SNF settings following acute hospitalizations are readmitted, which is associated with higher mortality and higher cost of care (Burke et al., 2016). CMS has designated 30-day readmissions from in-patient rehabilitation, measured at nearly 12%, as a national quality indicator. Of patients rehospitalized, 50% repeat this cycle of readmission within an 11-day period (Ottenbacher et al., 2014). As a result, significant focus must be placed on effective strategies to reduce readmissions from SNFs to foster the systemic improvement of outcomes, cost, and overall care.

CMS has identified the causes of 30-day readmissions ranging from heart failure and sepsis to pulmonary, gastrointestinal, and metabolic disorders. Additional causes of readmission may include falls, seizures, and other neurological conditions. Telehealth is particularly well suited to addressing the breadth of readmissions causes in SNF settings. (See Box 19.1)

Therefore, thoughtfully designed and seamlessly integrated telehealth solutions present a promising opportunity to reduce all-cause readmissions within SNF and to create successful transitions of care.

Heartbeat Health ("Heartbeat") is a nationwide, virtual cardiovascular care company that works with providers, patients, and payers to manage heart disease and its risk factors using digital tools. Heartbeat's mobile and web apps enable on-demand virtual consultations with providers, including internists and cardiologists, for patients and care team members. The integration of remote diagnostic results and clinical data into the Heartbeat platform allows for extensive remote evaluation and management of patients. To evaluate the potential of telemedicine benefits in skilled nursing settings, Heartbeat partnered with 13 skilled nursing facilities throughout the northeastern United States to provide a subset of its capabilities to over 3,500 beds and 40,000 patients during 12 months between 2019 and 2020. Heartbeat was able to provide a turnkey solution through its apps to each facility, which included:

- Telemedicine triage by internists and cardiologists,
- Structured and unstructured capture of patient information before a virtual visit,
- Provider entry and review of recommendations, diagnostics, and follow-up instructions after a virtual visit, and
- Referral and inclusion of additional specialists, such as cardiologists, when necessary.

Box 19.1

TELEHEALTH BENEFITS IN SNF SETTINGS

- Timely consultation for acute condition change with EPs or specialists outside of the facility, to triage care.
- Augment the existing facility staffing by filling in gaps in time or clinical expertise.
- Leverage skilled clinical team members at the facility to provide hands-on assistance to patients and providers providing remote consultation.
- Significantly more cost-effective than a single instance of patient rehospitalization.
- Create a bridge from triage to specialty care and begin the process of disease management while the patient is in a structured care setting.

Facilities, which anticipated a reduction in readmissions rates and related financial incentives, paid a monthly fee to Heartbeat for these services.

Across the SNFs, Heartbeat was able to augment existing skilled nursing staff by delivering both internal medicine and specialty medicine via remote care. Staff members at a facility were trained to identify and request consultations via the Heartbeat app for patients believed to need a transfer to a local ED. The app captured relevant information about the patient and the patient's condition as entered by a nurse or nursing director at the facility. The app matched the request to an available internist, or if necessary, a cardiologist, and a telemedicine visit would be initiated almost immediately within the app onto a device stationed at the requesting facility. The Heartbeat provider would triage the patient following established clinical guidelines, ordering diagnostics and requesting follow-up, or even a transfer to the hospital as necessary. This specific application of the Heartbeat telemedicine solution resulted in a 39% reduction in rehospitalizations across all patients over 12 months, compared with expected and chart-reviewed recommendations for hospitalization. The results corresponded to an estimated saving attributable to readmission reduction of $4.3 million over 12 months. As a result, Heartbeat continues to offer its services to these facilities while expanding its footprint nationally.

Beyond the reduction in rehospitalizations and its subsequent savings, Heartbeat was also able to identify patients with moderate to high cardiovascular risk during consults and to provide referrals to cardiologists within the platform. These patients began cardiovascular disease management programs while in a structured care setting, delivered virtually through the same app. In summary, the partnership between Heartbeat and 13 skilled nursing facilities successfully demonstrated at scale the ability for telemedicine to both decrease immediate readmission risk through provider triage and longer-term hospitalization risk through virtual cardiovascular disease management program delivery.

The expansion of telehealth in SNFs empowers providers to establish unique programs for care coordination with acute partners and payers under value-based care. Access to a telehealth program, staffed with EPs, provides SNFs with access to triage services to determine if a nonemergency change in condition requires an ED visit. Programs like this strengthen care coordination between the SNF and the acute partner and promote patient-centered care. As a result, both health care providers limit avoidable returns to the hospital, and the patient remains in the appropriate care setting. Furthermore, programs like this reduce transportation and geographical barriers often associated with providing access to care in the time of need.

HOME HEALTH AGENCIES

Medicare home health care provided in a person's home after a hospital or skilled nursing stay would be the logical setting for telehealth. Home health agencies (HHAs) share similar value-based risk for financial penalties as SNFs and hospitals related to hospital readmissions. Therefore, the goal is to manage changes in condition, adhere to the discharge plan of care, and avoid emergency transfers resulting in hospitalization. The visiting nurse's access to an EP for telehealth consultation before an ED transfer could result in continued treatment at home. The combination of using both telehealth and remote patient monitoring (RPM) allows providers face-to-face visits and continuous monitoring of key biometric parameters.

RPM enables patients to utilize technology that transmits health information from home to a remote software platform that is under regular monitoring. RPM allows patients to self-monitor vital signs with connected medical peripherals to gather critical diagnostic information such as blood pressure, weight, pulse oxygenation, temperature, glucose levels, and even heart and lung sounds. Vital signs readings then get transmitted to the RPM platform for ongoing management, which alerts medical professionals when patient readings breach acceptable parameters. RPM, coupled with integrated telehealth face-to-face access to care team members, provides advanced clinical oversight when access to care is limited.

Although some health systems implement telehealth programs within a HHA, widespread adoption has faltered due to limited CMS reimbursement, lack of EMR interoperability, and regulations that require onsite visits to bill Medicare (*The Promise and Potential for Telehealth in Home Health*, n.d.). EPs have the potential to serve homebound patients but would need to lobby with home care agencies to mitigate current regulatory challenges in this space.

INDEPENDENT AND ASSISTED LIVING

Both independent living and assisted living offer housing arrangements that provide various services to support an older person's ability to live independently (Table 19.1)

A 2015 report published by Argentum, a national association representing providers of senior living, presents a comprehensive profile of the older adult living in these communities (*Senior Living Resident Profile*, n.d.). The report identifies the top chronic conditions of this population as cardiovascular disease (46%), diabetes (7%), and depression (18%). A goal of senior living providers is to keep those living in their communities healthy and independent as long as possible. Therefore, chronic care management could be delivered through telehealth with the advantage of convenience, immediate access for changes in condition, and reduced visits to the ED. Some IL and AL organizations are beginning to collaborate with EPs to establish a virtual immediate care center to provide services traditionally received at primary care centers or EDs.

PALLIATIVE CARE AND HOSPICE

Palliative care and hospice both offer comfort care, symptom relief, and psychosocial support; however, there are significant differences between them. Hospice expenses are completely covered by Medicare if patients meet eligibility criteria, which includes a prognosis of six months or less and excludes any treatment other than end-of-life symptom management. Palliative care, on the other hand, can begin at diagnosis of a terminal disease and includes curative interventions; payment varies by insurance plans (*Hospice vs. palliative care: What's the difference? | VITAS*, n.d.). Opportunities for use of telehealth are more favorable for patients receiving palliative care since some private insurance and Medicare Advantage plans are more likely to pay for

Table 19.1 INDEPENDENT LIVING AND ASSISTED LIVING

Independent Living	Assisted Living
• Offers hospitality services such as: ▪ Housekeeping ▪ Laundry services (excludes personal laundry) ▪ Transportation ▪ Activities and ▪ Dining services (Up to 3 meals/day at additional cost)	• Offers hospitality services such as: ▪ Housekeeping ▪ Laundry services ▪ Transportation to doctor appointments ▪ Activities and ▪ Dining services (3 meals/day with no additional cost)
Medical/Nursing Services: • Does not provide nursing or medical care. • Some communities may have physician clinics onsite.	**Medical/Nursing Services:** • Assists with activities of daily living (ADLs), i.e., bathing, dressing, doing personal laundry. • Medication management • 24-hour access to caregivers and medical personal ▪ Provision of nursing care is dependent on state regulations and vary throughout the United States.

telehealth visits. The primary goal of palliative care is to "improve quality of life for both the patient and the family, regardless of diagnosis" (Rome et al., 2011). Adding the EP to the palliative care team provides an additional dimension to the quality of life for the patient by potentially avoiding an ED visit through a triage consultation. Although palliative care occurs more often in the hospital setting, this is changing as the continuum of care has evolved with changes in health care delivery models. Skilled nursing facilities are developing palliative care programs. Given the absence of onsite physicians, the role of the EP can prove to be a valued team member.

TECHNOLOGY AND OOH CARE

While care team members and patients in the OOH care settings benefit from integrated telehealth, these care settings have limited interoperability compared to the acute care health systems. OOH care settings remain heavily dependent on faxing, in part due to the slow adoption of electronic health records (EHR) and lack of interoperability. The Healthcare Information and Management Systems Society, Inc. (HIMSS) describes interoperability as "the ability of devices, software, and information systems to connect within or outside the boundaries of healthcare organizations to exchange and access patient data with the purpose of addressing health issues of individual patients and the population in general" (*Interoperability in healthcare*, n.d.). Interoperability, especially with telehealth solutions in OOH care settings, is poised for growth, which will provide clinicians with a longitudinal care record to better triage care needs and chronic disease management. Comprehensive telehealth in the OOH care setting requires more than just access to the video component. The most comprehensive telehealth systems will include interoperability with EHRs and diagnostic equipment to connect the care team with real-time clinical information.

The use of artificial intelligence (AI) and clinical decision support (CDS) is improving the use of structured and unstructured data stored in the EHR to predict changes in conditions, facilitate better care, and support transitions of care. Alerts generated through its use suggest to the nurse specific assessments and, depending on the outcome, prompt a physician telehealth encounter. Telehealth would allow intervention before further decline or change occurred. By having EHR integration consisting of admit discharge transfer (ADT), diagnosis, allergies, clinical notes and assessments, medication lists, vital signs, advance directives, and laboratory results, the physician has access to a comprehensive view of the patient health record. Also, telehealth platforms integrated with RPM provide an additional assessment using real-time data. Without integration, remote clinicians would need to access the EHR and streaming medical device independent of the telehealth platform requiring multiple displays or computers to view all this information at one time. Telehealth interoperability helps to ensure clinical data from various systems is available to the care team and provides a comprehensive view of the patient to support remote clinical decisions.

CONCLUSION

As health care advances, telehealth is providing a gateway to improve care coordination and the delivery of health care across all OOH care settings. The 2020 COVID-19 pandemic has demonstrated the value of telehealth as access to OOH face-to-face assessments was prohibited or extremely limited. EPs are uniquely qualified to manage OOH change in conditions through their ability to triage a patient's health status, quickly extending the care team to oversee patient care without geographic barriers. EPs, along with telehealth programs in the OOH care settings, are poised to improve the quality of care by managing patients in place in the most appropriate care setting. The future of health care and access to large pools of health data will increase the use of CDS tools using artificial intelligence (AI) to assist with ongoing health care. AI will be used to predict a decline in health sooner, thereby assisting clinicians with data-driven proactive care capabilities. Expanding CDS in OOH care settings will help onsite care team members to improve resource management and provide focused care sooner for those in need. Utilizing telehealth and CDS to expand the interaction between OOH onsite care team members and EPs can significantly enhance health care delivery. With telehealth platforms transitioning to mobile-ready applications, EHR interoperability, connectivity to medical peripherals, and CDS, OOH care can easily be expanded to any care team member without barriers.

In the post-COVID-19 crisis, OOH providers, having experienced the tremendous value of telehealth, have the opportunity to begin investing in technology so that when regulations catch up to medical practice they will be prepared.

KEY TAKEAWAYS

➢ Physician reimbursement for telehealth in OOH care settings will support telehealth and RPM for ongoing care management across all OOH care settings to deliver virtual care when needed.

➢ Telehealth provides an extension to all care team members and removes barriers commonly associated with access to care in OOH care settings.

➢ Through use of a well-designed telehealth program, the role of ED physicians has evolved to triage change in condition in OOH care settings beyond the walls of the ED.

➢ Interoperability and connected medical peripherals, coupled with telehealth, provide remote care team members with the health and diagnostic information needed to provide remote patient-centered care.

➢ OOH settings need to overcome barriers such as initial investment, ongoing costs, staff training, regulations, and reimbursement challenges before embracing the concept of telehealth as a viable care option.

REFERENCES

Burke, R. E., Whitfield, E. A., Hittle, D., Min, S. joon, Levy, C., Prochazka, A. V., et al. (2016). Hospital readmission from post-acute care facilities: Risk factors, timing, and outcomes. *Journal of the American Medical Directors Association*, 17(3): 249–255.

CMS finalizes policies to bring innovative telehealth benefit to Medicare Advantage | CMS. (n.d.). Retrieved September 7, 2020, from https://www.cms.gov/newsroom/press-releases/cms-finalizes-policies-bring-innovative-telehealth-benefit-medicare-advantage.

Home | Provider Data Catalog. (n.d.). Retrieved June 28, 2021, from https://data.cms.gov/provider-data/?redirect=true

Home health quality measures | CMS. (n.d.). Retrieved August 28, 2020, from https://www.cms.gov/Medicare/Quality-Initiatives-Patient-Assessment-Instruments/HomeHealthQualityInits/Home-Health-Quality-Measures.

Home Health Value-Based Purchasing Model | CMS Innovation Center. (n.d.). Retrieved August 28, 2020, from https://innovation.cms.gov/innovation-models/home-health-value-based-purchasing-model.

Home Health VBP | CMS. (n.d.). Retrieved August 26, 2020, from https://www.cms.gov/Medicare/Quality-Initiatives-Patient-Assessment-Instruments/Value-Based-Programs/Other-VBPs/HHVBP.

Hospice vs. palliative care: What's the difference? | VITAS. (n.d.). Retrieved September 9, 2020, from https://www.vitas.com/hospice-and-palliative-care-basics/about-palliative-care/hospice-vs-palliative-care-whats-the-difference.

IMPACT Act of 2014 Data Standardization & Cross Setting Measures | CMS. (n.d.-a). Retrieved August 26, 2020, from https://www.cms.gov/Medicare/Quality-Initiatives-Patient-Assessment-Instruments/Post-Acute-Care-Quality-Initiatives/IMPACT-Act-of-2014/IMPACT-Act-of-2014-Data-Standardization-and-Cross-Setting-Measures.

IMPACT Act of 2014 Data Standardization & Cross Setting Measures | CMS. (n.d.-b). Retrieved August 13, 2020, from https://www.cms.gov/Medicare/Quality-Initiatives-Patient-Assessment-Instruments/Post-Acute-Care-Quality-Initiatives/IMPACT-Act-of-2014/IMPACT-Act-of-2014-Data-Standardization-and-Cross-Setting-Measures.

Interoperability in healthcare. (n.d.). Retrieved September 14, 2020, from https://www.himss.org/resources/interoperability-healthcare.

Keehan, S. P., Cuckler, G. A., Poisal, J. A., Sisko, A. M., Smith, S. D., Madison, A. J., et al. (2020). National Health Expenditure Projections, 2019-28: Expected Rebound In Prices Drives Rising Spending Growth. *Health Affairs (Project Hope)*, 39(4): 704–714.

Medicare Advantage growth higher for 2020 | ForeSee Medical. (n.d.). Retrieved September 7, 2020, from https://www.foreseemed.com/blog/medicare-advantage-growth-2020.

Medicare nursing home compare overview. (n.d.). Retrieved August 31, 2020, from https://www.medicare.gov/NursingHomeCompare/About/howcannhchelp.html.

Morley, M., Bogasky, S., Gage, B., Flood, S., & Ingber, M. J. (2014). *Medicare Post-Acute Care Episodes and Payment Bundling*, 4(1), E2.

Nation's Older Population to Nearly Double. (n.d.). Retrieved June 28, 2021, from https://www.census.gov/newsroom/press-releases/2014/cb14-84.html

Ottenbacher, K. J., Karmarkar, A., Graham, J. E., Kuo, Y. F., Deutsch, A., Reistetter, T. A., et al. (2014). Thirty-day hospital readmission following discharge from postacute rehabilitation in fee-for-service medicare patients. *Journal of the American Medical Association*, 311(6): 604–614.

Pozniak, A., Turenne, M., Mukhopadhyay, P., Morefield, B., Slanchev, V., Linehan, K., et al. (2018). *Evaluation of the Home Health Value-Based Purchasing (HHVBP) Model First Annual Report Evaluation of the HHVBP Model 2017 Annual Report.*

The promise and potential for telehealth in home health. (n.d.). Retrieved September 3, 2020, from https://mhealthintelligence.com/features/the-promise-and-potential-for-telehealth-in-home-health.

Proportion of skilled nursing VBP losers grows as 77% receive medicare payment cuts—Skilled Nursing News. (n.d.). Retrieved August 13, 2020, from https://skillednursingnews.com/2019/12/proportion-of-skilled-nursing-vbp-losers-grows-as-77-receive-medicare-payment-cuts.

Research shows shortage of more than 100,000 doctors by 2030 | AAMC. (n.d.). Retrieved August 25, 2020, from https://www.aamc.org/news-insights/research-shows-shortage-more-100000-doctors-2030.

Rome, R. B., Luminais, H. H., Bourgeois, D. A., & Blais, C. M. (2011). The role of palliative care at the end of life. *Ochsner Journal*, 11(4): 348–352.

Scott, B. C., & Eminger, T. L. (2016). Bundled payments: Value-based care implications for providers, payers, and patients. In *American Health and Drug Benefits*, 9 (9): 493–496). Engage Healthcare Communications, Inc. www.AHDBonline.com

Senior Living Resident Profile: Key national and state demographics, demographics, diagnoses, adverse events, and types of assistance needed. (n.d.). Retrieved June 28, 2021, from https://www.argentum.org/wp-content/uploads/2018/09/Senior-Living-Resident-Profile-WhitePaper.pdf

The Affordable Care Act: A brief summary. (n.d.). Retrieved August 26, 2020, from https://www.ncsl.org/research/health/the-affordable-care-act-brief-summary.aspx.

The skilled nursing facility value-based purchasing (SNF VBP) Program | CMS. (n.d.-a). Retrieved August 13, 2020, from https://www.cms.gov/Medicare/Quality-Initiatives-Patient-Assessment-Instruments/Value-Based-Programs/SNF-VBP/SNF-VBP-Page.

The skilled nursing facility value-based purchasing (SNF VBP) Program | CMS. (n.d.-b). Retrieved August 26, 2020, from https://www.cms.gov/Medicare/Quality-Initiatives-Patient-Assessment-Instruments/Value-Based-Programs/SNF-VBP/SNF-VBP-Page.

20

Remote Physiologic Monitoring

KSENYA K. BADASHOVA, TENAGNE HAILE-MARIAM, AND ROBERT JARRIN ▪

INTRODUCTION

Remote physiologic monitoring (RPM) can be broadly defined as the process of collecting and transmitting a patient's clinical information to a remote care provider and is fundamental to the practice of distance-based clinical care. Most RPM systems use digital technologies and secure virtual platforms to capture and transmit physiologic data from a patient who is located outside a customary health care setting. Data sources can be numerous and may vary from descriptive logs such as patient and caregiver reports to high fidelity digital readouts from connected sensors, wearables, and medical devices. Some monitoring systems employ clinical decision support (CDS) or have built-in "intelligence" that flags and escalates abnormal results for expedited review. Systems can be designed to provide patient data with increasing granularity without physical proximity, thereby allowing clinicians to provide effective and timely monitoring, feedback, and therapeutic interventions.

RPM permits early recognition of acute exacerbations in patients with chronic diseases. Ongoing monitoring can result in more timely interventions, such as medication dosing changes, mitigating morbidity, and conserving resources that might be needed if the disease state should worsen. Remote clinicians can adjust the type and frequency of RPM data that is collected to more reliably assess and appropriately elevate a patient's level of care. Although there is more experience in the use of RPM in the management of patients with chronic diseases, it is utilized to monitor patients with both chronic and acute illness after they are discharged from hospital with associated decreases in the rate of hospital readmissions. More recently, RPM, in conjunction with telehealth and home visits, is being used to increase inpatient bed capacity by facilitating the delivery of in-patient-level care to patients residing outside of traditional hospital settings, such as their primary residences (including home and assisted living facilities) and in underused commercial spaces such as hotels or even repurposed out-patient clinical facilities and office spaces (*Additional background*, 2020). Advances in data transmission technologies, coupled with increasingly available, affordable, and portable connected medical devices, have improved the utility of RPM to diagnose, monitor, and treat more complex and dynamic medical conditions. Similarly, improvements in RPM protocols and platforms will improve a clinician's ability to determine the appropriate level, timing, and type of care that can be delivered along the continuum of illness severity. All of these advances, especially when they are integrated with programs that support the integration of patient care between the in-patient and out-patient environment, can be expected to improve quality and decrease cost. They will also allow EDs and EM clinicians to initiate and monitor care of patients who are not physically in the ED and play a more meaningful role in providing ongoing distance-based medical care. It is therefore apt to discuss RPM in the context of current and potential paradigms for providing emergency telehealth.

IMPLEMENTATION MODELS

RPM is typically implemented in a synchronous (real-time transmission) or asynchronous (store-and-forward) model. Either model allows clinicians to review and act on data as soon as the information is received or on an intermittent basis. In all cases, predetermined thresholds or algorithms can be used to identify critical values and escalate such findings for real-time clinical review. An extreme example of continuous RPM with synchronous transmission and immediate clinical decision making is used in tele-intensive care (Tele-ICU programs). Such programs differ significantly from less resource-intensive home-based RPM programs that allow for intermittent (e.g., daily or weekly) review of data and clinical interventions. In either model, the collected data must be delivered in a manner that allows the clinician to provide timely, appropriate, and actionable care. Tele-ICU is a robust field of practice and will be introduced only briefly below. Rather, we will focus on implementation models that can be used for patients that do not need prolonged, ICU-level care.

Chronic Disease Management

RPM that provides for intermittent monitoring is applicable in a variety of clinical conditions that are amenable to less frequent evaluation and intervention. Patients with chronic diseases, as well as those with an acute illness, can be monitored in this manner. In patients with chronic diseases, early markers for worsening disease, such as acute weight gain in patients with congestive heart failure (CHF), can be identified through the transmission of daily weight measurements taken on a connected scale. This data is trended to provide for early identification and treatment of exacerbations before the patient's condition worsens and sometime before the patient has noticeable symptoms. Use of RPM has been associated with decreased mortality and hospitalizations in CHF (Klersy, 2009) and chronic obstructive pulmonary disease (COPD) patients (Segrelles Calvo, 2014). A systematic review and thematic synthesis of patient experience with chronic disease RPM programs has demonstrated increases in patient satisfaction as well as clinical outcomes (Walker, 2019). These benefits are listed in Box 20.1.

Box 20.1

BENEFITS OF CHRONIC CONDITION RPM

Enhanced patient understanding of their condition
Earlier action by clinicians in response to the collected data
Increased patient certainty of when to seek medical attention
Reduction in hospitalizations and clinic visits
Increased confidence in shared decision making
Increased sense of safety in remaining independent at home
Reduced anxiety about their medical condition

RPM that provides for intermittent monitoring is also invaluable for distance-based care in situations when data transmission is technically limited due to a variety of constraints such as poor connectivity or lack of appropriate devices.

Management of Acute Illness

RPM has been less utilized in the care of patients with acute illnesses. The COVID-19 pandemic, with the resultant influx of affected patients who overwhelmed EDs and hospitals across the nation, has provided opportunities to implement RPM programs. Early in the pandemic, it became clear that patients who were asymptomatic and stable on presentation could later develop silent hypoxia, dyspnea, and respiratory failure within days or weeks of their initial presentation. Admitting each COVID-19 patient to the hospital for observation and monitoring was unfeasible, while discharging patients without appropriate follow-up was equally impractical. RPM provided the opportunity to continue monitoring discharged patients through the critical period to ensure proper escalation. (See Figure 20.1.) As devastating as it has been, the COVID-19 pandemic has shown how RPM can facilitate appropriate utilization and coordination of clinical and community-based resources to meet patient care needs safely.

A study conducted in Minnesota enrolled 3,701 patients after tele-urgent care or ED visits into the COVID-19 RPM program. Of the 1,496 patients flagged for abnormalities by RPM, 4.58% were escalated to the ED and 3.9% followed up in clinic (Annis, 2020). Another study enrolled patients discharged from the Massachusetts General–Brigham system after a COVID-19-related admission into a portal-based RPM program. Patients reported daily pulse oximetry, temperature readings, and their responses to a brief symptom-related questionnaire. The authors reported a decrease in the need for ED or hospital readmission among enrolled patients (Gordan, 2020).

Aalam et al. reported a COVID-19 RPM program that was initiated on patients who were discharged from the ED with the ability to self-report daily pulse oximeter, temperature readings, and responses to a short survey (see Figure 20.1). A tiered escalation response for nonresponding patients and those with indications for worsening in their clinical condition flagged them for further follow-up (Aalam, 2021).

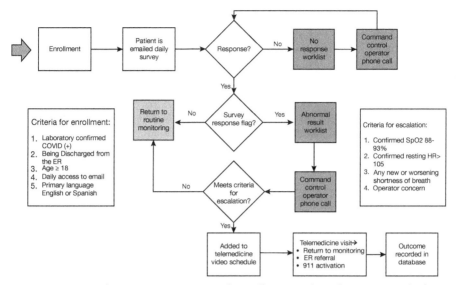

Figure 20.1 Example RPM program protocol, enrollment, and escalation criteria (Aalam, 2021). Reprinted with permission.

Home-based Hospitalization Programs

Experience has been accumulating for providing care that is usually reserved for hospitalized patients to those who can remain in their homes. A randomized controlled trial (RTC) of 91 adults admitted through the ED to home care versus inpatient care for various acute conditions showed reduced cost, shorter length of stay, fewer imaging and laboratory studies, and lower 30-day readmissions in the hospital in the home (HITH) patient population (Levine et al., 2018). A meta-analysis of 61 RCTs of hospital-level care for home-based patients showed reduced mortality, readmission rates, and costs, with higher patient satisfaction ratings (Caplan et al., 2012). In addition to good outcomes and satisfaction data, these programs allowed for decreased utilization of traditional hospital beds.

The COVID-19 pandemic has led to the expansion of programs that provide care for patients with clinical care needs that are traditionally provided within hospitals to receive care in other settings. The programs are not limited to patients who are in the ED, but the very nature of the pandemic and its resultant overcrowding of hospitals resulted in patients spending more time in EDs than previously. Therefore, in addition to programs such as those that showed the utility of ED-based RPM for traditional ED patients, benefit has been shown for the ED as a launching pad for patients to receive hospital-level care in nontraditional settings. For example, under the COVID-19 public health emergency (PHE), the Centers for Medicare and Medicaid Services (CMS) instituted the Acute Hospital Care At Home (AHCAH) program, which allowed for patients who are admitted to the hospital to receive hospital-level care outside of the "four walls" of the hospital. Such regulatory waivers enabled reimbursements by CMS that provide opportunities for EPs to further incorporate RPM into their practice. These programs initiated under the COVID-19 PHE are being applied to a variety of conditions ranging from acute infections such as cellulitis to acute exacerbations of chronic illness such as COPD.

As a result, EM clinicians can play a crucial role in identifying appropriate patients, and the ED can serve as a hub for enrolling patients into AHCAH and initiating the necessary RPM. With appropriate institutional support, they can collaborate with clinicians from other specialties to not only enroll patients, but to oversee continued RPM in patients whose care extends into, for example, nonconventional hours and weekends when the ED might be able to provide a higher level of response than is afforded by other specialties. EM clinicians participating in the care of patients within accountable care organizations (ACOs) have the added opportunity to collaborate with primary care teams to optimize individual treatment plans and respond to data from RPM within predetermined parameters. RPM can thus be integral to reducing adverse patient outcomes through prompt identification and response to data and information that portends a patient's clinical decompensation. EM-based clinicians can be utilized to connect patients with other physicians via telemedicine visits or, if needed, initiate patient transfer to a higher level of care through an ambulance or other transportation service.

Patient care coordination that is based out of the ED for discharged patients who require RPM provides an ideal opportunity to orchestrate medical care and treatment plans through interdisciplinary information sharing and collaboration. Under such programs, RPM can be used to optimize quality of care and bridge gaps in transitions of care. EDs can also provide an ideal platform for coordinating RPM and information transfer needs given the long history of EM practitioners' experience with receiving and evaluating RPM data. The pandemic has opened numerous opportunities for all physicians to utilize RPM and can help EM play an increased role in enrolling and monitoring patients in RPM programs in coordination with other physicians and the whole patient care team.

MANAGEMENT OF CRITICALLY ILL PATIENTS (TELE-ICU)

Monitoring a patient's physiologic parameters in real time, continuously, allows remote clinicians to assist in the management of critically ill inpatients. Generally, continuous real-time remote monitoring is utilized when there exists a central infrastructure and the technology enabling trained, dedicated clinicians to manage, interpret, and respond in collaboration with bedside clinicians in the ICU or ED. Telecritical care or Tele-ICU deserves its own complete description that is beyond the scope of this chapter. However, EM clinicians should be aware of this model, as it can be applied to the ED in the setting of ED boarding. ED boarding signifies that patients who are admitted to the medical ward or intensive care unit remain in the ED for extended periods due to limitations in hospital capacity. This results in a form of "hybridized" care by EM and in-patient clinicians. As pressure is placed on ICU bed capacity, many EDs have witnessed a surge in the number of ICU patients with prolonged ED stays. In these cases, EM clinicians or intensivists, either in the hospital or located offsite, may use continuous RPM technologies and telehealth to care for critical patients in the ED. A recent retrospective study showed decreased mortality in medical ICU (MICU) boarders in the ED when they were enrolled in RPM and electronic intensive care unit (TeleICU) care protocols (Kadar, 2019). Continuous RPM for "just-in-time" interpretation portends a high level of patient acuity that can be resource intensive. Clinicians and facilities must determine when continuous patient monitoring programs are applicable for their situation, institution, and patients.

OPERATIONS OVERVIEW

In the last few years, RPM has grown exponentially in its breadth of application as well as the number of companies providing services. Purchasing remote monitoring equipment and services accounts for only a small fraction of the implementation process. Launching an RPM program successfully takes an immense amount of preliminary research and preparation.

Before setting up RPM, a needs assessment should be conducted to identify the type of program that would be most beneficial. Identifying and involving stakeholders is key to success. Administrators, health care providers, health IT personnel, and patients should all be involved in optimizing the service and ensuring long-term program viability. The needs assessment should consider whether acute or chronic care monitoring is of greater benefit to the organization. In the primary care setting, chronic care monitoring may provide the greatest value for patients with difficult to manage chronic diseases that could benefit from touchpoints between clinic visits. It is best to separate patients by condition as each requires tracking of different symptoms and physiologic parameters, and some may require multiple devices. Acute care focuses on short-term monitoring for conditions such as COVID-19 or pneumonia, identifying who could benefit after discharge, as well as enhancing transitions back to primary care and identifying postsurgical complications early. After choosing the monitoring approach and patient population, treatment goals must be set. Establishing baseline metrics is essential to identifying decompensating patients and intervening in a timely manner. Notification and escalation protocols must be developed to guide patient treatment plans. Workflows for clinicians managing the RPM platform must be created. Finally, graduation goals should be outlined for short-term monitoring programs. Patient engagement dictates the success or failure of the program. Ensuring patients have internet access and are open to using technology is essential to success. The initial implementation should be limited to a small sample size to allow for reassessment, adjustment, and optimization of the program prior to broad application in clinical practice. However, incrementally scaling the program is just as important as starting with a small patient population. A scaling process helps the program grow out of the pilot phase and gain momentum, while allowing for program reevaluation and adjustment as it gradually expands and fully integrates into the workflow.

PLATFORMS AND VENDORS

The process of selecting and contracting a suitable vendor with an appropriate platform is imperative to the success of an RPM program. Once the mission and goals of the RPM program are envisioned, the search for a vendor may commence. A vendor should be selected based on the expertise and experience that complement the needs of the patient population, as well as the mission and goals of the program as they will play an integral part through the launch and beyond.

The American Medical Association (AMA) has released a digital health implementation playbook that identifies six central variables essential to vendor appraisal (See Box 20.2.) The six variables are business, information technology, security, usability, customer service, and clinical validation (Digital Health Implementation Playbook Step 4: Evaluating the Vendor, n.d.). When evaluating the business, the funding sources, financial stability, and affiliations should be considered. The business model, product cost, reimbursement rates, risk sharing, and support for payment program participation should also be considered (Digital Health Implementation Playbook Step 4: Evaluating the Vendor, n.d.). A vendor's information technology division should be examined to ensure it is compatible with the electronic health records (EHRs) and platforms providers and patients will be using. The security systems in place are of outmost importance, as confidential information will be exchanged and transmitted regularly. The usability or the ease of navigating the system is critical for clinician and patient participation. A well-designed platform minimizes disruptions in clinician workflow and maintains high patient compliance. Knowing the target patient population, especially their level of digital and health literacy, helps predict the challenges they may face. The vendor's ability to provide customer support during and after program implementation is important to review. Specifically, attention should be directed to the extent of support offered for employee and provider training, data analysis, patient education, and training. The vendor must understand regulatory requirements as well as their obligations to help facilitate appropriate insurer payment. Customer reviews posted regarding experience with the vendor and the platform can provide helpful insights. Lastly, AMA recommends examining clinical validation by reviewing any clinical outcomes from previous programs and published peer-reviewed research. Vendor selection for RPM takes time, and program implementers should not rely only on information provided by the vendor; it is important to speak with current customers, project managers, and customer service representatives to gain a better understanding of the product and services offered. This is a long-term relationship that, when chosen carefully and thoughtfully, can provide the tools needed to build a successful RPM program.

EQUIPMENT MANAGEMENT

Some of the most common connected devices used to monitor patients' physiologic parameters include blood pressure, heart rate, blood oxygen levels, temperature, and weight, all of which are an essential part of RPM. Emerging technologies are multiparameter biosensors, often in patch or mini-device formats, that can continuously collect and transmit a variety of physiologic parameters. CMS coverage and payment of some RPM services require medical devices that automatically transmit physiologic data from patients to the provider and do not allow patient self-reported data from unconnected traditional medical devices. Thus, ensuring the patient has the necessary equipment and the knowledge of how to use it appropriately is of outmost importance. The clinician can order RPM equipment for delivery to the patient's home or provide it directly to the patient in clinic or at the ED. Patient education on proper device use is offered in various forms, including in-person training,

Box 20.2

KEY COMPONENTS OF VENDOR APPRAISAL FOR RPM PROGRAM (DIGITAL
HEALTH IMPLEMENTATION PLAYBOOK STEP 4: EVALUATING THE VENDOR, N.D.)

BUSINESS:

- Organizational overview—tenure, funding source, financial stability, affiliations, notable customers, etc.

- Impact to program ROI—product cost, business model, reimbursement rates, risk sharing, support payment program participation, etc.

INFORMATION TECHNOLOGY:

- Ability to integrate with your current IT landscape, particularly your EHR system

- Cost, process, and timeline associated with integration and product updates

- Ensure the data elements of most importance to your clinicians and patients can be captured[14]

SECURITY (APPENDIX D.3)

- HIPAA compliance and process for ensuring protection of confidential patient information Liability and process

- Liability and process for managing potential security breaches

USABILITY:

- User experience of device and interface for patients and care team members

- Patient and care team engagement metrics

- Ability to engage with and encourage participation from patients

- Degree to which this technology/vendor will reduce disruption to existing workflow

CUSTOMER SERVICE:

- Level of support available to practice during and after implementation—staff training, patient education, project management, data analysis and insights, etc.

- Degree of technical support available to patients

CLINICAL VALIDATION:

- Documented clinical outcomes

- Published peer-reviewed research

video instruction, and virtual assistance. Ensuring the patient can properly use the device is fundamental to high-quality monitoring. Once the patient completes the RPM program the equipment is returned to the provider or vendor for destruction or sanitization, repackaging, and reuse. Some vendors include equipment and equipment management in their RPM package.

Uptake of consumer health related digital devices by the general public can predate proof of utility cost-effectiveness. Nonetheless, such advances, especially as they relate to the monitoring of clinical characteristics such as vital signs, weight, exercise, and even "sleep hygiene," hold promise as beneficial to increasing availability, adoption, and even clinical utility as part of RPM platforms. A publication by Natarajan and colleagues showed that physiologic data obtained from Fitbits worn by patients with COVID-19 might serve to predict need for hospitalization (Natarajan, 2020).

HUMAN RESOURCES

Implementing an RPM program is not an easy feat. It requires a multidisciplinary group capable of identifying needs, creating a vision, designing the workflow, developing a budget, negotiating contracts, building and training a provider team, choosing a platform, working closely with a vendor, gauging success, and scaling appropriately. The core teams necessary to undertake such a project include a primary team, an administrative team, and an implementation team.

The primary team is involved in developing and managing all facets and phases of the project such as creating the business model, the implementation plan, and the daily workflows. This team thrives from the diversity of representatives at the front lines, administration, and IT. A diverse team ensures a multifaceted approach in system development and problem solving. The administrative team focuses on funding, resource allocation, contract negotiation, and budget approval. Practice owners, partners, chairs, directors, and upper management review and authorize the financial aspects of the project. The implementation team is responsible for the execution of everyday tasks that drive the program. They are the people out in the field who enroll and educate the patients, review data, escalate care, and maintain the platforms used for monitoring and providing technical support. The data collection, monitoring, and escalation is conducted by designated health care providers in small offices or by clinicians at call centers at larger institutions. Together the teams form an interdisciplinary unit that can establish and perfect an RPM program.

FINANCIAL CONSIDERATIONS

Return on Investment (ROI) is a measure that determines the quality of the investment. It is the ratio of net profit from the investment over the cost of the initial investment. The ROI depends on the RPM model, population size, cost of devices, cost of vendor/platform, cost of clinicians, and support staff reimbursement rates. While a number of calculators take inputs on number of patients monitored to estimate annual revenues from existing CPT* codes related to RPM, it is important to consider the use case, staffing model, technology, patient base, and other practice factors. Calculating ROI on RPM is not straightforward and requires consideration of the investment, risk, and returns required to have a successful program.

Originally, CMS made determinations on coverage and payment policies for RPM starting in 2018, under the Medicare Physician Fee Schedule Final Rule. Over the years, CMS has expanded payment policies to include several remote monitoring codes, including most recently in 2021 (*Final policy, payment, and quality provisions . . .*, 2020). Previously, RPM was limited to patients with chronic conditions, in the 2021 Physician Fee Schedule (PFS) proposed rule (85 FR 50118), CMS clarified that the services may be extended to patients with acute conditions as well. CMS further specified that RPM services were typically restricted to "established patients" or patients who have been evaluated by the clinician who recommends RPM as part of a treatment plan. However, during the public health emergency, this restriction was lifted allowing new and established patients for the duration of the COVID-19 pandemic to ensure adequate access to care for all patients.

RPM services must be reported by a physician or nonphysician provider who may bill separately for evaluation and management (E/M) services (i.e., physician assistants, nurse practitioners, certified nurse specialists, and certified nurse-midwife). Some of the intraservice work involved in RPM may be performed by clinical staff or auxiliary personnel under the general supervision of the billing provider so long as they perform such services within their scope of practice as allowed by law, regulation, facility policy, level of education, and licensure.

RPM devices used for physiologic monitoring must be a medical device as defined by the Food and Drug Administration (FDA) and must digitally transmit the patient data. Importantly, CMS clarified that patients cannot manually enter data to satisfy this requirement as data must be automated from the device. In order to bill for the device(s) and monitoring solution, patients must be monitored for at least 16 days over a 30-day period. CMS also waived this requirement during the public health emergency for patients with a COVID-19 diagnosis or for those suspected of having the illness, and instead required "at least two days of data collected" in those situations. CPT* code 99453 may be billed once at the onset of RPM for each episode of care and covers patient education and setup, and CPT* code 99454 may be billed every 30 days for the supply of equipment and transmission of data. A treatment plan must be formed at the onset of enrollment, the completion of which necessitates graduation from the program. Treatment and management services are billed under CPT* codes 99457 (initial 20 minutes) and 99458 (each additional 20 minutes) in a calendar month of monitoring.

CMS stipulated that at least part of the 20 minutes of "interactive communication" must be via live, real-time, synchronous audio conversation, which may be further enabled by video interaction over the course of the billing period of monitoring to report services under CPT* code 99457. Every additional 20-minute increment of "interactive communication" has the same live, real-time, audio conversation stipulation and may be billed under CPT* code 99458.

Similar to telehealth, RPM technologies allow caregivers to evaluate their remote patients from a remote location (Table 20.1). However, despite the notable similarities from a systems and operations standpoint, telehealth and RPM are considered two distinct services. Until recently, CMS did not reimburse RPM services and incorrectly categorized remote and virtual care services under the moniker of "telehealth." However, CMS has distinguished RPM, stating it is not subject

Table 20.1 CPT Codes

CPT Code	Description
	Digitally Stored Data Services
99091	Collection and interpretation of physiologic data (e.g., ECG, blood pressure, glucose monitoring) digitally stored and/or transmitted by the patient and/or caregiver to the physician or other qualified health care professional, qualified by education, training, and licensure/regulation (when applicable) requiring a minimum of 30 minutes of time, each 30 days
	Remote Physiologic Monitoring Treatment Management Services
99453	Remote monitoring of physiologic parameters(s) (e.g., weight, blood pressure, pulse oximetry, respiratory flow rate), initial; setup and patient education on use of equipment
99454	Device(s) supply with daily recording(s) or programmed alert(s) transmission, each 30 days
99457	Remote physiologic monitoring treatment management services, clinical staff/physician/other qualified health care professional time in a calendar month requiring interactive communication with the patient/caregiver during the month; first 20 minutes
99458	Remote physiologic monitoring treatment management services, clinical staff/physician/other qualified health care professional time in a calendar month requiring interactive communication with the patient/caregiver during the month; additional 20 minutes

to arduous regulatory limitations such as permissible originating sites or the use of telehealth place of service codes.

Other codes have also been introduced for remote and non-face-to-face services that include interprofessional consultations, online digital eVisits, and patient self-reported blood pressure management. These codes, in addition to temporary HCPCS (Healthcare Common Procedure Coding System) codes established by CMS, and other non-face-to-face codes, including care management service codes, form the growing volume of digital medical service codes that offer coverage and payment for remote services. In the future, it is expected that other innovative areas of digital medical services will be reflected in new codes. Eventually, payment, particularly for professional services rendered through artificial intelligence, software as a medical device, and clinical decision support, should become more common.

CONCLUSION

Innovation is most pronounced in times of need. The COVID-19 pandemic propelled the development of various models of RPM to increase hospital capacity and to place a safety net for stable discharged patients at risk of decompensation. The Department of Health and Human Services (HHS) issued waivers that CMS implemented and then tweaked reimbursement policies for telehealth and RPM, thereby enabling providers to incorporate RPM into their practice. Various opportunities have opened to EM, including participating in HITH programs, working closely with ACOs, and creating short-term RPM programs for patients with acute conditions.

Emergency telehealth platforms can utilize RPM to receive, transmit, analyze, and prioritize patient information. These platforms can be expected to improve both out-of-hospital and in-hospital clinical care and lead to improved outcomes and patient satisfaction. Fundamental to coordinating and providing timely and meaningful interventions is the ability to access and evaluate actionable data. For RPM to be of utility, it is important that the clinical resources to provide appropriate patient care are in place and that critical information from RPM and subsequent clinical care are properly integrated into the continuum of a patient's records. Likewise, the ability to integrate and utilize RPM systems and data is an essential component of emergency telehealth programs.

Developing an RPM program is a challenging and multifaceted task that can be pursued in various ways, including working with a vendor that facilitates device distribution and manages the virtual platform. Technological advancements in conjunction with patient-centered care make RPM an integral part of health future.

KEY TAKEAWAYS

➢ RPM should present useful and actionable data on a continuous or intermittent basis that is evaluated and triggers a clinical response that is robust enough to meet the patient's needs in a timely and appropriate manner.

➢ The breadth, depth, and timing of RPM data, and the communications platforms utilized to transmit that data, should match the patient's clinical needs and acuity.

➢ Although RPM device requirements are dictated by CPT° codes, payment policies vary according to insurer.

➢ Setting up an RPM program is no easy feat and requires significant human capital, research, and investment.

➢ The ROI depends on the RPM model, population size, cost of devices, cost of vendor/platform, cost of clinicians, and support staff reimbursement rates.

REFERENCES

Aalam, A. A. (2021, January 20). Remote patient moniotring for ED discharges in the Covid-19 pandemic. *Emergency Medicine Journal*, 1–3.

Additional background: Sweeping regulatory changes to help U.S. healthcare system address COVID-19 patient surge. (2020, March 30). Retrieved January 31, 2021, from cms.gov: https://www.cms.gov/newsroom/fact-sheets/additional-backgroundsweeping-regulatory-changes-help-us-healthcare-system-address-covid-19-patient.

Annis, T. P. (2020). Rapid implementation of a COVID-19 remote patient monitoring program. *Journal of the American Medical Informatics Association*, 27(8): 1326–1330.

Caplan, G. A., Sulaiman, N. S., Mangin, D. A., Aimonino Ricauda, N., Wilson, A. D., & Barclay L. (2012). A meta-analysis of "hospital in the home." *Medical Journal of Australia*, 197(9): 512–519. doi:10.5694/mja12.10480

Digital Health Implementation Playbook Step 4: Evaluating the vendor. (n.d.). Retrieved from www.ama-assn.org: https://www.ama-assn.org/practice-management/digital/ digital-health-implementation-playbook-step-4-evaluating-vendor.

Final policy, payment, and quality provisions changes to the Medicare physician fee schedule for calendar year 2021. (2020, December 1). Retrieved January 29, 2021, from www. cms.gov: https://www.cms.gov/newsroom/fact-sheets/final-policy-payment-and-quality-provisions-changes-medicare-physician-fee-schedule-calendar-year-1.

Gordan, W. J. (2020). Remote patient monitoring program for hospital discharged COVID-19 patients. *Appl Clin Inform*, 11(5): 792–801.

Kadar, R. B. (2019). Impact of telemonitoring of critically ill emergency department patients awaiting ICU transfer. *Critical Care Medicine*, 47(9): 1201–1207.

Klersy, C. D. (2009). A meta-analysis of remote monitoring of heart failure patients. *Journal of the American College of Cardiology*, 54(18): 1683–1694.

Kumar, S. M. (2013). Tele-ICU: Efficacy and cost-effectiveness approach of remotely managing the critical care. *The Open Medical Informatics Journal*, 7(1): 24–29.

Levine, D. M., Ouchi, K., Blanchfield, B., Diamond, K., Licurse, A., Pu, C. T., & Schnipper, J. L. (2018). Hospital-level care at home for acutely ill adults: A pilot randomized controlled trial. *Journal of General Internal Medicine*, 33(5): 729–736. doi:10.1007/ s11606-018-4307-z

Natarajan A, S. H. (2020, November 30). Assessment of physiological signs associated with COVID-19 measured using wearable devices. *NPJ Digital Medicine*, 3.

Neuman, M. D. (2014). Association between skilled nursing facility quality indicators and hospital readmissions. *JAMA*, 312(15): 1542.

Segrelles Calvo, G. G. (2014). A home telehealth program for patients with severe COPD: The PROMETE study. *Respiratory Medicine*, 108(3): 453–462.

Walker, R. C. (2019). Patient expectations and experiences of remote monitoring for chronic diseases: Systematic review and thematic synthesis of qualitative studies. *International Journal of Medical Informatics*, 124: 78–85.

21

Direct-to-Consumer or On-Demand Telehealth

ADITI U. JOSHI AND SYLVAN WALLER ■

INTRODUCTION

Direct-to-consumer (DTC) telehealth refers to directly marketing on-demand telehealth visit options to consumers. Whether using telephone or video chat, patients can speak with a clinician and get care, advice, and prescriptions for their medical concerns almost immediately. DTC telehealth allows increased patient access and engagement. The modalities through which consumers can seek this on-demand care have evolved significantly over the last few years to include asynchronous interactions, such as short message services (SMS), voice, and video.

DTC telehealth typically occurs in one of three contexts: (1) with an existing health care provider; (2) with a different clinician from the same health care organization; or (3) with an entity outside of the organization from which the patient has an existing relationship. Outside entities could be labeled as private-sector DTC telehealth companies that are contracted by a health system, an insurance company, or charge a fee for service (Welch, 2017). Currently, the private sector has been most visible in creating platforms for DTC telehealth and is often cited as being the purveyor of this health care modality. Their model allows patients to easily create an account and seek medical care through a patient's modality of choice (text, voice, video) from any state in which the company has licensed clinicians. Most companies have remote clinicians covering multiple states and cover a large geographic area.

While DTC service initially focused on low-acuity urgent care needs, recently, a number of start-up companies have developed platforms catered to providing a specific service, such as prescriptions for birth control or treatments for erectile dysfunction (see Table 21.1).

As telehealth has grown, however, clinics, hospitals, and larger health care systems have also started creating or offering digital health solutions to their patients, members, and employees. Organizations are recognizing the benefits of access, customer loyalty, and branding that on-demand care utilizing a local telehealth physician can bring. This chapter further outlines how to develop a DTC telehealth program and considerations for implementation.

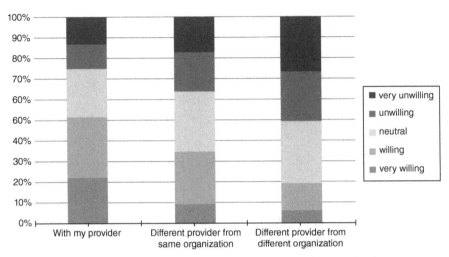

Figure 21.1 Willingness to use telemedicine. From Patient preferences for direct-to-consumer telemedicine services: a nationwide survey (Welch, 2017).

TYPES OF CONSUMER TELEHEALTH OFFERINGS

Aside from large companies marketing directly to consumers, institutions and physician networks can set up their own offerings for on-demand DTC services. Clinician staffing for the service can be supplied by local clinicians, clinicians associated with the health system, or contracts with existing regional or national provider groups. DTC telehealth markets directly to consumers who can engage with their choice of clinician over telehealth. These services are typically targeted to acute care and primary care. On-demand is a modality that surgeons may also use to triage known patients with postoperative complaints, as well as a term that sometimes describes the immediate request for a consultation from another physician for assistance in decision making.

Acute Care DTC Telemedicine

DTC telehealth is a natural fit for patients seeking immediate care for an acute problem. This clearly represents how many health consumers often think of telehealth—a patient at home initiating a call to a physician for an acute issue. Consumers often need clear guidance as to which common complaints are appropriate for telehealth

Table 21.1 EXAMPLES OF SPECIALITY ON-DEMAND TELEHEALTH SERVICES

Specialty Services	Example Service Providers
Women's Health, menopause, fertility	Hers, Olympya, Rory, Kindbody, Carrot Care
Men's Health, fertility	Hims, Lemonaid, Roman, Bright
Behavioral Health	Talkspace, Lifestance, Cerebral
Cardiology	HeartBeat Health
Teleintesivist	Advanced ICU, Caregility, Eagle

evaluations. These typically include respiratory infections, sprains, rash, urinary tract infections, and other complaints that may present to urgent care centers (UCCs). However, it is hypothesized that most complaints can be successfully evaluated, or at least triaged, over telehealth, allowing for patients to be seen more quickly than may be possible at their primary care, UCC, or emergency department (ED). These visits may also help patients with clarification on a previous diagnosis, disease progression, and whether or not a higher level of care is necessary at that moment.

A study funded by the Rand Corporation in 2016 found that the availability of DTC telehealth has increased utilization by patients who may not have otherwise sought health care for their immediate problem without this mode of access and subsequently, may be increasing costs (Uscher-Pines, 2016). However, DTC telehealth has increased access to care for patients (Uscher-Pines, 2016). It is still unclear whether this increased access will save the health system money over time by providing patients with earlier interventions and prevention of more expensive care associated with late presentation of disease. Employer programs using DTC for employee triage to decrease health care costs are another strategy that might show longer term cost benefits (Teledoc Health, 2020).

Primary Care DTC Telemedicine

Telehealth can also be used by primary care providers (PCPs). Consumers most commonly use DTC telehealth in primary care for acute exacerbations of chronic diseases, quick checkups on blood pressure or medication effects, clarification of lab or radiology results, or to initiate long term care. The use of DTC telehealth empowers patients to manage their health and may lead to better chronic disease management, which may help avoid emergent ED visits (Totten, 2019). Frequent consumer-initiated telehealth visits may also allow for more rapid titration of medication dosing, better medication adherence, and improved disease surveillance. These programs are especially useful for integrated delivery networks, accountable care organizations (ACOs), or employer-based health plans seeking to decrease ED and return visits for chronic disease conditions. For example, within an integrated delivery network, ED clinicians should be aware of the availability of telehealth by PCPs and encourage it as a route for follow-up care.

PROGRAMMATIC CONSIDERATIONS

Needs Assessment

Implementing a new technology is a good opportunity to reassess the needs of patients in the community to create the most impactful and successful interventions. Some examples one needs to consider include the rate of medication adherence, prevalent diseases and risk factors, the number of clinicians servicing a geographic area, the number and type of care centers, and resources for patient care. More specific to DTC programs, a critical assessment of community resources available to enable patients with immediate or same-day services should be completed. Some factors that DTC telehealth can impact include access to same-day appointments and same-day lab testing. Improvement in these resources through DTC telehealth could impact urgent care center utilization and local ED wait times. Hospitals are required to do this type of needs assessment and may also be able to incorporate local, regional, and national level reports to aid this type of research (Martin, 2012).

Program Scope

Implementation of a DTC telehealth program should be informed by the needs assessment and targeted to accomplish specific and measurable goals. Some examples include (1) improve access for existing patients measured as time to next available appointment; (2) reduce the cost to acquire a new patient; (3) build brand loyalty measured in return visits or use of services across multiple departments, or public ratings, or (4) reduce employee health costs. The goals will determine the type of staffing, platform, and programs offered. Emergency medicine practitioners can serve an important role in many of these service offerings and goals due to their ability to manage acute unscheduled care without a prior patient relationship. If information systems are in place, ED groups can support staffing, create linkages to in-person care, and coordinate care for follow-up. It is worth remembering that some of these goals may change over time and mapping future goals will be necessary to expand any program.

Financial Considerations

Creating a DTC telehealth program takes a tremendous amount of upfront resources. There may be significant costs related to selecting, licensing, and implementing a DTC telehealth platform. Additionally, creating an implementation team, patient and clinician facing support services, clinician training, and marketing may require investments in capital and dedicated personnel. The scope of services and the level of integration of the DTC platform with practice management systems will determine if the DTC program will be profitable. In some cases, the downstream impact of the DTC program related to new referrals, new procedures, and brand loyalty, though difficult to measure, may still justify the investment. Many health care organizations that have implemented DTC telehealth have found that it takes time to build traction with the service, establish the right price point, and build awareness (Wicklund, 2019). Reimbursement for telehealth expanded significantly during the COVID-19 pandemic, potentially increasing revenue opportunities.

Operations and Staffing

Telehealth implementations are typically more complex than anticipated. DTC telehealth is considered to be a quick and accessible consumer friendly service. It requires nimble operational staff that includes clinicians, program management, registration staff, marketing, billing, compliance, IT, and quality assurance. It is important to have in place a system to manage patient and clinician technical support, whether it is managed in-house or by the telehealth platform vendor. Change management, assessing an organization's readiness, developing champions for the program, and getting staff buy-in and support, is critical to success. The operations team will need to work closely with the telehealth platform partner for implementation and ongoing success.

Program scope and available hours will impact the staffing requirements for the DTC telehealth offering. The simplest model would be to completely outsource the services to the selected telehealth platform vendor. In this case, a white labeled telehealth platform would be made available to consumers who receive care from the telehealth company's contracted clinicians licensed in the appropriate state. These services may be available 24/7, but the organization will have minimal control over the clinicians, their qualifications, and how they practice. An organization would work with the platform company to capture testing at local facilities and downstream referrals.

If an organization has clinician and budgetary capacity, it can work with the platform vendor to route calls to the available clinician within the health care organization. A hybrid model may exist, where the telehealth platform company's clinicians cover after-hours or overflow visits. This allows the organization to protect its brand and further control local testing, referrals, and practice.

DTC TELEHEALTH TECHNOLOGIES

Selecting a telehealth platform is dependent on organizational goals and program scope. A number of companies offer telehealth platforms, usually including a web and mobile app consumer interface. Typically, they will offer comprehensive implementation, integration, training, marketing, and technical support. Some vendors also offer clinician staffing services.

Technology

Technology has become the most commoditized component of telehealth and can be utilized via the electronic health record (EHR) or through a stand-alone telehealth platform. Many EHR products now include a telehealth module or functionality into their products. This can be a viable option depending on cost and on whether the system has robust functionality to meet the program scope. The biggest challenge with EHR-based telehealth solutions is that some products do not have a direct-to-consumer front end, a mobile application, or integrations with existing EHRs. They may be offered through the patient portal, which makes them more difficult to access for nonestablished patients. However, for clinicians, this may provide the simplest and most integrated experience. Stand-alone telehealth solutions have the telemedicine component, whether voice, video, text, or email as well as e-prescribing functionality and embedded documentation modules catered to making telehealth documentation efficient. Almost every vendor provides white labeling and customization of the front end. Some level of integration with the EHR is available,

Table 21.2 CONSIDERATIONS FOR CHOOSING TELEHEALTH PLATFORM VENDOR PARTNER

Increase revenue	Cut costs
Fee for service/cash	Insurance reimbursement
Reduce the cost of care overall for a specialty group, DRG, or ACO	Reduce avoidable admissions to the hospital
Subscription or concierge model?	Out-patient care or in-patient care, or both

often through HL-7 or continuity of care documents (CCD). It is important to note that telehealth vendor registration modules will require integration with the practice management system if a medical record number match is desired or to streamline insurance billings. Otherwise, many implementations are set up in parallel with the main practice management system, with the telehealth platform collecting registration information and utilizing fee for service billing (Table 21.2).

Cost and Business Models

The cost of implementing a DTC telehealth platform depends on a number of factors. There are typically one-time costs for implementation, and then ongoing licensing, maintenance, and support fees. The recurring costs may change with volume of visits or users. Marketing support and training may be included or at an additional expense.

The other cost to consider is related to staffing. Whether using in-house clinician capacity or outsourcing to the vendor's clinician group, staffing remains a significant cost. DTC telehealth is an on-demand service; therefore, there are fixed costs of being available when there may be low demand. Consideration should be given to the per consult fees associated with using the platform only versus outsourcing the visits to the vendor group. While telehealth services are becoming more broadly reimbursed by government and private payers, keep in mind that systems integration may drive a decision to use a fee for service or a cash model for DTC visits. There may be other costs associated with nonclinical staffing as well. For example, you may need a project manager and IT liaison to work with the platform provider for implementation and beyond.

Many health systems and large medical groups have elected to provide these services by having the patient pay directly before the visit with a credit card. In these models, they charge enough to cover the cost of the service (license fees from the technology platform and the access fees from the clinical visits), while trying to keep the costs low so that patients will use the service.

In the model where a system or clinic is focused on reducing cost or reducing avoidable admissions, the system or clinic may pay for the entire cost of the service and benefit by reducing utilization of expensive specialty or primary care services. Some organizations cover employees to use the service, increasing engagement with the service and potentially decreasing the referral rate to higher level of care. In models where a visit is reimbursed through a global payment or ACO model, no direct payment from the patient occurs and the costs are offset by reducing expenses.

Several telehealth companies provide specialty services contracts with health systems and medical groups using a subscription model or recurring monthly fee. These models typically provide specialty services, such as for hypertension or heart failure, to the patient for ongoing chronic diseases management and may result in lower overall total cost of care for these conditions (Totten, 2019).

User Experience

Both the patient and clinician are users of the DTC telehealth platform. The better platforms have designed an efficient user experience and workflow that uses the technology to scaffold the encounter and improve communication between patient and clinician. The ability to push and pull data into an EMR is an important component that improves the user experience, cuts down on duplication of work, and improves quality and patient safety. The DTC telehealth platform is often considered a "digital" front door to a health care organization. It is important that the look and feel of the web and mobile interfaces are simple, attractive, and memorable. Consistent branding will help consumers identify the organization and trust the care they receive. Ideally, the service clearly identifies the clinicians who are available for visits, including their affiliations and qualifications. DTC services that leverage their own clinicians from the practice tend to have higher patient satisfaction (Welch, 2017). This also allows patients to have a more seamless experience, since local clinicians understand local geography, traffic patterns, and driving distance, and can more easily send patients to the most appropriate brick-and-mortar services with a warm hand-off. Consult pricing, streamlined complaint resolution, online technical support, and convenient hours also impact the patient experience.

QUALITY ASSURANCE AND METRICS FOR SATISFACTION

Once a program has been implemented, it is imperative to have systems in place that ensure quality and safety. Given that DTC telehealth is on-demand, consumer facing, and serves as a digital front door to a health care organization, there are some specific considerations for monitoring DTC telehealth programs (Table 21.3).

Antibiotic stewardship and adherence to clinical guidelines are areas of particular interest in DTC telehealth. Due to concerns related to disrupting the medical home, scrutiny has been applied in these areas to assure that the DTC telehealth services meet quality standards. A number of studies have examined this issue; however, it is important to consider that guideline adherence for in-person care is generally low and highly variable. As many of the common DTC telehealth complaints revolve around antibiotics prescriptions, an antibiotic stewardship program can monitor clinician practice patterns and intervene as necessary. Previous studies have noted that there may be an increase in antibiotic prescribing and a lack of standardization in history and physical examination (Schoenfeld, 2016). However, others have shown that there was better stewardship when compared to ED visits (Halpren-Ruder, 2019). Physicians can also be evaluated for their adherence to telehealth clinical guidelines and their referral patterns to ED/UCCs. While there are no specific

Table 21.3 QUALITY ASSURANCE METRICS IN DTC

User Experience	Technology	Clinical
Patients: Resolution or follow-up for complaint; Escalation to in-person care by venue (PCP, ED, UCC); Satisfaction;	System downtime; missed calls/requests; dropped calls, response time to clinician, to technical support; Number of technical support calls; visit length; network issues; video or audio transmission problems impacting visits	Antibiotic stewardship: evaluation, and comparison of antibiotic prescribing rate in various setting (telehealth, DTC, PCP office, UCC, ED)
Complaint resolution; time to visit from time of request		
Clinician: Ability to adequately assess patient concern; difficulty of handing patient off to in-person care; visit length		Clinical Guideline Adherence: evaluation and comparison of guideline adherence in various settings (telehealth, DTC, PCP office, UCC, ED)
System: increased geographic patient reach; patient loyalty; new referrals, ratings		

telehealth clinical guidelines, existing guidelines can be tailored to telehealth visits. The use of guidelines can also be helpful to clarify for clinicians the possible scope of practice over telehealth and can support training and reeducation.

CONCLUSION

Creating a successful DTC telehealth program requires understanding the landscape of telehealth as a whole, knowing the system and community health needs, and planning a program based on those requirements. DTC telehealth is expanding by health care organizations that have created their programs for employees and existing patients, and seek to increase access to communities in surrounding population areas. As national and local DTC telehealth models continue to grow, there needs to be a sustained movement to ensure access and quality.

KEY TAKEAWAYS

> ➤ An organizational and community needs assessment can help define the program scope for a DTC telehealth service.
> ➤ The telehealth platform can be licensed from a stand-alone vendor or as part of some electronic health record systems.
> ➤ Cost considerations for DTC telehealth include platform fees, clinical staffing, administrative support, marketing, quality assurance, and training.
> ➤ Clinical staffing can occur via health care organizations' own clinical capacity, in partnership with the telehealth platform vendor as a hybrid model, or completely outsourced.

> ➢ Evaluating the user experience of DTC telehealth programs is important to improve both clinician and patient experiences that impact satisfaction and brand loyalty.
> ➢ Quality assurance mechanisms should be in place for patient experience, technology, and clinical metrics

REFERENCES

Halpren-Ruder, D. (2019, July). Quality assurance in telehealth: Adherence to evidence-based indicators. *Telemedicine and e-Health*, 25(7): 599–603.

Martin, C. (2012). Telehealth Program Developer Kit. Retrieved December 7, 2020, from California Telemedicine and eHealth Center: https://www.nrtrc.org/content/article-files/Business%20Plans/2012%20Program%20Developer%20Kit%20-%20Part%201.pdf.

Schoenfeld, A. J. (2016, May 1). Variation In quality of care provided during commercial virtual visits in urgent care: A standardized patient audit study. *JAMA Internal Medicine*, 176(5): 635–642.

Teledoc Health. (2020, September). *Case Studies*. Retrieved December 7, 2020, from Teledochealth.com: https://assets.ctfassets.net/l3v9j0ltz3yi/vzun4FkkQDMLoISvsRpPx/a7289a068fec3d582c55dfff71553b74/Hamilton_Health_Hub_Employer_Clinic_Case_Study.pdf.

Totten, A. M. (2019). *Telehealth for acute and chronic care consultations*. Agency for Healthcare Research and Quality. Rockville, MD: AHRQ Publication No. 19-EHC012-EF.

Uscher-Pines, L. (2016, March 23). Access and quality of care in direct-to-consumer telemedicine. *Telemedicine and e-Health*, 22(4): 282–287.

Welch, B. H. (2017, November 28). Patient preferences for direct-to-consumer telemedicine services: a nationwide survey. *BMC Health Services Research*, 17(784).

Wicklund, E. (2019, August 22). *Direct-to-consumer telehealth requires careful planning, preparation*. retrieved December 7, 2020, from mHealth Intelligence: https://mhealthintelligence.com/news/direct-to-consumer-telehealth-requires-careful-planning-preparation.

22

Telehealth Facilitates Value-Based Care in Emergency Department Settings

DEBORAH ANN MULLIGAN, KRISTA DROBAC,
AND ROBERT SHESSER ■

INTRODUCTION

There is a broad consensus among policymakers and health care stakeholders that medical care needs to shift from the current fee-for-service paradigm to alternative models that encourage the development of "value-based" systems that can achieve better outcomes at lower cost. A series of "new" payment models, including pay for performance, shared savings, bundled payments, and global capitation, have been developed and implemented in a limited manner, but emergency medicine is still practiced primarily in a fee-for-service environment (Farmer & Brown, 2017; Pines, McStay, George, Wiler, & McClellan, 2016; Arkwright, Edwards, & Mattison, 2018). As alternative models become more widely adopted, emergency physicians (EPs) should provide leadership by coordinating with physician-colleagues and health systems in developing new patient management systems to help shift acute unscheduled care into evolving payment models.

> Without the participation and leadership of EPs, emergency department (ED) visits will most likely decrease, and EPs may not be considered intrinsic to a comprehensive, holistic patient management model.

New skills relating to coordination of patient care will need to be developed and incorporated into emergency medicine residency training programs. The increased use of telehealth needs to be integrated into emergency medicine's "new" value-based, coordinated care model.

TENETS OF VALUE-BASED CARE

Value-based care is patient access to timely, appropriate care that is coordinated across specialties and focused on improving outcomes rather than increasing the volume of services. Measures of the effectiveness of value-based care include patient satisfaction, access to care (including specialists), appropriateness of the setting of care, timeliness of care, unplanned admissions, care coordination, and overall resource stewardship.

Telehealth software platforms can help providers understand important industry benchmarks and foundational data, including emergency department length of stay, cost, volume, quality, and patient statistics. A successful approach to meeting these benchmarks must include a strategy for managing a population's acute, unscheduled care needs. Multiple venues and formats exist for the management of unscheduled needs, including physician offices, retail clinics, urgent care centers, freestanding EDs, traditional hospital EDs, and emergency telehealth encounters. The goal of a value-based, population health strategy is to efficiently link a patient to the most appropriate level of care for their needs.

Traditionally, the hospital ED has provided most after-hours needs for populations. People use the ED for many different conditions and health concerns, which represent varying levels of severity. Some of these conditions include both adult and pediatric acute injury and illness, acute episodes of chronic illnesses, mental health needs, substance abuse issues, and prescription refills. However, as ED costs in a fee-for-service environment are higher (for a variety of reasons) than some of the alternatives listed above, multiple management strategies have been advocated to direct appropriate patients toward the lower cost alternatives that are still appropriate for their disease severity.

As alternative payment models grow and integrated health systems develop management pathways that provide a more flexible response to unscheduled medical concerns, it is almost certain that emergency telehealth will support new management paradigms. As these systems have yet to fully mature, the use cases for telehealth applied to emergency care are somewhat limited and currently tend to support fee-for-service operations more than value-based care.

The COVID-19 pandemic has been a catalyst for the application of telemedicine in the evaluation of urgent/emergent complaints. Although most new telemedicine programs begin in a fee-for-service mode, once patients, payers, and providers have seen how effectively urgent complaints can be evaluated with telehealth visits and how much unnecessary expense can be avoided, it is certain that telehealth will become a mainstay in the management of urgent complaints in future value-based systems.

OPPORTUNITIES IN VALUE-BASED CARE

Just as COVID-19 has catalyzed new ED or EP-based telehealth services, virtually every other medical specialty has quickly moved many of their "cognitive" visits to telehealth. In some ways, the progress made by other specialties has narrowed emergency medicine's telehealth opportunities and provides a wake-up call for EPs. EPs must now move quickly to develop programs that can be funded either by traditional fee-for-service billings or by another "risk-taking entity" such as an insurance company, hospital, or accountable care organization (ACO).

There are several use cases in which emergency telehealth could contribute to cost savings in value-based care models, utilizing telehealth to direct patients to the most appropriate and cost-efficient care setting.

Triage and treatment: A telehealth encounter used to make a triage determination as to the optimal timing and location a patient should be seen. Conceptually, this extends existing nurse telephone triage systems that have already been developed by both insurance companies and integrated delivery systems. Such systems have been shown to reduce costs and be acceptable to patients (American College of Emergency Physicians, 2021).

A value-driven, highly coordinated response leveraging telehealth could be created for a number of disease states. COVID-19 has created the need to reduce the number of patients with clear-cut respiratory complaints in offices, urgent care centers, and perhaps hospital EDs. For example, an initial telemedicine visit from home would allow a clinician to determine if a patient's clinical condition was safe for outpatient testing. The patient could then go to a "comprehensive" outpatient specimen collection facility. Once a patient is in the ED waiting area, tele-triage could be used to assess and care for appropriate patients to decrease wait times, left without being seen, and time of exposure (see Chapter 15). EP-based telehealth services can facilitate public health mitigation strategies during the pandemic by increasing social distancing. These services can be a safer option for both ED clinicians and staff, as well as patients, by reducing potential infectious exposures. If coordinated, they can reduce the strain on health care systems by minimizing the surge of patient demand on facilities and reduce the use of personal protective equipment (PPE). Any number of telehealth follow-ups can be arranged to contextualize the patient's results, identify patients who could benefit from remote monitoring, and follow the patient until recovery.

Consultation: There are currently three well-established specialty use cases for a telehealth consultation by an out-of-hospital specialist to a hospital ED. These are teleradiology, teleneurology (stroke) (see Chapter 8), and telepsychiatry (see Chapter 9). Although the consultant is not an EP, this model should result in cost savings and increased efficiency, thereby making it adaptable to a VBC model. Such consultations can reduce unnecessary transfers, potentially reduce unnecessary admissions, and enhance ED throughput by providing faster access to certain specialists.

The advent of COVID-19 has catalyzed a new use case for telemedicine, the "internal consultation", where certain specialty clinicians who formerly would see a patient in-person now perform a teleconsult for ED patients. This practice was initially spurred by specialist reluctance to see patients before the advent of rapid SARS-CoV-2 test results, the need to reduce the use of personal protective equipment, and the need for timely consultations. Specialties that were early adopters of this practice in the George Washington University Hospital ED included the specialties of Psychiatry, Neurology, and Rheumatology.

The use of telemedicine for specialty consultation in the ED will almost certainly grow in the post-COVID-19 era and extend to most specialties. Specialty physicians have now become more comfortable with telehealth and, at least during business hours, a greater number will be seeing telehealth visits in the outpatient setting. An ED consultation can be easily added and integrated into their workflow more efficiently than seeing the patient in person. The ability to obtain an "internal" telemedicine visit with a specialist could lead to fewer admissions and quicker specialty follow-up that will be of great benefit for value-based care (see Chapter 12).

ONGOING CARE FOLLOWING PATIENT DISCHARGE FROM THE EMERGENCY DEPARTMENT

Payers have recognized that postdischarge patient management and care coordination are essential to avoiding unnecessary admissions, readmissions, and return visits to the ED. The American College of Emergency Physicians has developed the Acute Unscheduled Care Model (AAUCM; American College of Emergency Physicians, 2020) as a way for EPs to more directly participate in Medicare's advanced alternative payment models by accepting some financial risk for their admission and discharge decisions on Medicare beneficiaries. This program was initially oriented toward patients with certain diagnoses (e.g., syncope, chest pain, abdominal pain, and altered mental status) that have a high variability of ED admission rates among different hospitals.

The program rewards physicians for reducing costs by:

1. Reducing hospital in-patient and observation stays
2. Enhancing the ability of EPs to avoid unnecessary postdischarge care
3. Avoiding post-ED visit adverse events

This proposed program uses a retrospective reconciliation methodology and the combination of claims data and provider-reported metrics. Providers would receive admission/observation reduction targets, and those who meet or exceed these targets without an increase in postdischarge events would receive an additional payment from Medicare.

Clearly, the advent of this type of program would change the very nature of the "traditional" ED visit that results in the binary outcomes of admission or discharge. In both instances, the EP generally passes that responsibility for the patient to another physician upon ED discharge. The need for ongoing, active EP involvement in discharged patients is another good use case for a telehealth encounter.

The AAUCM makes no mention of a "toolkit" that allows EPs to safely discharge "borderline" admissions. The two elements of this toolkit are an ED-based care coordinator and the use of telehealth services for ED follow-ups by the EP group where responsibility for follow-up care cannot be easily transitioned to a primary care provider. As the AAUCM was developed before the COVID-19-related loosening of telehealth regulations, it asks Medicare to develop a waiver such that EPs could provide and bill for one telehealth encounter with the patient in their home.

EM AND ACCOUNTABLE CARE ORGANIZATIONS

The Affordable Care Act (ACA) and subsequent Obama-era legislation developed several programs that were designed to accelerate the move from volume to value. The ACA permitted the development of ACOs that are designed to deliver health care in a more coordinated, efficient manner to a defined population (American College of Emergency Physicians, 2015). The population is most frequently Medicare recipients, but could include Medicaid or commercially insured patients according to regional relationships and the maturity of the ACO. An ACO can be organized by an integrated delivery system, hospital, or hospital system, physician organizations of various types, or a community health center. The role of the EP within an ACO will depend primarily on the nature of the organization that sponsors the ACO and the relationship of the EP to that organization.

Five different ACO models can be developed. The details of each are beyond the scope of this chapter. However, the essence is that Medicare calculates the historical costs for caring for patients associated with ACO physicians (generally primary care), and the total cost of care in subsequent years is compared to the historical costs. The ACO models differ in whether there is any downside risk and the amount of the bonus available when the ACO reduces costs. There are also a variety of quality metrics that the ACO must meet to qualify for the bonus.

There are no universally applicable models that describe emergency medicine's participation in an ACO, and even less is known about how telemedicine could enhance EP participation. The range of possibilities would differ according to the ACO's organization and the relationship of the EM group to both the ACO and hospital. As with the AAUCM, the use of telemedicine by the ED group to monitor more closely certain "borderline" discharged patients could improve care and patient satisfaction while decreasing costs.

CONCLUSION

It is highly likely that as our health system evolves, future iterations will attempt to manage patients' emergent/urgent needs in a more integrated and comprehensive manner than today's highly "siloed" system. New management configurations may open opportunities for EPs to play an active management role in ways other than the current face-to-face encounter in the ED. EPs should place themselves at the information crossroads of future systems that will allow them to continue to add value in this important function.

KEY TAKEAWAYS

> ➤ Use of emergency telehealth can support emerging value-based initiatives in various ways to reduce costs, improve outcomes, and facilitate patient satisfaction.
> ➤ Follow-up care after discharge from the emergency department can facilitate continuity of care and bridge the time between the EP caring for the patient and the hand-off to a PCP.
> ➤ Emergency telehealth consults conducted in advance of an ED visit could direct a patient to a more appropriate care venue or initiate an outpatient testing regimen that could avoid an in-person visit entirely.
> ➤ "Internal" specialty consultation via telehealth could help improve ED throughput, reduce unnecessary admissions, and speed up needed specialty evaluations.

REFERENCES

American College of Emergency Physicians. (2021). Acute Unscheduled Care Model (AUCM). Enhancing appropriate admissions. Accessed February 27, 2021, at https://aspe.hhs.gov/system/files/pdf/255906/ProposalACEP.pdf.

American College of Emergency Physicians. (2015, November). The role and value of the emergency department in an accountable care organization.

Arkwright, B. T., Edwards, J., & Mattison, J. (2020). Making telehealth a strategic asset to achieve efficiency. *Telehealth and Medicine Today* Audio File November 2018.

Farmer, S., & Brown, N. A. (2017). Value-based approaches for emergency care in a new era. *Annals of Emergency Medicine*, 69(6): 684–686.

Halamka, J., & Cerrato, P. (2020). The digital reconstruction of health care. *NEJM Catalyst Innovations in Care Delivery*, 1(6).

Pines, J. M., McStay, F., George, M., Wiler, J. L., & McClellan, M. (2016). Aligning payment reform and delivery innovation in emergency care. *American Journal of Management Care*, 22(8): 515–518.

Schaye, V., Reich, J. A., Bosworth, B. P., Stern, D., et al. (2020). Collaborating across private, public, community, and federal hospital systems: Lessons ;learned from the Covid-19 pandemic response in NYC. *NEJM Catalyst Innovations in Care Delivery*. 1(6).

23

Tele-Ultrasound

ELIZABETH DEARING AND KEITH BONIFACE ■

INTRODUCTION

Medical imaging has made significant advancements in the past half-century. Ultrasound in particular has seen marked improvements in image quality as well as affordability and accessibility of machines. Despite these advances, access to ultrasound imaging has not grown at the same rate due to lack of trained providers who are able to acquire and/or interpret ultrasound images. Tele-ultrasound is an emerging field that can bridge the gap and provide increased access to this important imaging modality in remote or lower-resource settings.

ULTRASOUND AND THE RISE OF POINT-OF-CARE ULTRASOUND

Ultrasound has the benefit of being relatively low-cost compared to other imaging modalities, and it is noninvasive, increasingly portable, and does not produce ionizing radiation. Given these benefits, point-of-care ultrasound (POCUS) has long been used by clinicians at the bedside to aid in diagnosis as well as to increase the safety of bedside procedures. In a typical ultrasound examination in North America, a trained nonphysician sonographer obtains the ultrasound images and a radiologist interprets the images obtained. The interpretation is then relayed to the patient by the bedside clinician. POCUS differs from this traditional workflow because the bedside clinician both performs and interprets the ultrasound study, and the results are integrated into the care of the patient, all in real time. POCUS uses portable ultrasound machines at the bedside of patients to answer specific clinical questions, guide procedures, and monitor response to therapy.

Many medical specialties currently employ POCUS to care for patients. Emergency medicine and trauma surgery have been at the forefront of incorporating POCUS into clinical practice, beginning with the Focused Assessment with Sonography in Trauma, or FAST, exam in the 1980s. As ultrasound machines found their place in emergency departments (EDs) for the evaluation of trauma patients, it became clear that ultrasound could improve the accuracy and efficiency of diagnosis and treatment in many clinical conditions. With smaller, more portable machines and improving resolution, POCUS has been increasingly utilized for a broad range of indications, as it has generally been shown to reduce length of stay in the ED and improve patient safety and outcomes. Additionally, ultrasound guidance for central line placement in the internal jugular vein has been shown to improve safety and quality when compared to landmark-based catheterization and is recommended in clinical practice (Brass, Hellmich, Kolodziej, Schick, & Smith, 2015; Saugel, Scheeren, & Teboul, 2017). The American College of Emergency Physicians (ACEP) requires competency in point-of-care ultrasound in 11 clinical applications for all residents in emergency medicine. POCUS has also been used globally by emergency physicians and other specialties, who may not have ready access to diagnostic imaging, especially cross-sectional imaging, to improve patient care in resource-limited settings. The use of POCUS continues to spread to other specialties, including internal medicine, pediatrics, and family medicine, in order to provide improved care for patients in both in-patient and out-patient settings.

HISTORY OF TELE-ULTRASOUND

Tele-ultrasound is a subset of telemedicine that uses technology to remotely interpret ultrasound studies and/or guide acquisition of ultrasound images. Tele-ultrasound has evolved from necessitating that the radiologist be in the same hospital as the sonographer to allow them to be connected only through a broadband connection. In addition, this technology has allowed ultrasound to develop from asynchronous interpretation of technician-acquired images to synchronous guidance and real-time interpretation.

The National Aeronautics and Space Administration (NASA) has been at the forefront of telemedicine and tele-ultrasound in its efforts to provide care to crew members that may be in space for extended periods of time without direct access to health care providers or diagnostic testing. The International Space Station (ISS), launched in 1998, is equipped with a space-adapted ultrasound machine, the only diagnostic imaging available on the ISS due to technical constraints for other forms of imaging. Additionally, trauma has been noted to be one of the highest risks for the crew's health, and ultrasound has been proven helpful in diagnosing injury in these patients (Sargsyan et al., 2005). Because of advances in transmission speed, real-time consultation can assist crew members in performing ultrasound in space, with guidance and interpretation by physician sonographers at Mission Control. Ultrasound experts on the ground provide just-in-time training to astronauts who were not medically trained prior to deployment and then used cue cards to help refresh the remote sonographer memory of the views desired, as well as guide communication to improve images (Sargsyan et al., 2005; Chiao et al., 2005; Fincke et al., 2005).

Cardiology and obstetrics also began to use tele-ultrasound in the 1990s to improve patient care in rural and remote areas. Many of these studies began to use tele-ultrasound to guide referrals from remote areas to tertiary care centers, in addition to increase capacity for local care by reducing transfers (Sobczyk, Solinger, Rees, & Elbl, 1993). In one study, echocardiography was performed on pediatric patients up to 250 miles away from the tertiary care center in Louisville, Kentucky and reviewed by the pediatric cardiologists. Even with the poorer technology in 1991–1992 as compared to today, they showed that 83% of the studies gave accurate diagnostic impressions and only 2% resulted in an inappropriate clinical decision. Tele-ultrasound has also proved valuable in low- and middle-income countries where other cross-sectional imaging modalities may be limited and expensive to maintain their programming.

ROLE OF TELE-ULTRASOUND

The rapid evolution of ultrasound technology, as well as the shrinking size of ultrasound equipment and decreasing price point, has led to the expansion of ultrasound equipment from out of the radiology department to other in-patient and office-based settings. However, a significant limitation to the dissemination of clinical ultrasound is the lack of trained providers. The majority of physicians are not competent in ultrasound, primarily because they lack exposure or training inasmuch as currently ultrasound education is integrated into just a few medical specialties. Additionally, until recently, undergraduate medical education did not include exposure to ultrasound. These factors have created a large population of physicians without skills in the acquisition and interpretation of ultrasound. Sonographers could help add to the workforce of people teaching image acquisition, although their radiology role does not include the interpretation of images to direct patient care.

As ultrasound equipment becomes more accessible, the goal should therefore be to increase the number of trained clinicians, specifically the number of credentialed clinicians who are able to both perform ultrasound exams and make clinical decisions based on their acquired images. Ultrasound-trained clinicians traditionally include sonographers, radiologists, ultrasound-trained physicians, or other health care providers (e.g., advanced practice providers or APPs); however, their training programs vary. The ultrasound expert must complete certain requirements in order to be considered competent in ultrasound. The standards for competency are based on the provider role and the overseeing organization (e.g., American Registry for Diagnostic Medical Sonography (ARDMS) for sonographers, American College of Radiology (ACR) for radiologists). On the other hand, POCUS credentialing is a local process and varies in its requirements (e.g., type of exam, prerequisite training) from institution to institution. Increasing the number of competent and credentialed providers is the ideal but is not necessarily realistic since this requires additional training and time that may not be available.

Ultrasound is moving into U.S. in-patient and out-patient clinical settings as more clinicians gain training and credentialing. Its utility has led to greater use in remote sites that may have sonographers with less experience than these traditional settings. The number of trained clinicians could therefore also be enhanced by increasing familiarity with ultrasound image acquisition. Experienced sonographers need only be trained in how to transfer images and connect to the tele-ultrasound expert in order to help increase access to care. Tele-ultrasound can help to increase the competence of local providers, regardless of the experience level of sonographers, and improve the decisions of local clinicians for the tertiary care of their patients. The addition of expert tele-ultrasound consultation can prevent the need to transfer the patient to another location that provides comprehensive ultrasound services, enabling the patient to be taken care of near home. For experienced sonographers, the addition of centrally located experts in cardiology, maternal-fetal medicine, congenital heart disease, and other specialties can improve the level of care provided locally by leveraging the expertise of these tele-ultrasound experts over multiple remote sites.

Still, it can be difficult to staff remote locations with experienced sonographers due to lack of availability of trained clinicians. Tele-ultrasound can help to bridge the gap to provide competent care at the remote site with a less experienced sonographer; however, appropriate training and oversight are necessary. Initially, a combination of didactics and hands-on training is important. To ensure the quality of the training, clinicians continue developing their skills after their initial training by receiving continued support and feedback on their images. The type and degree of initial training, as well as ongoing support, depend on the background of the clinician and the goal of training (Table 23.1).

TECHNOLOGY

Generally, tele-ultrasound can be divided into asynchronous and synchronous. In asynchronous tele-ultrasound (also known as store and forward), the expert image interpreter reviews the ultrasound images at some time after image acquisition onsite. This can be accomplished using email, cloud storage systems, and online picture archiving and communication systems (PACS). This is the most common method of connecting two sites, as it requires the least bandwidth and can be done without requiring both clinicians to be available simultaneously. This is a significant advantage given the differences in time zones that are encountered in global health. A disadvantage of asynchronous tele-ultrasound is that there are no opportunities to either augment a technically limited exam by adding extra views or improve existing views with real-time direction (as the patient may no longer be with the sonographer when the images are reviewed remotely). Asynchronous tele-ultrasound requires more repeat examinations than synchronous tele-ultrasound, but overall, even with less robust technology, some studies have shown that store-and-forward technology has similar accuracy to synchronous tele-ultrasound in low-risk patients (Malone et al., 1997; Fuentes, 2003).

At its most basic, synchronous, or real-time, tele-ultrasound consists of a video stream of the ultrasound image data and a voice communication between the two sites. This can be augmented with a video stream from a camera displaying the probe positioning to aid the tele-ultrasound consultant in improving and optimizing the view. This technology can be very helpful if the person acquiring the ultrasound images does not have significant ultrasound experience. This was initially commercially packaged for POCUS in the Tempus Pro™, a telemedicine solution designed for out-of-hospital use by paramedics. As technology has evolved (both ultrasound technology and wireless connectivity), the newest generation of hand-held ultrasound devices has integrated solutions to help connect the remote sonographer to the tele-ultrasound consultant. Devices such as the Clarius™, Butterfly IQ™, and Philips Lumify™ have the capability to stream the ultrasound image along with a video stream from the camera of the smart phone or tablet connected to the ultrasound probe to the consultant. However, synchronous tele-ultrasound requires more

Table 23.1 TRAINING FOR TELE-ULTRASOUND PROVIDERS

	Initial Instruction	Hands-on Instruction	Additional Instruction	Quality Assurance/Image Review	Ideal Providers
Just-in-Time Training	Brief didactic (e.g., 20 min)	Brief initial hands-on scanning session; instruction from guidance by expert in real time	"Cue cards" or image guides/videos showing ideal views	Real-time guidance with expert	Ideal for nonphysicians/APPs and for focused/specific examination
Training for Image Acquisition only	Variable depending on background of clinician	Variable depending on background of clinician		Real-time guidance or delayed image review with feedback	Ideal for sonographers or other clinicians with ability to acquire images but without education for interpretation and application
Training for Credentialing Providers	Detailed didactics	Multiple scanning sessions with expert or with expert review of images		Delayed review of acquired images with feedback given by expert reviewer	Ideal for physicians/APPs to incorporate in clinical practice and decision making

robust connectivity and simultaneous availability of both the remote sonographer and the centralized tele-ultrasound consultant. In the near future, we can expect that technology will continue to evolve and overcome some of these identified barriers, such as access to high-bandwidth connectivity and availability of computer software and hardware, to increase implementation of synchronous tele-ultrasound. (Adambounou, et al., 2012; Popov, Popov, Kacar, & Harris, 2007).

In fact, significant advancements in technology and telecommunications have already been made in the past few decades due to improvement in data transmission and bandwidth, making tele-ultrasound increasingly more feasible. Prior studies have found that a minimum transmission rate of 384 kbit/s is necessary for diagnostically acceptable images (Brebner, Ruddick-Bracken, & Brebner, 1999; Brebner et al., 2000; Chan et al., 1999). Newer technology has allowed the use of WiFi and cellular networks to transmit data, making synchronous or real-time data sharing and guidance feasible (Pian et al., 2013). Access to broadband has also continued to grow globally. Still, a recent study showed that a third of participants in a study in sub-Saharan Africa may lack internet access or the bandwidth necessary to make data sharing in either an asynchronous or synchronous manner possible (Shokoohi et al., 2019). While this is becoming less of an issue over time, consideration of internet connectivity in the remote site should guide the use of asynchronous or synchronous protocols.

The equipment necessary includes not only the ultrasound machine but also the software to transmit images and videos and, if using synchronized guidance, simultaneously perform two-way audio transmission. When use of tele-ultrasound began, users had to have a computer at each location in order to transmit data (Fuentes, 2003). Systems for synchronous tele-ultrasound were pieced together with available equipment and software to transmit not only the ultrasound data but also audio for guidance. The cost of such systems and for the high-speed access lines for transmission in the past could be prohibitive. However, this technology has become more affordable. Newer cart-based and hand-held ultrasound systems have the ability to transmit images directly from the ultrasound machine to an image archival system. In addition, many ultrasound machines and systems are now designed with telecommunications as an integral part with live-streaming of the video feed (Figure 23.1). Without live-streaming availability, researchers have also studied the use of images recorded on a mobile phone or video camera, with relatively high subjective quality reported. Mobile phones, as well as laptops, have been used to receive and view image remotely (Marsh-Feiley, Eadie, & Wilson, 2018). Also available are cloud-based storage systems to allow easy sharing for clinical care as well as image review.

CLINICAL USES OF TELE-ULTRASOUND

Intensive care units (ICUs) are a unique setting where tele-ultrasound may have a growing role. Fully 11% of the ICU beds in the United States are covered by tele-ICU of some form or another (Lilly et al., 2014). Tele-ultrasound is a small incremental step over the connectivity already utilized in tele-ICU, given the presence of camera streams of the patient and bedside clinician to the centrally located expert already involved in a patient–physician relationship. This existing technological and consultative capacity has paved the way for including tele-ultrasound in the ICU, especially

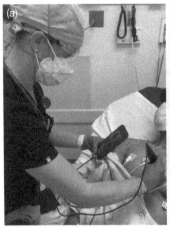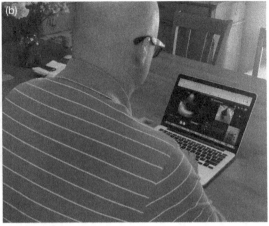

Figure 23.1 Synchronous tele-ultrasound. A provider performs a cardiac ultrasound on a patient (A) while receiving real-time feedback on image acquisition as well as interpretation by an ultrasound expert (B).

given ultrasound's demonstrated role in the assessment of shock and dyspnea (Lichtenstein & Meziere, 2008; Shokoohi et al., 2015). This tele-ultrasound guidance of both physicians and nurses in the ICU has been used to evaluate the heart, lungs, and bladder, and has been demonstrated to produce diagnostic quality images that can answer the clinical question at hand, leading to improved patient care (Olivieri et al., 2020; Becker et al., 2017; Levine et al., 2016).

Similarly, in less densely populated regions of the country, critical access hospitals play a key role in the health care safety net. Some EDs and clinics are staffed with advanced practice providers practicing under a delegation agreement with a remote physician. Tele-ultrasound between the local clinician–sonographer and the remote physician can help streamline the differential diagnosis and rule in or rule out serious causes of illness and injury.

In global health, tele-ultrasound programs have existed for years, especially in the realm of maternal-fetal medicine and cardiology (Britton et al., 2019). These programs have brought knowledge of centrally located specialists to a larger number of clinical sites and patients who may otherwise never have been able to "see" a specialist because of geographic and/or financial limitations. In recent years, the World Health Organization (WHO) has focused on the lack of specialists and clinicians by "task shifting," or the redistribution of tasks from highly qualified health workers to health workers with shorter training and fewer qualifications. The goal of this process is to make more efficient use of available health care workers and provide increased access to essential health services that otherwise would be in shortage. Tele-ultrasound can impact this task shifting, and support of the remote health care worker/sonographer can improve access to the important diagnostic tool of ultrasound. The WHO has specifically supported the task shifting of antenatal ultrasound to midwives as long as appropriate training and mentoring systems are in place (WHO Reproductive Health Library, 2016). Other clinical providers include paramedics in the prehospital setting (Boniface, Shokoohi, Smith, & Scantlebury, 2011) and military special operations forces (Hampton, Vasios, & Loos, 2016).

In addition to task shifting from physicians to nonphysicians, the use of ultrasound at the bedside by clinicians to answer focused clinical questions has significant impact in austere medical environments. In East Africa, one group has trained physicians, midwives, and clinical officers in the use of point-of-care ultrasound and has provided them with asynchronous tele-ultrasound support for varied populations, such as 18 Delta special forces medics, physicians and nurses on cruise ships, and clinicians at U.S. embassies around the globe (Boniface et al., 2019).

IMPLEMENTATION OF A TELE-ULTRASOUND PROGRAM

Case Study

A 67-year-old male with a history of congestive heart failure, chronic obstructive pulmonary disease, and lung cancer presented to a rural ED with shortness of breath. Initial vital signs demonstrated a temperature of 100.4 degrees F, blood pressure 89/43, heart rate 109, respiratory rate (RR) 22, and pulse oximetry 95% on room air. In the ED, the patient received a bolus of crystalloid, with mild improvement in blood pressure. Laboratory evaluation was significant for a leukocytosis to 13.4 and a lactate level of 3.5. Antibiotics for presumed sepsis were initiated.

The patient became increasingly more short of breath, with RR of 26. The advanced practice provider (APP) caring for the patient, concerned that the patient may now have fluid overload due to the IV fluids, obtained a chest X-ray, which did not show overt heart failure or pneumonia. The differential diagnosis also included pulmonary embolism and pericardial effusion; however, there were no echocardiography technicians available overnight. Computed tomography was considered, but the patient was unable to lay flat.

The APP had some ultrasound experience but did not feel comfortable acquiring adequate images and interpreting the scans. Utilizing an established tele-ultrasound connection, the APP was able to get real-time guidance from an ultrasound-trained emergency physician at a tertiary care center who guided probe movements to optimize the images and diagnose a large pericardial effusion with evidence of pericardial tamponade. An emergent pericardiocentesis was performed successfully, which stabilized the patient until the on-call cardiologist arrived to take over management.

Tele-ultrasound programs have several requirements (Table 23.2) but generally rely on equipment and procedures that are already in place. Large tertiary care centers can work with more rural or resource-limited settings locally, regionally, nationally or internationally in order to provide higher-level care to areas that may not necessarily have access to that level of care. Alternatively, rural or resource-limited areas may initiate an agreement with a larger center to provide higher-level care to their patients without the need to travel long distances. The distance between the two sites can therefore vary greatly. Emergency physicians have been at the forefront of POCUS and POCUS education of other providers, including residents, students, nurses, and paramedics. Emergency physicians in the United States generally have many of the components for tele-ultrasound in place and could therefore easily set up a tele-ultrasound program with a more resource-limited or rural location locally, regionally, nationally, or internationally.

Table 23.2 IMPLEMENTATION REQUIREMENTS OF A TELE-ULTRASOUND PROGRAM

Requirements		Additional Considerations
Establish program based on need with agreement between sites	May be initiated by expert or by remote site	Can be used for locations with limited access to care or to help guide need for transfers to larger centers
Ultrasound machine	Cart-based or hand-held	Consider exam types and need for advanced functions when purchasing machine
Telecommunications	Internet and/or WiFi for image transmission	Synchronous tele-ultrasound possible with higher bandwidths
Image archival system and computer for image review	Encrypted online or cloud-based database with one- or two-computer system	May be limited by machine as well as connectivity
Providers	Physicians, APPs, sonographers, other health professionals (e.g., nurses, paramedics)	Depends on availability of providers at remote site
Ultrasound expert	Credentialed ultrasound provider	Must maintain credentialing with hospital and/or credentialing board
Training	Initial training for acquiring and/or interpreting images	Ongoing training, image review/quality assurance for exams performed

ADDITIONAL CONSIDERATIONS/BARRIERS

The implementation of tele-ultrasound requires the following additional considerations.

Privacy

Tele-ultrasound programs should protect patient privacy and abide by relevant regulations such as the Health Insurance Portability and Accountability Act (HIPAA). Ultrasound images should include protected health information (PHI) such as name, medical record number (MRN), and date of birth. Including this information is important for data storage as part of a patient's medical record. Encryption of data is necessary to protect patient information when sending images or patient information remotely. Recently, the lack of security of some sites that store diagnostic medical imaging was discovered (Gillum, 2019). Real-time guidance also brings up the issue of data privacy with regards to communication platforms. There are specific third-party communications platforms that offer HIPAA-compliant software. As we continue to expand our ability to transmit images and videos and provide real-time guidance with patient care, it is imperative that we take precautions to protect the patient's health care information.

Cost

One of the major changes in ultrasound technology in the past two decades is the affordability of machines. Although more comprehensive machines can still cost hundreds of thousands of dollars, smaller and more portable machines designed for the point-of-care market have become significantly more affordable. Refurbished machines offer another more affordable option, as these machines can cost less than new machines and provide adequate image quality and machine functionality. Additionally, smaller hand-held machines have become increasingly more affordable, costing less than 10% of the cost of a cart-based system. The type of examinations performed should be considered in addition to price. In general, more expensive ultrasound machines have more functionality. For example, a remote echo program would likely need a more expensive machine for detailed imaging and specialized functions (e.g., ECG tracing, pulse-wave Doppler). POCUS providers, on the other hand, generally do not require many advanced functions and are able to use simpler, and therefore cheaper, machines. Overall, the decreasing price of ultrasound equipment has increased access to ultrasound in clinical care. All the same, the machine and functionality should be appropriate for the desired ultrasound examination.

Need for Interpreters

Tele-ultrasound can be utilized in both rural and resource-limited settings within the United States and abroad. When dealing with locations around the world, language interpreters are a consideration, especially for synchronous examinations, but also for ensuring clarity of the final report from the tele-ultrasound expert.

Medical Licensing

Tele-ultrasound falls under the umbrella of telemedicine with regard to licensing. In general, the physician/provider must be licensed where the patient is located for the ultrasound examination.

Reimbursement

For care in the United States, the Centers for Medicare and Medicaid Services (CMS) will reimburse both the originating site and the distant site practitioners for defined telehealth services, but these vary depending on the state. Only a few states have policies that specifically define reimbursement for store-and-forward ultrasound applications and generally only cover a technical fee for performance of the ultrasound in these cases (Center for Connected Health Policy, 2018). Telemedicine is a growing field in the United States, and policies are constantly changing. Thus, additional reimbursement may be provided in the future, especially for synchronous tele-ultrasound exams. For originating sites outside the United States that are not supported by grant funding or donated services, a contract between the centrally located tele-ultrasound expert and the remote site would define payments for both the operator performing the scan and the consultant guiding and interpreting the ultrasound.

CONCLUSION

Improvements in ultrasound technology have transformed ultrasound machines from being large and immobile to small and portable, with significantly improved image resolution. Several companies now offer hand-held or tablet-based ultrasound systems in addition to larger portable machines. Improvements in connectivity have led to improved image transmission, including in real time, with similar image quality between sites.

The affordability and portability of newer ultrasound systems may ultimately democratize access to POCUS. While this possibility seems like a positive overall, it raises serious concerns about the quality of care provided when there is greater availability of an ultrasound tool than of skilled providers with ultrasound training who understand its clinical applications and limitations.

Tele-ultrasound is one way to ensure quality of care as more machines than ultrasound experts are deployed throughout clinical settings around the globe. Task shifting from remote experts to local physician and nonphysician clinicians who perform ultrasound under synchronous or asynchronous direction can help provide access to the valuable diagnostic and therapeutic capabilities of ultrasound while ensuring quality of care.

Tele-ultrasound continues to grow and aid in medical care in a broad range of clinical sites—from rural America to cruise ships and from remote global sites to space. The advancements in ultrasound technology, in combination with its benefits as a medical imaging modality, have led to the increasing use of tele-ultrasound in health care.

KEY TAKEAWAYS

- ➤ Ultrasound has become an integral part of clinical care, with the benefits of being noninvasive, increasingly portable, cost-effective, and avoiding ionizing radiation.
- ➤ Tele-ultrasound systems can be developed in both asynchronous and synchronous connections, depending on resources, technology infrastructure, and provider availability.
- ➤ Tele-ultrasound can help provide necessary care to facilities that may not have providers trained in ultrasound image acquisition or interpretation.
- ➤ Synchronous tele-ultrasound provides rapid and real-time assistance, which helps expedite patient care.

REFERENCES

Adambounou, K., Farin, F., Boucher, A., et al. (2012). Système de télé-expertise échographique temps réel et de télédiagnostic échographique temps différé. Étude pilote au Togo [System of telesonography with synchronous teleconsultations and asynchronous telediagnoses (Togo)]. *Médecine et Santé Tropicales*, 22(1): 54–60.

Becker, C., Fusaro, M, Patel, D., Shalom, I., Frishman, W., & Scurlock, C. (2017). The utility of teleultrasound to guide acute patient management. *Cardiology in Review*, 25: 97–101.

Boniface, K. S., Shokoohi, H., Smith, E. R., & Scantlebury, K. (2011, June). Tele-ultrasound and paramedics: real-time remote physician guidance of the Focused Assessment With Sonography for Trauma examination. *American Journal of Emergency Medicine*, 29(5): 477–481.

Boniface, K. S., Raymond, A., Fleming, K., Scott, J., Kerry, V. B., Haile-Mariam, T., et al. (2019, April). The Global Health Service Partnership's point-of-care ultrasound initiatives in Malawi, Tanzania and Uganda. *American Journal of Emergency Medicine*, 37(4): 777–779.

Brass, P., Hellmich, M., Kolodziej, L., Schick, G., & Smith, A. F. (2015). Ultrasound guidance versus anatomical landmarks for internal jugular vein catheterization. *Cochrane Database of Systematic Reviews*, 1(1): 1–169.

Brebner, J. A., Ruddick-Bracken, H., Brebner, E. M., et al. (1999). Low-bandwidth tele-ultrasound. *Journal of Telemedicine and Telecare*, 5: S75–S76.

Brebner, J. A., Ruddick-Bracken, H., Brebner, E. M., et al. (2000). The diagnostic acceptability of low-bandwidth transmission for tele-ultrasound. *Journal of Telemedicine and Telecare*, 26(6): 335–338.

Britton, N., Miller, M. A., Safadi, S., et al. (2019). Tele-ultrasound in resource-limited settings: A systematic review. *Frontiers in Public Health*, 7(244): 1–13.

Center for Connected Health Policy. (2018, Fall). State telehealth laws and reimbursement policies. (Fall 2018). Accessed Septermber 13, 2019, at https://www.cchpca.org/telehealth-policy/state-telehealth-laws-and-reimbursement-policies-report.

Chan, F. Y., Whitehall, J., Hayes, L., et al. (1999). Minimum requirements for remote realtime fetal tele-ultrasound consultation. *Journal of Telemedicine and Telecare*, 5(3): 171–176.

Chiao, L., Sharipov, S., Sargsyan, A. E., Melton, S., Hamilton, D. R., McFarlin, K., et al. (2005). Ocular examination for trauma: Clinical ultrasound aboard the International Space Station. *Journal of Trauma*, 58(5): 885–889.

Fincke, E. M., Padalka, G., Lee, D., Van Holsbeeck, M., Sargsyan, A. E., Hamilton, D. R. et al. (2005). Evaluation of shoulder integrity in space: First report of musculoskeletal US on the International Space Station. *Radiology*, 234(2): 319–322.

Fuentes, A. (2003). Remote interpretation of ultrasound images. *Clinical Obstetrics and Gynecology*, 46: 878–881.

Gillum, J., Kao, J., & Larson, J. (2019). Millions of Americans' Medical images and data are available on the internet. Anyone can take a peek. *Propublica*. Accessed September 20, 2019, at https://www.propublica.org/article/millions-of-americans-medical-images-and-data-are-available-on-the-internet.

Hampton, K. K., Vasios, W. N., & Loos, P. E. (2016). SOLCUS: Update on point-of-care ultrasound in special operations medicine. *Journal of Special Operations Medicine: A Peer Reviewed Journal for SOF Medical Professionals*, 16(1): 58–61.

Levine, A. R., Buchner, J. A., Verceles, A. C., et al. (2016). Ultrasound images transmitted via FaceTime are non-inferior to images on the ultrasound machine. *Journal of Critical Care*, 33: 51–55.

Lichtenstein, D. A., & Mezière, G. A. (2008). Relevance of lung ultrasound in the diagnosis of acute respiratory failure: The BLUE protocol. *CHEST*, 134(1): 117–125.

Lilly, C. M., Zubrow, M. T., Kempner, K. M., et al. (2014). Critical care telemedicine: Evolution and state of the art. *Critical Care Medicine*, 42(11): 2429–2436.

Malone, F. D., Nores, J. A., Athanassiou, A., Craigo, S. D., Simpson, L. L., Garmel, S. H., & D'Alton, M. E. (1997). Validation of fetal telemedicine as a new obstetric imaging technique. *American Journal of Obstetrics and Gynecology*, 177(3): 626–631.

Marsh-Feiley, G., Eadie, L., & Wilson, P. (2018). Telesonography in emergency medicine: A systematic review. *PLoS One*, 13(5): e0194840.

Olivieri, P. P., Verceles, A. C., Hurley, J. M., Zubrow, M. T., Jeudy, J., & McCurdy, M. T. (2020, July). A pilot study of ultrasonography-naïve operators' ability to use tele-ultrasonography to assess the heart and lung. *Journal of Intensive Care Medicine*, 35(7): 672–678.

Pian, L., Gillman, L M., McBeth, P. B., Xiao, Z., Ball, C. G., Blaivas, M., et al. (2013). Potential use of remote telesonography as a transformational technology in underresourced and/or remote settings. *Emergency Medicine International*, 28: e986160.

Popov, V., Popov, D., Kacar, I., & Harris, R. D. (2007). The feasibility of real-time transmission of sonographic images from a remote location over low-bandwidth Internet links: A pilot study. *American Journal Roentgenology*, 188(3): W219–W222.

Sargsyan, A. E., Hamilton, D. R., Jones, J. A., et al. (2005). FAST at MACH 20: Clinical ultrasound aboard the International Space Station. *Journal of Trauma—Injury, Infection and Critical Care*, 58(1): 35–39.

Saugel, B., Scheeren, T. W. L., & Teboul, J. L. (2017). Ultrasound-guided central venous catheter placement: A structured review and recommendations for clinical practice. *Critical Care*, 21(1): 225.

Shokoohi, H., Raymond, A., Fleming, K., et al. (2019). Assessment of point-of-care ultrasound training for clinical educators in Malawi, Tanzania and Uganda. *Ultrasound in Medicine and Biology*, 45(6): 1351–1357.

Shokoohi, H., Boniface, K. S., Pourmand, A., et al. (2015). Bedside ultrasound reduces diagnostic uncertainty and guides resuscitation in patients with undifferentiated hypotension. *Critical Care Medicine*, 43(12): 2562–2569.

Sobczyk, W. L., Solinger, R. E., Rees, A. H., & Elbl, F. (1993). Transtelephonic echocardiography: Successful use in a tertiary pediatric referral center. *Journal of Pediatrics*, 122(6): S84–S88.

WHO Reproductive Health Library. (2016, November). WHO recommendations on antenatal care for a positive pregnancy experience. The WHO Reproductive Health Library. Geneva: World Health Organization.

24

Emerging and Innovative Technologies

AHMAD A. AALAM, SAM P. TARASSOLI, DAMIEN J. DRURY,
ELIAS G. CARAYANNIS, AND ANDREW C.MELTZER ■

INTRODUCTION

While telemedicine—the remote diagnosis and treatment of patients using tele-communications technology—has existed in some form for decades, modern tele-medicine began with the widespread availability of video chat on home computers and mobile phones. Over time, these video communications became tailored spe-cifically for telemedicine applications by integrating scheduling, privacy, billing, and documentation. Yet, the widespread acceptance of telemedicine among both clinicians and patients remained low during the past decade. Despite the theoretical advantages of remote care, technical issues, poor digital literacy, privacy concerns, and low awareness, among other challenges, remained for clinicians and patients, in addition to institutional inertia and low investment by health care organizations.

But in 2020, the COVID-19 pandemic accelerated the adoption of telemedicine in all fields of medicine. The need to socially distance, as well as a series of emer-gency waivers by the Centers for Medicare and Medicaid Services (CMS), reduced the regulatory restrictions on telehealth and pushed telemedicine into the main-stream of health care. Within 12 months, telemedicine has been transformed from a niche practice to a core component of nearly all specialties, including emergency care. With this massive expansion, digital technology that is well established in other industries has been incorporated into telehealth to improve diagnosis and therapies. In 2021, telehealth, a broader term than telemedicine, is being used to describe a set of services utilizing telecommunications technology; no longer a simple doctor–patient video chat, it is remote care that incorporates cutting-edge digital tools from across the technological spectrum, including advanced computing, social media platforms, and artificial intelligence (AI) to improve health care delivery beyond the walls of the clinic room (see Figure 24.1). In this chapter, we discuss how these inno-vative technologies have impacted, and will further enhance, emergency telehealth.

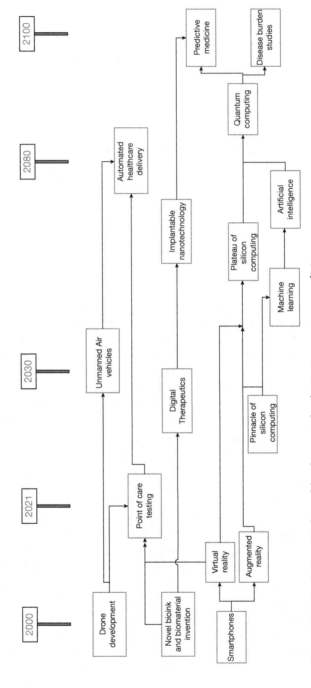

Figure 24.1 Prediction timeline of developing technologies in emergency medicine.

TELEHEALTH IN EMERGENCY CARE

Emergency care is a broad category of medicine but is unified around the vision of providing acute and unscheduled care. The lack of appointments and the time-dependent nature of the care separate this field from other specialties. Emergency care is care for anyone and at any time. Incorporating telehealth removes the rigid requirement of the emergency department (ED) space. Thus, emergency telehealth is care for anyone, at anytime *and anywhere*. The benefit is to provide care on-demand without limitations as to time or space.

MONITORING MULTIPLE PATIENTS

In the ED, multiple patients must be managed simultaneously across often large treatment facilities with varying acuity. While one patient is being treated, others must be monitored and updated. There is opportunity for remote care within the same department or hospital. In the ED, telemedicine video monitors, combined with advanced computer algorithms, can provide contextually relevant data for multiple patients at the same time. Real-time relevant guidelines and clinical prompts can be delivered to clinicians during emergency situations. One randomly controlled simulation study found that errors and deviations from guidelines in pediatric arrest were significantly reduced when augmented reality (AR) video displays were used to communicate with clinicians (Siebert et al., 2017).

PROVIDING DIRECT THERAPY

While traditional telemedicine allows for remote diagnosis, the video interface itself can serve as a source of therapy. The use of immersive virtual reality (VR) video may provide relief for a patient experiencing pain or anxiety (Schmitt et al., 2010; Hoffman et al., 2014). A study conducted in the ED at George Washington University Hospital found a significant drop in patients' pain score, anxiety, and anger levels after using VR for up to 20 minutes (Sikka et al., 2019). VR used alone or in addition to traditional ED pharmacological therapies can help manage patients in distress.

IMPROVING PROCEDURAL SKILLS

The use of video communication in emergency telehealth provides a natural extension to using AR applications to assist patient care. Via AR, the video can be analyzed and clinical decision tools can be integrated to make a diagnosis or assist with procedures. AR has been used to assist with neurosurgery (Davis et al., 2016) and could likewise be used for ED-based procedures. Other studies have shown the benefits of AR procedural training, which include increased availability (McGrath et al., 2017), decreased costs (Kleinert et al., 2015), and improved outcomes (Grantcharov et al., 2004; Schout et al., 2010). A fully immersive interface as experienced with VR offers greater access to simulation scenarios which enable clinicians to prepare for real-life emergency situations (Lloyd, 2018).

WORKING WITH SPECIALISTS

The use of video telemedicine to communicate between a clinician and their patients can be extended to video communication between an emergency medicine (EM) clinician and other stakeholders, such as nurses, specialists, hospital administrators, and prehospital paramedics. In addition to real-time communication, asynchronous telemedicine, also known as store-and-forward telemedicine, allows video imaging, examination results, or clinical evaluation to be stored for review at a later time. Store-and-forward is most commonly used by out-patient specialties, such as dermatology (Chuchu et al., 2018), where it has been shown to increase efficient use of clinician time by allowing data to be gathered prior to clinician review, enabling quicker synthesis and decision making. For ED clinicians, store-and-forward may lead to more effective referral or consult requests to other specialties in an asynchronous manner (Muir et al., 2011). Future changes are likely to involve increased volume and quality of available data, coupled with the integration of other technologies. Indications continue to expand for asynchronous emergency telehealth (Winburn, 2018), especially with emerging technologies that support forwarding a hologram of an incident resulting in injury, for example, or transmission of a VR evaluation for the patient to complete at home.

MONITORING POST-DISCHARGE

The capability to perform remote diagnostic testing involves more than video appointments with patients; it can also occur on a continuous basis via wearable devices (Vegesna et al., 2017). Wearable devices integrate into mobile health apps on smart phones to monitor heart rate, blood pressure, activity level, glucose monitoring, and more. These monitoring devices often connect with other devices as part of the internet of medical things (IoMT) and present an opportunity to improve care after ED discharge by integrating with established patient health data, sending alerts to providers, and providing communication with emergency services (Al-khafajiy et al., 2019). It is not uncommon for a patient to present to the ED now after remote patient monitoring (RPM) alerts the patient to conditions such as atrial fibrillation (Perez et al., 2019) or warning signs of major depression (Huckvale et al., 2019; *How Facebook AI. . .*, 2020).

REMOTE PATIENT MONITORING TO PREVENT ED VISITS

RPM technologies show great potential for improving coordination of post-ED care, decreasing the number of ED attendances via earlier detection of acute events (such as falls) and preventing ED readmissions (Bashi et al., 2017; UK-DOH, 2011). (For further detail on RPM, see Chapter 20.) Home remote monitoring technology refers

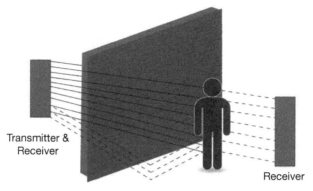

Transmitter &
Receiver

Receiver

Figure 24.2 Demonstration of the multipath effects in space and through objects.

to smart devices within the home which monitor the occupants while both assisting them and detecting critical events. The volume of use cases is huge: from fall prevention and detection to charting gradual changes in behavior, such as decreased activity levels, or increased nighttime bathroom visits that prompt early intervention (Liu et al., 2016).

One emerging passive RPM technology that shows great promise is radio-frequency-based health monitoring. The advancement in wireless technology, coupled with the proliferation of the IoMT, has enabled technology providers to look beyond communication-only devices and instead explore applications such as human sensing. When wireless signals move across space, they interact with physical bodies and express wave-related changes like reflection and diffraction, which leads to phenomena better known as "multipath effects." Multipath effects provide useful information about the physical characteristics of the space, such as human body location and certain activities (see Figure 24.2; Fang et al., 2016).

Multipath effects have been tested across a wide range of applications, ranging from sensing whole-body movement to breathing and heart rate (Adib et al., 2015). Current models require expensive specialist equipment to reach accurate measures; thus, more affordable technology will be necessary to achieve wider adoption (Tan, 2019). This opens the door to a new era of passive and contactless RPM that could be integrated with AI processing capabilities to understand advanced disease processes and prevent adverse health events early on.

DIGITAL THERAPEUTICS

The expansion of telehealth has been associated with an expansion of digital therapeutics (DTs). The capability of DTs complements telehealth, and they often have the ability to collect biomarkers via wearable devices or RPM, analyze data with advanced software, and display data on mobile apps. More powerful computers may warrant quicker and more effective diagnosis by recognizing early symptoms and signs and highlighting any "red flags" (Simon et al., 2019). In addition to managing ED patients, powerful computing with adaptive software such as artificial intelligence (AI) or machine learning (ML) holds promise for other aspects of ED functions, such as bed management, ambulance direction, and resource allocation.

DTs differ from traditional devices in several areas, and regulating DTs requires a more flexible approach to patient safety and efficacy compared to traditional devices and therapeutics. For example, DTs often use adaptive computing technology such as AI or ML, in which a feedback loop improves accuracy and effectiveness over time. In these cases, the initial accuracy may be very different than once used by millions of participants. A second categorical distinction between traditional therapeutics and DT is the need for connection with other platforms. DTs are less effective in isolation. The internet of things (IoT) or more specifically the IoMT ecosystems, augment and multiply the power of individual DTs. A third distinction between DTs and traditional therapies is the vigilant need for cybersecurity (see Chapter 7). With the increased volume of personal information, and increased connectivity to health care databases and devices, a security lapse can have major consequences for the individual patient and potentially other patients in the same connected system. A malicious or unintentional hack may reveal protected health information (PHI), cause device malfunctions, or sabotage a whole connected health system. Several recent high-profile cyberattacks into hospital systems have highlighted these concerns (Collier, 2020). The media has underscored fears of cyberattacks on devices such as implantable defibrillators or automated medication delivery systems. To address safety issues, the Food and Drug Administration (FDA) has created a novel Digital Health Center of Excellence (FDA, 2021) (https://www.fda.gov/medical-devices/digital-health-center-excellence) to coordinate the regulatory process associated with DTs.

DIGITAL BIOMARKERS

Digital biomarkers include electronic medical records, genetic data, and patient-generated data obtained from wearable devices and mobile applications. In one study, the data being collected had been increasing at a rate of 48% annually (Stanford Medicine, 2017). Large amounts of validated digital biomarkers may accurately predict disease and diagnose existing medical conditions in ways not currently possible with the traditional annual checkup. An example of a device with medical applications is the Apple Watch™, which has been shown effective at diagnosing atrial fibrillation (Turakhia et al., 2019). Other digital biomarkers may help ED clinicians more easily understand longitudinal health data about their patients, thus avoiding unnecessary admissions or workup. In order to make sense of digital biomarkers, powerful computing capabilities will be needed to analyze the data.

ARTIFICIAL INTELLIGENCE AND MACHINE LEARNING

AI will become increasingly integrated in medicine and wider society. Machine learning as a subdivision of AI works by studying, understanding, and comparing data to discover common patterns and explore variations. AI is already in use for smart digital document management in organizing and interrogating electronic notes in order to make them more accessible and searchable to ED clinicians (Amisha et al., 2019). When coupled with quantum computing, AI and ML can help to triage multiple casualties in a major trauma scenario through early trend recognition. In the future, EDs will rely on AI on a daily basis, receiving actionable insights such as red-flag symptom alerts, in combination with risk profiles based on lab tests and imaging, suggesting diagnosis and augmenting a clinician's decision-making process. This will decrease errors and increase efficiency by furnishing the EP with key data and applicable guidelines to optimize management.

DRONES AND AERIAL VEHICLES

Sometimes, communication and monitoring are not enough, and patients need actual physical equipment to help them. Drones or unmanned aerial vehicles (UAVs) are remote-controlled vehicles that can rapidly deliver a payload (Newcome, 2004). Although they were initially developed for military purposes, they may be a useful technology in emergency medicine (Rodriguez et al., 2006). One of the first instances of the use of a drone in a medical disaster was in the Philippines to monitor 2013 Typhoon Haiyon (Rosser et al., 2018). The surveillance provided information about the number of wounded so that hospitals could better prepare. In the future, drones can be incorporated with robotic technology and reduce the needed staff on the ground in high-risk environments (Harnett et al., 2008).

The speed of drones and similar aerial vehicles has made them an attractive choice for emergency medical deliveries. Proof-of-concept systems have been around for over a decade for delivery of vaccines (Mendelow et al., 2007) and for sending other emergency medicines and equipment (i.e., for point-of-care testing; Frontières, 2014). Delivery of automated external defibrillators (AEDs) has been simulated in the Netherlands and demonstrated delivery within a 2-kilometer radius within two minutes (Husten, 2014). Other simulations have found that drones strategically placed in a city can reach more than 90% of the population in less than 60 seconds, more rapidly than a traditional ambulance (Pulver, Wei, & Mann, 2016). In the future, drones may safely and autonomously carry patients to hospital or medical staff to emergency scenes.

SOCIAL MEDIA

Social media has been another effective mechanism to engage ED patients. Social media facilitates two-way communication and drives patient engagement and health literacy. Analysis of social data may also inform ED clinicians on patients' social circumstances, interests, concerns, and beliefs. Privacy and data stewardship concerns complicate the use of these technologies. However, many patients are willing to share their social media data with their ED physician (Padrez et al., 2016).

CONCLUSION

Emergency telehealth will continue to grow in scope and complexity through existing and developing technologies to provide emergency care. This trend will be magnified by integration across technologies in a human-centered IoMT eco-system. These new applications will supplement the current established telehealth tools and expand into new populations, including the elderly and underserved groups. VR and AR could replace video as the standard technology for vir-tual visits, enabling ED clinicians to provide care remotely through a variety of interfaces that simulate or augment traditional doctor–patient interactions. ML and AI will take part in everyday ED procedures and will become the corner-stone of electronic medical record (EMR) development. Improved information management will lay the ground for better implementation of DT in the setting of the expected wide implementation of quantum computing to support interpreting images, diagnosing conditions, and initiating patient management. With the ex-panded use of wearables, emergency clinicians may be able to effectively intervene prior to the ED visit and prevent acute exacerbation of illness. These interventions may transform the practice of emergency care and emergency telehealth. Over time, emergency clinicians may well find the mix of front-door presentations shifting as a response.

KEY TAKEAWAYS

- ➤ The structure of emergency health care services will evolve to better accommodate widespread use of telehealth modalities via centralization of services through hub-and-spoke models.
- ➤ The use of AI and ML will improve clinician decision making in the ED by providing contextually relevant information.
- ➤ Live video use will develop beyond its existing single channel, encompassing AR and VR, mobile, and social.
- ➤ The volume of available data from both personal devices and health care-specific remote monitoring devices will continue to grow as well as the IoMT ecosystem associated with each patient.
- ➤ Novel telehealth use cases such as analgesic adjuncts, digital phenotyping, and virtual reality training will be expanded and implemented across the wider emergency medicine field.

REFERENCES

Accenture. (2018). Retrieved from Digital Health Tech Vision 2019 | Accenture: www.accenture.com/healthtechvision.

Adib, F., Mao, H., Kabelac, Z., Katabi, D., & Miller, R. (2015). Smart homes that mon-itor breathing and heart rate share on. *CHI '15: Proceedings of the 33rd Annual ACM Conference on Human Factors in Computing Systems.*

AHA. (2020). Retrieved from Using Remote Patient Monitoring Technologies for Better Cardiovascular Disease Outcomes Guidance at https://www.heart.org/-/media/files/about-us/policy-research/policy-positions/clinical-care/remote-patient-monitoring-guidance-2019.pdf?la=en.

Al-khafajiy, M., Kolivand, H., Baker, T., Tully, D., & Waraich, A. (2019). Smart hospital emergency system via mobile-based requesting services. *Multimedia Tools and Applications*, 78(14), 20087–20111.

Amisha, Malik, P., Pathania, M., & Rathaur, V. (2019). Overview of artificial intelligence in medicine. *J Family Med Prim Care*, 8(7), 23–28.

Asch, J. M., Asch, D. A., Klinger, E. V., Marks, J., Sadek, N., & Merchant, R. M. (2019). Google search histories of patients presenting to an emergency department: an observational study. *BMJ open*, 9(2), e024791.

Bashi, N., Karunanithi, M., Fatehi, F., Ding, H., & Walters, D. (2017). Remote monitoring of patients with heart failure: an overview of systematic reviews. *Journal of medical Internet research*, 19(1), e18.

Burkholder, T. W., Bellows, J. W., & King, R. A. (2018). Free open access medical education (FOAM) in emergency medicine: the global distribution of users in 2016. *Western Journal of Emergency Medicine*, 19(3), 600.

Cadogan, M., Thoma, B., Chan, T. M., & Lin, M. (2014). Free Open Access Meducation (FOAM): the rise of emergency medicine and critical care blogs and podcasts (2002–2013). *Emergency Medicine Journal*, 31(e1), e76–e77.

Carley, S., Beardsell, I., May, N., Crowe, L., Baombe, J., Grayson, A., . . . & Body, R. (2018). Social-media-enabled learning in emergency medicine: a case study of the growth, engagement and impact of a free open access medical education blog. *Postgraduate medical journal*, 94(1108), 92–96.

Collier B, Horgan S, Hones R, Shepherd L. The implications of the COVID-19 pandemic for cybercrime policing in Scotland: A rapid review of the evidence and future considerations. *The Scottish Insitute for Policing Research.* May 2020 (1).

Chuchu, N., Dinnes, J., Takwoingi, Y., Matin, R. N., Bayliss, S. E., Davenport, C., . . . & Williams, H. C. (2018). Teledermatology for diagnosing skin cancer in adults. *Cochrane Database of Systematic Reviews*, (12).

Davis, M. C., Can, D. D., Pindrik, J., Rocque, B. G., & Johnston, J. M. (2016). Virtual interactive presence in global surgical education: international collaboration through augmented reality. *World neurosurgery*, 86, 103–111.

Dexheimer, J. W., & Borycki, E. M. (2015). Use of mobile devices in the emergency department: A scoping review. *Health informatics journal*, 21(4), 306–315.

de la Torre Díez, I., Cosgaya, H. M., Garcia-Zapirain, B., & López-Coronado, M. (2016). Big data in health: a literature review from the year 2005. *Journal of medical systems*, 40(9), 1-6.

Dilsizian, S. E., & Siegel, E. L. (2014). Artificial intelligence in medicine and cardiac imaging: harnessing big data and advanced computing to provide personalized medical diagnosis and treatment. *Current cardiology reports*, 16(1), 441.

Fang, B., Lane, N. D., Zhang, M., Boran, A., & Kawsar, F. (2016, June). BodyScan: Enabling radio-based sensing on wearable devices for contactless activity and vital sign monitoring. In Proceedings of the 14th annual international conference on mobile systems, applications, and services (pp. 97–110).

FDA. (2021). *Digital health center of excellence*. Retrieved from https://www.fda.gov/medical-devices/digital-health-center-excellence.

Follmann, A., Ohligs, M., Hochhausen, N., Beckers, S. K., Rossaint, R., & Czaplik, M. (2019). Technical support by smart glasses during a mass casualty incident: a randomized controlled simulation trial on technically assisted triage and telemedical app use in disaster medicine. *Journal of medical Internet research*, 21(1), e11939.

Frontières, M. S. (2014). *Innovating to reach remote TB patients and improve access to treatment.* Retrieved from Médecins Sans Frontières: https://www.msf.org/papua-new-guinea-innovating-reach-remote-tb-patients-and-improve-access-treatment.

Glass. (2020). Retrieved from https://www.google.com/glass/start.

Google AR & VR. (2020). Retrieved from https://arvr.google.com.

Google Cardboard. (2020). Retrieved from https://arvr.google.com/cardboard.

Grantcharov, T. P., Kristiansen, V. B., Bendix, J., Bardram, L., Rosenberg, J., & Funch-Jensen, P. (2004). Randomized clinical trial of virtual reality simulation for laparoscopic skills training. *Journal of British Surgery,* 91(2), 146–150.

Greene, J. (2013). Social media and physician learning: is it all twitter?. *Annals of emergency medicine,* 62(5), A11–A13.

Grock, A., & Paolo, W. (2016). Free open access medical education: a critical appraisal of techniques for quality assessment and content discovery. *Clinical and experimental emergency medicine,* 3(3), 183.

Harnett, B. M., Doarn, C. R., Rosen, J., Hannaford, B., & Broderick, T. J. (2008). Evaluation of unmanned airborne vehicles and mobile robotic telesurgery in an extreme environment. *Telemedicine and e-Health,* 14(6), 539–544.

Healthcare industry solutions & services—United Kingdom. (2020). Retrieved from IBM: https://www.ibm.com/uk-en/industries/healthcare#tab_2618884.

Hoffman, H. G., Meyer III, W. J., Ramirez, M., Roberts, L., Seibel, E. J., Atzori, B., . . . & Patterson, D. R. (2014). Feasibility of articulated arm mounted Oculus Rift Virtual Reality goggles for adjunctive pain control during occupational therapy in pediatric burn patients. *Cyberpsychology, Behavior, and Social Networking,* 17(6), 397–401.

Hölbl, M., Kompara, M., Kamišalić, A., & Nemec Zlatolas, L. (2018). A systematic review of the use of blockchain in healthcare. *Symmetry,* 10(10), 470.

How Facebook AI helps suicide prevention. (2020). Retrieved from https://about.fb.com/news/2018/09/inside-feed-suicide-prevention-and-ai.

Huckvale, K., Venkatesh, S., & Christensen, H. (2019). Toward clinical digital phenotyping: a timely opportunity to consider purpose, quality, and safety. *NPJ digital medicine,* 2(1), 1–11.

Husten, L. (2014). *Grad student invents flying ambulance drone to deliver emergency shocks.* Retrieved from Forbes at https://www.forbes.com/sites/larryhusten/2014/10/29/grad-student-invents-flying-ambulance-drone-to-deliver-emergency-shocks/?sh=4b59d9091bfc.

Kleinert, R., Wahba, R., Chang, D. H., Plum, P., Hölscher, A. H., & Stippel, D. L. (2015). 3D immersive patient simulators and their impact on learning success: a thematic review. *Journal of medical Internet research,* 17(4), e91.

Kohn, M. S., Sun, J., Knoop, S., Shabo, A., Carmeli, B., Sow, D., ... & Rapp, W. (2014). IBM's health analytics and clinical decision support. *Yearbook of medical informatics,* 23(01), 154–162.

Liu, L., Stroulia, E., Nikolaidis, I., Miguel-Cruz, A., & Rincon, A. R. (2016). Smart homes and home health monitoring technologies for older adults: A systematic review. *International journal of medical informatics,* 91, 44–59.

Lloyd, R. (2018, February). Simulation training in virtual reality. Retrieved from EMJ Blog: https://blogs.bmj.com/emj/2018/02/12/simulation-training-in-virtual-reality.

Marr, B. (2019). *The important difference between virtual reality, augmented reality and mixed reality.* Retrieved from Forbes at https://www.forbes.com/sites/bernardmarr/2019/07/19/the-important-difference-between-virtual-reality-augmented-reality-and-mixed-reality/?sh=20c7971335d3.

Mashamba-Thompson, Tivani P., and Ellen Debra Crayton. "Blockchain and artificial intelligence technology for novel coronavirus disease 2019 self-testing." *Diagnostics* 2020, 10(4), 198.

McGrath, J. L., Taekman, J. M., Dev, P., Danforth, D. R., Mohan, D., Kman, N., ... & Won, K. (2018). Using virtual reality simulation environments to assess competence for emergency medicine learners. *Academic Emergency Medicine,* 25(2), 186-195.

Mendelow, B., Muir, P., Boshielo, B., & Robertson, J. (2007). Development of e-Juba, a preliminary proof of concept unmanned aerial vehicle designed to facilitate the transportation of microbiological test samples from remote rural clinics to National Health Laboratory Service laboratories. *South African Medical Journal,* 97(11), 1215–1218.

Moore, G. E. (2006). Cramming more components onto integrated circuits, Reprinted from Electronics, volume 38, number 8, April 19, 1965, pp. 114 ff. IEEE solid-state circuits society newsletter, 11(3), 33–35.

Muir, J., Xu, C., Paul, S., Staib, A., McNeill, I., Singh, P., . . . & Sinnott, M. (2011). Incorporating teledermatology into emergency medicine. *Emergency Medicine Australasia*, 23(5), 562–568.

Munzer, B. W., Khan, M. M., Shipman, B., & Mahajan, P. (2019). Augmented reality in emergency medicine: a scoping review. *Journal of medical Internet research,* 21(4), e12368.

Newcome, L. R. (2004). *Unmanned aviation: A brief history of unmanned aerial vehicles.* 2004 American Institute of Aeronautics and Astronautics, Inc. (AIAA) Reston, Virginia

Oculus. (2020). *Oculus | VR headsets and equipment.* Retrieved from https://www.oculus. com.

One drop blood glucose monitoring kit. (2020). Retrieved from Apple: https://www.apple. com/shop/product/HMN02LL/A/one-drop-chrome-blood-glucose-monitoring-kit.

Padrez, K. A., Ungar, L., Schwartz, H. A., Smith, R. J., Hill, S., Antanavicius, T., . . . & Merchant, R. M. (2016). Linking social media and medical record data: a study of adults presenting to an academic, urban emergency department. *BMJ quality & safety,* 25(6), 414–423.

Perez, M. V., Mahaffey, K. W., Hedlin, H., Rumsfeld, J. S., Garcia, A., Ferris, T., . . . & Turakhia, M. P. (2019). Large-scale assessment of a smartwatch to identify atrial fibrillation. *New England Journal of Medicine,* 381(20), 1909–1917.

Perrin, A. (2015). Social media usage. Pew research center, 125, 52–68. Andrew Perrin. "Social Networking Usage: 2005-2015." Pew Research Center. October 2015. Available at: http://www.pewinternet.org/2015/10/08/2015/Social-Networking-

Poole, D., Mackworth, A., & Goebel, R. (1999). *Computational intelligence and knowledge.* Retrieved from www.cs.ubc.ca: https://www.cs.ubc.ca/~poole/ci/ch1.pdf.

Pulver, A., Wei, R., & Mann, C. (2016). Locating AED enabled medical drones to enhance cardiac arrest response times. *Prehospital Emergency Care,* 20(3), 378–389.

Rodriguez, P. A., Geckle, W. J., Barton, J. D., Samsundar, J., Gao, T., Brown, M. Z., & Martin, S. R. (2006). An emergency response UAV surveillance system. In AMIA Annual Symposium Proceedings (Vol. 2006, p. 1078). American Medical Informatics Association.

Rosser Jr, J. C., Vignesh, V., Terwilliger, B. A., & Parker, B. C. (2018). Surgical and medical applications of drones: A comprehensive review. JSLS: *Journal of the Society of Laparoendoscopic Surgeons,* 22(3).

Schmitt, Y. S., Hoffman, H. G., Blough, D. K., Patterson, D. R., Jensen, M. P., Soltani, M., . . . & Sharar, S. R. (2011). A randomized, controlled trial of immersive virtual reality analgesia, during physical therapy for pediatric burns. *Burns*, 37(1), 61–68.

Schout, B. M., Ananias, H. J., Bemelmans, B. L., d'Ancona, F. C., Muijtjens, A. M., Dolmans, V. E., . . . & Hendrikx, A. J. (2010). Transfer of cysto-urethroscopy skills from a virtual-reality simulator to the operating room: a randomized controlled trial. *BJU international*, 106(2), 226–231.

Siebert, J. N., Ehrler, F., Gervaix, A., Haddad, K., Lacroix, L., Schrurs, P., . . . & Manzano, S. (2017). Adherence to AHA guidelines when adapted for augmented reality glasses for assisted pediatric cardiopulmonary resuscitation: a randomized controlled trial. *Journal of medical Internet research*, 19(5), e183.

Sikka, N., Shu, L., Ritchie, B., Amdur, R. L., & Pourmand, A. (2019). Virtual reality-assisted pain, anxiety, and anger management in the emergency department. *Telemedicine and e-Health*, 25(12), 1207–1215.

Simon, G., DiNardo, C. D., Takahashi, K., Cascone, T., Powers, C., Stevens, R., ... & Chin, L. (2019). Applying artificial intelligence to address the knowledge gaps in cancer care. *The Oncologist*, 24(6), 772.

Social Media | Oxford Dictionary| Oxford Dictionary. (2020). Retrieved from https://www.lexico.com/definition/social_media.

Solenov, D., Brieler, J., & Scherrer, J. F. (2018). The potential of quantum computing and machine learning to advance clinical research and change the practice of medicine. *Missouri medicine*, 115(5), 463.

Stanford Medicine 2017 Health Trends Report. (2017). Retrieved from https://med.stanford.edu/content/dam/sm/sm-news/documents/StanfordMedicineHealthTrendsWhitePaper2017.pdf.

Tan, S. (2019). *Towards ubiquitous sensing using commodity WiFi.* Florida State University Libraries.

Tanguay, A., Dallaire, R., Hébert, D., Bégin, F., & Fleet, R. (2015). Rural patient access to primary percutaneous coronary intervention centers is improved by a novel integrated telemedicine prehospital system. *The Journal of emergency medicine*, 49(5), 657–664.

Thelen, S., Czaplik, M., Meisen, P., Schilberg, D., & Jeschke, S. (2016). Using off-the-shelf medical devices for biomedical signal monitoring in a telemedicine system for emergency medical services. In Automation, Communication and Cybernetics in Science and Engineering 2015/2016 (pp. 797-810). Springer, Cham.

Turakhia, M. P., Desai, M., Hedlin, H., Rajmane, A., Talati, N., Ferris, T., ... & Perez, M. V. (2019). Rationale and design of a large-scale, app-based study to identify cardiac arrhythmias using a smartwatch: The Apple Heart Study. *American heart journal*, 207, 66–75.

UK-DOH. (2011). Whole system demonstrator programme. UK Government.

Vegesna, A., Tran, M., Angelaccio, M., & Arcona, S. (2017). Remote patient monitoring via non-invasive digital technologies: a systematic review. *Telemedicine and e-Health*, 23(1), 3–17.

Ventola, C. L. (2014). Medical applications for 3D printing: current and projected uses. *Pharmacy and Therapeutics*, 39(10), 704.

Winburn, A. S., Brixey, J. J., Langabeer, J., & Champagne-Langabeer, T. (2018). A systematic review of prehospital telehealth utilization. *Journal of telemedicine and telecare*, 24(7), 473–481.

Yash Chavda, D. (2018). *3-D printed emergency medicine training.* Retrieved from www.emra.org: https://www.emra.org/emresident/article/3-d-printed-training.

Zhang, P., White, J., Schmidt, D., & Lenz, G. (2017). *Applying software patterns to address interoperability in blockchain-based healthcare apps.* Retrieved from https://arxiv.org: https://arxiv.org/abs/1706.03700.

COVID-19 Emergency Telemedicine Solutions

The COVID-19 pandemic has dramatically forwarded the use of telemedicine with many creative applications; Emergency Medicine staff were heavily involved in many of these. Early on, direct-to-consumer encounters were performed to screen patients for referral for COVID testing centers and expedite testing appointments. Many facilities screened presenting ED patients in an outside tent for COVID symptoms and then evaluated, tested, treated, and discharged mildly symptomatic patients via telemedicine. Some hospitals used teletriage to screen and sometimes treat ED patients to help decompress ED overcrowding and long wait times. During the pandemic, Centers for Medicare & Medicaid Services (CMS) has allowed for the virtual supervision of residents and advanced care providers, both for many inhouse patient care services, as well as virtual house calls. Remote patient monitoring via telemedicine has occurred both in the home as well as rural facilities. In Augusta, Georgia, the academic hospital created an ED to rural small hospital telemedicine hybrid program. The premise was to try and safely avoid transfers during the time of critical COVID overflow to their much larger center. With the virtual assistance of ED faculty who had more experience due to large volumes of patients, considerably ill and hypoxic COVID patients were effectively managed at small, rural hospitals.

CASE

A 52 year old woman presents to a small, 25 bed, rural hospital ED with dyspnea and hypoxia. Initial ED workup suggests COVID infection. PCR nasal swab for COVID-19 is performed but will not result for a day. A telemedicine consult to assist in management is placed to the closest large medical center about 100 miles away. A baseline assessment and intake note is generated by the hub ED attending. The patient is admitted and managed by the hospitalist and ED physicians in the rural hospital. The COVID test returns positive the next day. The hub emergency physicians round 1-2 times daily via mobile telemedicine (nicknamed Robo Doc by the rural site staff) making additional lab tests, imaging, oxygen delivery, and medication recommendations for this the patient as she moves through her illness. She worsens as anticipated, but is able to remain at the rural site despite high flow oxygen delivery requirements, advanced CT imaging, antiviral, antibiotic and steroid treatment. She starts improving after 6 days and after another 5 days, with physical therapy for deconditioning, is able to be discharged home.

This telemedicine model allows patients to remain in the community with family close by. The hub, which was over capacity with ill patients, was able to avoid another transfer and extended admission for an extended time or even altogether. The spoke was able to bill for the entire admission, including critical care.

If patients deteriorated beyond the rural sites' resources (e.g. intubation or vasopressors) during their hospitalization, there was always a failsafe contingency for immediate transfer to the hub, no questions asked. But every day that patients were able to be cared for at the spoke, was one less day they would have occupied the overcrowded hub. With several spokes recruited, there were typically about 10 to 15 simultaneous, remotely managed patients who would historically have immediately been transferred on initial presentation.

There are several other EM-related telemedicine applications used during the ongoing COVID pandemic (Please see the below resources for more details).

Jaffe T. Telehealth use in emergency care during coronavirus disease 2019: a systematic review Journal of the American College of Emergency Physicians Open. 2021 Jun; 2(3): e12443. Retrieved at https://www.ncbi.nlm.nih.gov/pmc/articles/PMC8087945/

Medicare Telemedicine Health Care Provider Fact Sheet. https://www.cms.gov/newsroom/fact-sheets/medicare-telemedicine-health-care-provider-fact-sheet Mar 17, 2020

COVID-19: Rapid Application of Technology for Emergency Department Tele-Triage: An Information Paper, American College of Emergency Physicians, https://www.acep.org/siteassets/covid-19---rapid-application-of-technology-for-emergency-department-tele-triage.pdf May 22, 2020

New CMS Telehealth Guidance: What You Need to Know. https://www.acep.org/corona/COVID-19-alert/covid-19-articles/new-cms-telehealth-guidance-what-you-need-to-know/ March 17, 2020

Shaheen E et al. ACEP COVID-19 Field Guide, Telehealth and Tele-Triage https://www.acep.org/corona/covid-19-field-guide/triage/telehealth-and-tele-triage/ September 8, 2020

EMERGENCY TRIAGE, TREAT, AND TRANSPORT (ET3) MODEL

In March 2021, CMS announced the start of an ongoing 5-year trial to determine the feasibility of EMS telemedicine support to guide redirection of selected patients to destinations other than an emergency department (ED). Traditionally, emergent EMS transport was only reimbursed for ambulance transport to certain destinations, usually EDs. But these are costly visits, and frequently a level of care far higher than required for the complaint. It is felt that it would be more efficient if other care facility options were available. These alternate sites would include agreed-upon lower acuity facilities such as urgent care clinics, primary care offices, or community mental health centers, or even no transport determination. Many facility agreements must be in place to ensure the right patients get to the right place at the right time. It is presumed that this project will redirect patients to more appropriate and lower cost options than automatic transport to already overcrowded EDs.

More information is available at the CMS website https://innovation.cms.gov/innovation-models/et3.

Tables, figures, and boxes are indicated by *t, f,* and *b* following the page number.